Health Informatics

(formerly Computers in Health Care)

Kathryn J. Hannah   Marion J. Ball
Series Editors

Springer
New York
Berlin
Heidelberg
Hong Kong
London
Milan
Paris
Tokyo

Health Informatics Series
(formerly Computers in Health Care)

Series Editors
Kathryn J. Hannah   Marion J. Ball

(continued after index)

Marion J. Ball   Kathryn J. Hannah
Susan K. Newbold   Judith V. Douglas
Editors

Nursing Informatics

Where Caring and Technology Meet

Third Edition

Forewords by Sue Karen Donaldson
and Ulla Gerdin

With 26 Illustrations

Springer

Marion J. Ball, EdD
Vice President, Clinical Solutions
Healthlink, Inc.
Baltimore, MD 21210, USA
and
Adjunct Professor
Johns Hopkins University School
  of Nursing
Baltimore, MD 21205, USA

Kathryn J. Hannah, PhD, RN
Adjunct Professor, Department of
  CommunityHealth Sciences
Faculty of Medicine
The University of Calgary
Calgary, Alberta T2N 4N1, Canada

Susan K. Newbold, MS, RN
Doctoral Candidate
University of Maryland
Baltimore, MD 20742, USA

Judith V. Douglas, MA, MHS
Lecturer
The Johns Hopkins University
  School of Nursing
Baltimore, MD 21205, USA

Series Editors:

Kathryn J. Hannah, PhD, RN

Marion J. Ball, EdD

Cover illustration: L'Ambulance by Anais Coudour, France, 1870, from the National Library of Medicine. The principles of caring and technology, demonstrated by the Red Cross nurse as she ministers to the patient and represented by the tools at the left, are still vital components of nursing informatics today.

Library of Congress Cataloging-in-Publication Data
Nursing informatics: where caring and technology meet/Marion J. Ball . . . [et al.]—3rd ed.
    p.   cm.—(Health informatics series)
    Includes bibliographical references and index.
    ISBN 0-387-98923-4 (hard cover; alk. paper)
    1. Nursing informatics.   2. Information storage and retrieval systems—Nursing.   I. Ball,
Marion J.   II. Health informatics.
    [DNLM: 1. Computers.   2. Information Systems.   3. Nursing.   WY 26.5 N974 2000]
RT50.5.N87   2000
610.73´0285—dc21   99-046287

Printed on acid-free paper.

Printed in the United States of America.

9 8 7 6 5 4 3

ISBN 0-387-98923-4   SPIN 10915837

Springer-Verlag   New York Berlin Heidelberg
A member of BertelsmannSpringer Science+Business Media GmbH

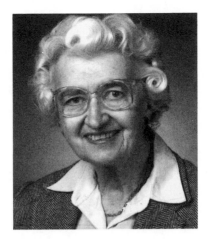

To Harriet H. Werley, RN, PhD, a seminal force in nursing informatics who challenged us in 1987 to use the term nursing informatics *as the title of our book*

Foreword

At the Johns Hopkins University School of Nursing, our mission is "to improve health care and advance the profession through research, practice, service, and education . . . and provide a positive and innovative force in the evolution of the nursing profession and changing healthcare system."

To transform professional education for the twenty-first century, we are rapidly building on the school's information technologies and establishing an informatics infrastructure. Our intent is to foster faculty resources and to use advanced information technology to communicate healthcare information to nurses, other health professionals, and consumers. We are working to extend the School of Nursing's reach beyond its on-site academic programs to the local, national, and global environment. Contributions such as books like this, now in its third edition, have helped us to mark the path and prepare the way.

Our goal is to provide leadership in educating nurses to be fully cognizant of and adept in using information technology tools as enablers to create and manage new knowledge. As knowledge workers, our nurses will be leaders, innovators, and clinical practitioners. Truly high tech and high touch, our graduates will transform the practice of health care, bringing the highest quality at the lowest cost. Like the contributors to this volume, they will be avid advocates and users of telematics, expert systems, robotics, and data mining. In the practice setting, they will use multimedia computer-based patient records systems. They will take advantage of Inter/ intra/extranet tools for distance and self-directed learning, for themselves and for their patients. We are now taking a giant step in this direction as the first school of nursing to propose a graduate professional doctoral degree in clinical nursing informatics, with special emphasis on the use of data for evidence-based practice and policy.

Still a relatively new field, informatics is critical to health care in the new millennium, as the chapters that follow make clear. Using state-of-the-art tools and creating robust infrastructures, informatics will create knowledge and translate research data into evidence-based care. Informatics will enable us to move theory into practice: to identify, measure, and track outcomes using patient data and case management to develop informatics-enabled clinical innovations. Informatics will allow us to practice as expert clinicians, to communicate as dedicated professionals, and to advance nursing science in areas such as genomics, which holds such incredible promise for future health care.

At Hopkins, we are dedicated to taking the lead in the new millennium. We are committed to developing the discipline of nursing, offering new avenues for certification, and preparing the nursing leaders we will need in the expanding knowledge area. We are prepared and ready to serve.

Sue Karen Donaldson, PhD, RN, FAAN
Dean and Professor of Nursing
School of Nursing
Professor of Physiology, School of Medicine
The Johns Hopkins University
Baltimore, MD, USA

Foreword

Today's patients enjoy an expanded role in health care—one that involves both opportunity and responsibility. Now at the center of the healthcare process, patients must embrace self-care, accepting more responsibility for their treatment and the environment in which it is administered. To aid them in this process, huge amounts of information on health, health symptoms, and specific diseases are now at their disposal. In most countries, patients also have the right to read their medical records, and patients in some countries actually own these records.

A new role for patients also signals a new role for nurses: to guide patients through this dense information flow. Nurses who accept this role must know about available sources for information and how to retrieve it. They must also be able to judge the accuracy and quality of the information, evaluate the information for the patient's specific situation, and help and guide patients through all necessary decisions.

Healthcare professionals today work in teams. To deliver high-quality, effective health care, team members share patient information and knowledge. The electronic patient record is a tool shared by all team members as a guide for daily decisions, quality assurance, and clinical and epidemiological studies. As a member of the professional team, the nurse has the same responsibilities as other team members to document patient assessments, nursing diagnoses, interventions, and outcomes. The nurse must be familiar with terminologies, data quality, the proper use of information technology, and the use and possibilities of electronic patient records and decision support systems.

Healthcare organizations are also subject to changes associated with the switch to the "information society." Because nurses are the major collectors and recorders of patient data in health care, their working environment is affected in many ways by this development. Nursing informatics is a skill and a competence that nurses must acquire in order to assume leadership roles in this new environment. Health care needs nurses on all levels of operation, and literacy in informatics is a prerequisite for nurses' career advancement in a modern healthcare delivery system.

Information technology is a tool that requires continuous development and maintenance. Nurses must make sure they have the skill and competence to assume leadership roles and influence system functionality, information content, and procedures. Nurses are good project managers, and with informatics competence, they can hold positions that impact both development and maintenance. Information technology constantly provides new possibilities. The nurse, with the patient at the center, must be able to judge system functionality in the context of needs and to judge costs in the context of their effects on operations, patient integrity, and data security.

As long as we can read and communicate with each other, mistakes are permitted only once. The modern nurse requires literature in nursing informatics that meets today's needs in health care. Distance learning, literature of good quality, and new pedagogic methods help nurses acquire necessary knowledge. Every one of the authors of this book has experienced the development of nursing informatics, and they now share their knowledge with other nurses. It is up to their audience to take it from here and gain control over future developments.

Ulla Gerdin, RN
Senior Project Manager
Swedish Institute for Health Services Development
Stockholm, Sweden

Series Preface

This series is directed to healthcare professionals who are leading the transformation of health care by using information and knowledge. Launched in 1988 as Computers in Health Care, the series offers a broad range of titles: some addressed to specific professions such as nursing, medicine, and health administration; others to special areas of practice such as trauma and radiology. Still other books in the series focus on interdisciplinary issues, such as the computer-based patient record, electronic health records, and networked healthcare systems.

Renamed Health Informatics in 1998 to reflect the rapid evolution in the discipline now known as health informatics, the series will continue to add titles that contribute to the evolution of the field. In the series, eminent experts, serving as editors or authors, offer their accounts of innovations in health informatics. Increasingly, these accounts go beyond hardware and software to address the role of information in influencing the transformation of healthcare delivery systems around the world. The series also increasingly focuses on "peopleware" and the organizational, behavioral, and societal changes that accompany the diffusion of information technology in health services environments.

These changes will shape health services in this new millennium. By making full and creative use of the technology to tame data and to transform information, health informatics will foster the development of the knowledge age in health care. As coeditors, we pledge to support our professional colleagues and the series readers as they share advances in the emerging and exciting field of health informatics.

Kathryn J. Hannah
Marion J. Ball

Preface

Nursing informatics has developed rapidly since the first edition of this book was published. Nursing has been a leader in integrating information technology into administration, education, research, and clinical care, while other health professions have lagged behind. Professional associations and schools of nursing have helped foster the discipline, establishing competencies and developing curricula.

As authors and editors, we believe that the nursing informatics literature has also helped to define the field and issues within it. This third edition of *Nursing Informatics: Where Caring and Technology Meet* reflects the most recent changes and supplements *Introduction to Nursing Informatics*, also published in this Springer series. As with the earlier editions, we asked a wide network of more than 40 contributors to represent as fully as possible the breadth and depth of nursing informatics expertise. Of the contributing authors, 23 have contributed to two editions, and seven to all three.

The third edition is structured differently than its two predecessors. As the field has evolved, it has begun to integrate the four basic nursing functions—clinical care, education, administration, and research. With this integration has come an acknowledgment of change as a constant in the profession and new roles as opportunities.

In this third edition, there are three sections. The first reviews the evolving discipline that is nursing informatics, with a special focus on professional education. The second focuses on enabling technologies in three areas—capabilities, approaches, and applications. The third section addresses emerging trends, and the appendices provide valuable information on nursing resources on the Internet and the World Wide Web.

What was "new" in the first two editions serves as the underlying framework for the third. Our contributors provide examples of integration in nursing practice rather than address it in theory. They report on advances in clinical nursing informatics to document the focus on patients, and they describe initiatives in telehealth, home care, and consumer informatics rather than discuss electronic networking in the abstract.

The truth is, nursing informatics has left its "baby steps" far behind. As a discipline, it is reaching maturity. Still, those of us who practice in this field have much to learn and much to do before we can transform health care.

We are fortunate to have the knowledge and the wisdom that our contributing authors provide in the pages that follow. Thanks to them, the third edition of *Nursing Informatics: Where Caring and Technology Meet* will guide us through this new millennium.

Marion J. Ball
Kathryn J. Hannah
Susan K. Newbold
Judith V. Douglas

Acknowledgments

As this volume documents, there is a place for nurse informaticians, who bring together caring and technology. There is also a place for those who give caring when technology can be of no assistance.

My heartfelt thanks to Charlene Cofill, Cathy Cummings, Rita Foster, Kathi Griffin, Karl Honse, Amy Jarboe, Mary Kirby, Shirley Mack, Barbara Ross, Christine Rover, Rita Russell, George Winer, Deidre Savage, and Antonio Quarles, all at the Arden Courts Alzheimer's Unit in Pikesville, Maryland. Special thanks to Mary Lindberg for her work on behalf of hospices and to Mary and Andre Thomas who volunteer their time through their church.

These are but a few of the army of incredibly kind and generous individuals who daily make the ill feel at ease and bring comfort to those in the last days of life.

To them all, we owe our deep regard and appreciation.

Marion J. Ball

We thank our husbands, John Ball, Rick Hannah, Paul Douglas, and Cree Newbold, for their continuing love and support. We want also to make special note of Jennifer Lillis and Mary Thomas for their patient and skillful help in bringing this volume into print.

Marion J. Ball
Kathryn J. Hannah
Susan K. Newbold
Judith V. Douglas

Contents

SECTION 1   AN EVOLVING DISCIPLINE

SECTION 2   ENABLING TECHNOLOGIES

Section 2.1   Capabilities

Section 2.2   Approaches

Section 2.3   Applications

SECTION 3   EMERGING TRENDS

APPENDICES

Content Array

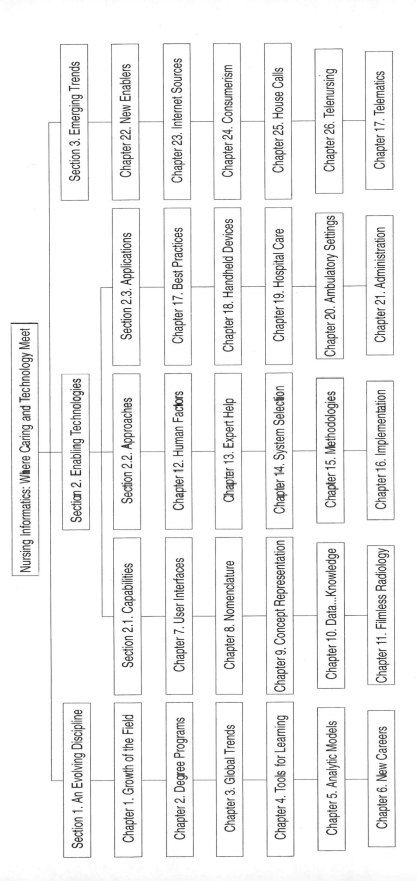

Nursing Informatics: Where Caring and Technology Meet

Section 1. An Evolving Discipline
- Chapter 1. Growth of the Field
- Chapter 2. Degree Programs
- Chapter 3. Global Trends
- Chapter 4. Tools for Learning
- Chapter 5. Analytic Models
- Chapter 6. New Careers

Section 2. Enabling Technologies

- Section 2.1. Capabilities
  - Chapter 7. User Interfaces
  - Chapter 8. Nomenclature
  - Chapter 9. Concept Representation
  - Chapter 10. Data...Knowledge
  - Chapter 11. Filmless Radiology

- Section 2.2. Approaches
  - Chapter 12. Human Factors
  - Chapter 13. Expert Help
  - Chapter 14. System Selection
  - Chapter 15. Methodologies
  - Chapter 16. Implementation

- Section 2.3. Applications
  - Chapter 17. Best Practices
  - Chapter 18. Handheld Devices
  - Chapter 19. Hospital Care
  - Chapter 20. Ambulatory Settings
  - Chapter 21. Administration

Section 3. Emerging Trends
- Chapter 22. New Enablers
- Chapter 23. Internet Sources
- Chapter 24. Consumerism
- Chapter 25. House Calls
- Chapter 26. Telenursing
- Chapter 17. Telematics

Section 1
An Evolving Discipline

Overview: New Directions in Nursing Informatics Education

MARION J. BALL

Over the past 15 years, in this new era of information and knowledge, we have seen significant curriculum changes in the area of nursing informatics (NI) education. Unlike the early days, when elementary courses outlined ways to incorporate enabling technologies into day-to-day nursing practice, nurses are now completing master's degrees and even doctorates in NI. As nurses have studied technology, technology has changed the way they study. Distance learning, telehealth, multimedia education, and the emphasis on continuous learning through conferences, courses, and workshops all contribute to the transition from traditional four-year programs to alternative nursing programs. New initiatives are introducing innovative ideas about NI education and the modalities used for it.

Informatics Courses: Trends and Objectives

In the coming years, more universities will develop educational programs in NI at the undergraduate, master's, and doctoral levels. Each level has a different objective, and each is developing programs at its own pace.

- Undergraduate programs aim to produce proficient users of information and information technology. Nevertheless, less than half of nursing schools currently offer informatics courses, a number that must continue to grow if students are to develop the basic computer competencies necessary for participation in NI specialty and interdisciplinary courses.
- Master's specialization programs in NI aim to produce nursing informatics specialists who can shape and manipulate information technology. Current programs are built around a core that emphasizes scientific inquiry, information management processes, data structures, and advanced nursing practice theory.
- Doctoral programs aim to produce NI scientists who can design innovative information systems, create models for system evaluation, make significant contributions to the research, and anticipate future nursing information requirements. Although doctoral programs offering prescribed curricula in NI are rare, more and more universities are allowing doctoral students to create their own course of NI study.

At all levels, there is a trend toward multimedia education, self-directed learning, and interdisciplinary study. All are valuable, but the interdisciplinary focus is particularly crucial, as it prepares the nursing informatician to think from other perspectives and collaborate with other disciplines to solve problems.

3

Continuing Education

Current projects in the United States reinforce the idea that NI education must be interdisciplinary and ongoing. Professional nursing organizations, informatics organizations, and universities sponsor a wide variety of continuing education opportunities. These include

- A very active Nursing Informatics Working Group (NIWG) sponsored by the American Medical Informatics Association (AMIA), an interdisciplinary organization
- NI educational sessions at the American Nurses Association's (ANA's) biennial convention
- The annual NI conference sponsored by the National League of Nursing's (NLN) Council for Nursing Informatics (CNI)
- The 13-month intensive course at Johns Hopkins, where new and challenging modalities of NI training are being developed

The international arena has also seen tremendous activity, well represented by the International Medical Informatics Association's (IMIA's) extremely active NI Special Interest Group. This association sponsors an excellent international NI conference every three years. Its 2000 meeting in New Zealand will address such issues as the history of NI, implementation and evaluation of health and nursing care systems, new approaches to the information technology (IT) needs of nurses and multidisciplinary teams, and future visions of the globally networked NI society. Every three years IMIA also sponsors MedInfo, an interdisciplinary international informatics conference.

Multimedia Education

Multimedia learning offers exciting possibilities to undergraduate and graduate nursing informatics students, as well as to nursing informaticians who recognize the importance of continuous learning. Computer-based multimedia, with its rich mixture of textual material, graphics, video, sound, and animation, open the door to abundant resources previously unavailable in books and classrooms. Existing and emerging examples of multimedia include

- Hypermedia and hypertext programs (like the World Wide Web)
- Multimedia databases
- Multimedia books
- Tutorials and problem-solving programs
- Virtual reality simulations and practice programs

Although software is still expensive to develop and content must be carefully regulated by nurses, the benefits of multimedia education can be significant. Computer-based multimedia ensures that learning is conducted at a time convenient to the student, offers access to diverse resources, provides quick feedback, and enables students to apply their learning to complex problems. Multimedia elements can also be used in patient education, a crucial advantage in the age of the empowered consumer. To realize these benefits, future research must develop effective tools for monitoring content, controlling cost, and evaluating and improving these programs.

Future Visions

Nursing informatics education will undergo more renovation in the coming decades. Course content will broaden and change. Large numbers of professionals trained in other disciplines (systems analysis and engineering, for instance) will continue to enter the field. The selection of educational software and Internet-based courses will grow. Nurses will become increasingly savvy in the business realm of their profession, with new courses pointing them toward jobs as chief information officers, senior administrators, chief executive officers, chief operations officers, and consultants. These trends will continue to expand the scope of the nursing profession, dissolving the remnants of nurses' menial task orientation and replacing it with a focus on managing the entire enterprise.

This new orientation is entirely appropriate. To meet the challenges of disease management, technology integration, evidence-based medicine, and the enlightenment of the consumer, nursing must play a key role in healthcare delivery, administration, and IT development and implementation. Because we face an enormous nursing shortage within the next five years, we will have to make effective and efficient use of existing talent by infusing a new set of IT tools. Education, in all its diverse forms, provides the foundation on which this effort will be built. Without it, nurse informaticians will be ill equipped to bring health care—and its enabling technologies—into the twenty-first century.

1
Nursing and Informatics

Marion J. Ball, Kathryn J. Hannah, and
Judith V. Douglas

Integrating computers into the practice of nursing is a challenge. As we embark on this new venture, we need to realize that nothing in life is easy. Change always elicits some fear, because it holds the unknown and unfamiliar. But if we remain complacent, viewing the glass as half full rather than half empty, we will miss the exciting opportunities that await the nursing profession in the twenty-first century. Our motto has always been, "don't wait for change . . . invent it!"

To understand where the nursing profession is today and where it is going in the near future, we first consider the external and internal forces that impact nursing. We then look at the new tools information technology is putting within our reach and explore how those tools, along with the emerging discipline of nursing informatics, will help us address those forces. We know that by the time this book is in print, there will be still more new approaches, new tools, and new applications available to the nursing profession.

Forces Impacting Nursing

Today, evolving standards of practice increase nursing accountability. The malpractice crisis has strengthened emphasis on complete and detailed nursing documentation. Changes in reimbursement methods are affecting nursing care delivery. Cost containment and consumerism place additional pressures on not only the individual nurse but also the entire nursing profession. The profession and its practitioners need to address, acknowledge, and prepare for the expanded and extended nursing roles created by advances in biomedical technology.

These external forces are exacerbated by internal pressures affecting the nursing environment. Hospital operations remain task oriented, systems do not promote practitioner accountability, and paperwork requirements have proliferated. These factors we cannot escape; we must confront them and master them. How do we do so? What are the new alternatives, the new tools available that allow us to address these forces? How can we grow in our profession and meet these challenges?

The change masters who have networked to produce this book will address these questions, repeatedly spiraling back to the host of issues and opportunities surrounding the use of computers in nursing care. Among the authors are nurses involved in every aspect of the profession, from clinical practice to education, from research to administration. They also include other professionals who have learned invaluable lessons in health care from the nursing profession and have lent their own special areas of expertise to nursing.

Information Technology Tools

No healthcare profession has more contact with the many aspects of patient care than does nursing. No other profession has more involvement with hospital information systems that touch all these aspects than does nursing. Unfortunately, until recently, nurses were not sufficiently involved in decisions regarding the selection and implementation of information systems or technology. As a result, many of the earlier systems in the marketplace and in hospitals have failed to meet nursing needs.

Nevertheless, there is little yield in dwelling on past failures—or even on the capabilities available at this exact moment in time. As Homer Warner, one of the United States' leading medical informaticians, has commented many times, "Let's not spend all our time and resources measuring how long it takes or how much it costs to get there with today's buggy. But let us get on with the job of building tomorrow's automobile and planning where to go with it." He means, of course, that we do not need to replicate. We do not need to study how we traveled with the old "horse and buggy" technology. Our challenge is to see how we can use new tools to innovate and transform.

In the mid-1980s, one of the authors (MJB) used to display one of the early laptop computers to her seminar audiences. Today, portable computers are part of the working world for health professionals. Nurses no longer need to stay tied to a large computer at a nursing station. Microchip technology allows us to augment as we innovate and transform, enabling us to access and enter information where it is needed—at the patient's bedside. Nurses no longer have to jot down vital signs and remember routine charting information until they can return to the nursing station to enter it. The tools go with the nurses who provide the care. There will be further transformation as we make innovative use of the tools available and cease to duplicate old manual methods of documentation.

Gradually, and with great effort, health care is implementing the computer-based patient record (CPR) concept across the continuum of care, from hospital to home care. Hospital information systems are being transformed into health information systems, and Web-enabled applications offer us exciting new capabilities. Building upon their traditional position at the center of patient care, nurses in the new millennium will play key roles in consumer health informatics, delivering and interpreting information. As health care becomes increasingly population and evidence based, nursing informatics will continue to be the discipline "where caring and technology meet" and will lead us toward the World Health Organization's vision of better health care for all.

Stages of Integration

Wherever we put new healthcare technology to use, we all pass through three defined stages before we become more or less comfortable with using the new technology. These three stages—substitution, innovation, and transformation—are classic diffusion steps in the adoption of computing and information technology.

Substitution

When we get a new tool into our hands, the only thing we can do with it at first is to try to do what we have been doing in a manual fashion. Maybe we can do it a little faster or a little more efficiently, but in effect, we are replacing a manual function with a new tool.

Over the past 25 years, we have remained in this first stage as we have introduced computers into health care. We brought computers into the admissions office, and we learned to type information into a terminal. By replacing typewriters, we could more easily disseminate the information and make changes without correction fluid. This made the task a bit easier, but we were only using part of the technology's capability.

Innovation

From substitution, we move into what is called the *innovation* stage. Here, we go beyond what we could do manually, using the computer to do things we could not do before. In this stage, the new technology begins to be diffused throughout health care. Computer systems become commonplace in large-scale health information systems, as they have in radiology, pharmacy, and clinical laboratories.

Transformation

It is true that other industries—airlines, travel, banking—are approaching the final stage of integration, the diffusion of the new tools, somewhat ahead of health care. This stage, called *transformation*, lies beyond substitution and innovation. It involves completely reinventing the way business is and can be done.

In the healthcare profession, the one area to have entered the transformation stage is radiology. Radiology practices today are a transformation of the processes in use as few as 10 years ago. Computerized axial tomography has given us the now-standard computed tomographic scan. Even the ways in which radiographic images (or X-rays) are read and reported are not at all similar to how they were done before new computerized capabilities were available. Every one of these instruments is based on a built-in computer.

When we look at the nursing profession and its practices, it is exciting to realize that we are navigating these phases together and that all of us are somewhere in this process. Since the second edition of this book, many of us have left the substitution stage and are entering into innovation. Nursing is becoming part of the revolution—not just the evolution—that is transforming the profession.

The Informatics Revolution

Clearly, nurses and all other healthcare professionals are having to learn new skills and approaches in order to leave the substitution stage of technology integration and enter the transformation stage. The learning process and the widespread use that follows are covered by the term *informatics*. The term *medical informatics*, in use for over 25 years, is becoming a widely used phrase with a more global definition that encompasses other healthcare professions.

Coined from the French word *informatique*, informatics includes all aspects of the computer milieu, from the theoretical to the applied. A recent attempt at a definition describes healthcare informatics as "the application of information technology to enhance the quality of care, facilitate accountability, and assist in cost containment" (Ball & Douglas, 1997). As the discussion of evolving definitions in Chapter 2 indicates, the field of informatics is continually undergoing self-analysis and redefinition in order to find its niche in our fast-changing world. The profession is now moving toward the next generation of nursing informatics, called *clinical nursing informatics*. This falls within the new clinical informatics paradigm (Ball et al., 1997) that must "integrate the processes of designing and redesigning [health care] with information sciences and information technology" (p. 18).

Here we cite one of the recent and most far-reaching attempts at a definition that includes nursing informatics, undertaken by Working Group 1 (WG1) of the International Medical Informatics Association (IMIA). According to WG1, health and medical informatics education is an inclusive term that covers nursing along with other professions. The recommendations prepared by WG1 clarify and set forth the knowledge and skills needed in health and medical informatics and specify learning outcomes within a robust and nonprescriptive framework.

To advance health and medical informatics education, WG1 plans to work with national societies and professional associations in harmonization efforts. This initiative merits the full participation of nursing informatics educators and specialists around the globe, and nursing is fortunately well represented in WG1.

Nursing Informatics

The part of informatics designed for and relevant to nurses has been labeled *nursing informatics*. This term and what it represents will become part of our entire professional vocabulary and practice. It combines all aspects of nursing—clinical practice, administration, research, and education—just as computing holds the power to integrate all four aspects.

Graves and Corcoran (1989) define nursing informatics as "a combination of computer science, information science and nursing science designed to assist in the management and processing of nursing data, information and knowledge to support the practice of nursing and the delivery of nursing care." Any use of information technologies by nurses in relation to the care of patients, the administration of healthcare facilities, or the educational preparation of individuals to practice the discipline is considered nursing informatics. This can include decision making, patient education, self-education, research, and administrative applications.

New Roles for Nurses

Developments in nursing informatics will continue to have a profound impact on how nursing is practiced. A side effect of the evolution of nursing informatics has been the growth of new roles for nursing, as discussed elsewhere in this volume. Such roles are developing in industry, research, systems development, nursing education, and nursing administration. Nurses, most notably those with bachelor's and master's degrees, are participating in the selection and implementation of systems for use at the bedside. Nurses also articulate the information needs of healthcare professionals and of clients in clinical practice settings to the system designers and engineers.

New roles are also evolving for nurses in the field of consulting. Hospitals are now beginning to hire nurse consultants to assist in the design and implementation phases as well as in the process of selecting computers. They are concerned not only with input into what the software should be but also with how healthcare professionals communicate with one another and with computing professionals. Furthermore, the understanding of data mining and expert systems use and their application to care is at the heart of evidence-based medicine and quality of care.

For the Clinical Nurse

Nurses with a vocation for direct patient care need not sacrifice their calling in order to participate in the information revolution in nursing. In fact, the reason that many nurses have ventured into the field of nursing informatics is a common vision of using information systems to enhance the practice of nursing and to benefit the patient by extending and improving health care, as their new roles illustrate.

Informatics will free nurses to assume the responsibility for planning holistic and humanistic nursing care for patients and their families, reviewing and examining nursing practice (quality assurance), applying basic research to innovative solutions to patient care problems, and devising creative new models for the delivery of nursing care. Hands-on, or "high-touch," care will remain the heart of the profession. Nurses in computer-aided patient care situations will become involved in administering some nontraditional therapies, such as hypnosis, therapeutic touch, acupuncture, biofeedback, and sonic vibration.

The advances in the use of information technology will necessitate a more scientific and complex approach to the nursing care process. Consequently, nurses will require better educational preparation and more inquiring and investigative approaches to patient care. Nurses will also need to be more discriminating users of information. No longer will nursing practice focus on the assessment and care planning phase; rather, it will emphasize the implementation phase. Thus, nurses will require an expanded repertoire of intervention skills as well as organizational management skills.

Based on the nurse's body of knowledge and professional judgment, autonomous nursing interventions are complementary to, not competitive with, physician-prescribed treatments. In this context, clinical nurse specialist training at the master's degree level offers nurses the opportunity to use increased knowledge and clinical practice skills at the bedside. This intensification of the role of bedside nurses provides alternate career paths for nurses who prefer patient care to administration, research, or education.

In the delivery of health care, nurses have traditionally provided the interface between the client and the healthcare system. They are now fulfilling this function in new ways as they move into a technologically advanced environment. With nursing informatics as a guide, nurses are identifying and developing new ways of using computers and information science as tools to support the practice of nursing. At the same time, computers and information science are facilitating a more sophisticated and expanded level of nursing practice. There is an interactive and synergistic effect between nursing informatics and nursing practice. The boundaries of nursing informatics are contiguous with those of nursing and, like them, dynamic and constantly changing.

Embracing Change

One key question remains: How do we get this new technology accepted by our colleagues? No hospital information system or standalone surgical software system will be installed successfully, no tool used effectively, unless there is an enormous amount of preparation and training. A diffusion pathway must be laid to bring something in that will completely revolutionize the way in which all of us practice our profession. If this pathway is never built, the attempt at computerization will be a failure. We do not have to guess at this. We have seen it happen.

As a profession, we have participated in government-funded investigations on the effect of hospital information systems on healthcare delivery in nursing practice. We are progressing beyond the clinical environment and moving professionally into the establishment of a bona fide research component. We will be looking at nursing practice and nursing education, assessing the problems and issues surrounding information technology, from implementation to ergonomics.

One of the biggest concerns now is that we provide strong master's and doctoral programs as well as superb bachelor's degrees in our nursing schools. The Johns Hopkins University School of Nursing is developing a doctoral program in clinical nursing informatics that will be a model for other programs. Nursing informatics needs to be incorporated into the curricula offered by all of our nursing schools. The National Library of Medicine has for years funded training programs in medical informatics, acting as a catalyst for change. Graduates of the first programs in nursing informatics are assuming leadership positions across the nation. With much work yet to do, the academic preparation of informatics nurse specialists remains critical, as chapters elsewhere in this section explain.

Awaiting the Future

Nursing informatics has arrived, and the baby has started to walk. In the process, nursing informatics has introduced new challenges and opportunities along with new computer applications. For nurses, it has created a new cadre of roles and a new vision of the nursing profession. Vendors of hospital information systems employ nurses as consultants now, as nursing liaison advisors to the data processing division. Nurses are becoming programmers, systems engineers, and systems analysts. We firmly believe that as computerization changes the profession, nursing will reappraise its value system and reward professionalism in a wide range of nursing duties not traditionally recognized. In sum, nursing will have greater diversity by virtue of employment opportunities in the health informatics field, leading to better health care worldwide.

We may ask ourselves, "Isn't this just individuals changing professions and leaving nursing?" Not quite, for it involves more. Systems analysts and engineers who come from nursing backgrounds practice their profession differently from those coming from an engineering or mathematics background. This holds tremendous advantages for nurses remaining in the more traditional nursing fields, for who understands the nursing process better than a nurse? Developers who understand the nursing profession and its needs, from abstract concepts to small details, are invaluable. Thus the evolution of professions—the hybridization of nurse and computer expert—is critical to effecting the transformation we anticipate.

What shape will that transformation take in the next five years? We will see more computer power become ubiquitous, voice input free our hands for patient care, and Web-enabled applications give us access to vast quantities of stored data and visual information. We will benefit from expert systems, data mining techniques, decision support systems, modeling systems, and nursing outcomes research. The greatest benefits, however, will not come from the individual tools, as powerful and as effective as they prove to be. Nursing will reap the most from the knowledge created from the information these new technologies make available. Computing will be a powerful utility, fueling our healthcare information systems just as electricity fuels our operating room lights and respirators.

In electronic terms, computing is the medium; information transformed into knowledge the message. This new medium of computing holds our future. It is our charge to use it well, to create the information-rich environment where patient care and the many functions that support it are of the highest quality. As a profession, nursing can do no less.

Questions

1. What are some of the forces impacting nurses today?
2. List and define the three stages of diffusion of new technology.
3. What role is industry playing in acknowledging the new discipline of nursing informatics?
4. Take a brief look into the future and give a description as to what you might be doing in your job 10 years from today. How does automation fit into this role?

References

Ball MJ, Douglas JV. Health care informatics: where caring and technology meet. *CommonHealth* 1997(Winter);18.

Ball MJ, Douglas JV, Hoehn BJ. Clinical informatics: a new paradigm. *M.D. Computing* 1997;14(1):18–23.

Graves JR, Corcoran S. The study of nursing informatics. *Image: Journal of Nursing Scholarship* 1989;21(4):227–231.

International Medical Informatics Association. IMIA Recommendations on Education in Health and Medical Informatics. http://www.imia.org/wg1 (October, 1999).

2
Academic Preparation in Nursing Informatics*

CAROLE A. GASSERT

Nursing informatics (NI) has become well established as a specialty within nursing and health informatics, the broader category of informatics practice. Nursing informatics practice focuses on the representation of nursing information and its management and processing within the health informatics community. It is one example of a domain-specific informatics practice. Medical, dental, and consumer informatics are other examples.

Informatics experts, including nurses, are being sought to help employers manage information more competitively. Increased recognition of the need for collecting and aggregating healthcare information has created exciting opportunities for nurses. They are crucial contributors to the development and implementation of the information structures and technology needed in today's healthcare environment.

Since the words "nursing informatics" first appeared in the literature in 1984, the field of practice has been named, defined, and recognized as a specialty by the nursing profession. Academic programs to prepare nurses within the field have also been developed. In addition, standards for the practice of nursing informatics have been written. Finally, a certification examination has been developed to credential as informatics nurses those individuals who demonstrate beginning levels of competency in NI.

The purpose of this chapter is to discuss the educational preparation of nurses in nursing informatics. Although the focus is on describing academic opportunities in NI, it is necessary to examine nursing informatics as a specialty, discussing its definition, specialty attributes, scope of practice, and standards as they influence academic program development.

---

*The views expressed in this chapter are solely those of the author and not necessarily those of the Health Resources and Services Administration, Department of Health and Human Services.

Evolving Definition of Nursing Informatics

Since the 1970s, nurses have been contributing to the design of information systems, consulting with healthcare agencies about selecting and using information technology, and helping to install and use information systems in hospitals. In 1992, their roles were professionally acknowledged when the American Nurses Association (ANA) recognized NI as an area of specialty practice in nursing (Milholland, 1992). Although many nurses practice in the specialty, others are still asking, "what is nursing informatics?"

The delineation of nursing informatics has been dynamic, changing to reflect growth within the field. As initially identified in the literature by Ball and Hannah (1984), NI was defined as the discipline of applying computer science to nursing processes. A year later, NI was described as a focus that uses information technology to perform functions within nursing (Hannah, 1985). This later definition was easily understood and therefore widely dispersed in nursing to explain the new practice area. Although useful, the definition failed to acknowledge NI activities beyond the use of computer applications.

Subsequent definitions represented a more widely delineated practice, including reference to a theoretical basis for practice. In 1988, Grobe described nursing informatics as "the application of the principles of information science and theory to the study, scientific analysis, and management of nursing information for purposes of establishing a body of nursing knowledge" (Grobe, 1988a, p. 29). A more widely disseminated and accepted definition appeared in a classic article that describes the study of nursing informatics. In their article, the authors define NI as "the combination of nursing science, information science, and computer science to manage and process nursing data, information, and knowledge to facilitate the delivery of health care" (Graves & Corcoran, 1989, p. 227). Computers are acknowledged as *tools* used in the NI field.

Both the Grobe definition and the Graves and Corcoran definition are important for three reasons. First, they more accurately describe the field, allowing such issues as information processing, language development, application of the systems life cycle, and usability to be identified as part of NI. Second, these definitions have implications for the content to be included in curricula used to prepare informatics nurses. Finally, these definitions serve as a foundation for the ANA's definition. The ANA scope of practice document states that nursing informatics "is the specialty that integrates nursing science, computer science, and information science in identifying, collecting, processing, and managing data and information to support nursing practice, administration, education, research and the expansion of nursing knowledge" (ANA, 1994, p. 3).

Specialty Attributes of Nursing Informatics

Designation of an interest area of nursing as a specialty is a multifaceted process (Panniers & Gassert, 1996). The following attributes must be demonstrated:

- A differentiated practice
- A research program
- Representation of the specialty by at least one organized body
- A mechanism for credentialing nurses in the specialty
- Educational programs for preparing nurses to practice in the specialty

Different focal points separate NI practice from other nursing specialties. Nursing informatics focuses on the structure and algorithms of information used by nurses in their practice, while other nursing specialties focus on the content of information used (Lange, 1997). In addition, informatics nurses focus on the processes of information management and the technology needed to effectively implement those processes.

Nurses have worked in informatics roles for more than two decades. Although the purchase and implementation of information technology in healthcare settings continues to demand considerable attention from informatics nurses, such activities do not define the entire domain of nursing informatics practice. Nursing language development, implementing NI educational programs, establishing telehealth systems, and solving systems usability issues are other examples of NI practice. These examples reflect the diverse and differentiated nature of NI practice.

By establishing a specific research program, nursing informatics has fulfilled a second attribute required for recognition as a specialty. When Schwirian (1986) proposed a research framework for NI, there was little reported scientific inquiry in the field. Since that time, however, an increasing number of NI researchers have reported their work at national and international conferences and in the literature. Recently, several authors have reported on the development of nursing language (Grobe, 1996; Henry et al., 1998; Martin & Norris, 1996; McCloskey et al., 1998; Ozbolt, 1996; Saba, 1997). Others have studied the impact of systems on patient care (Brennan, 1998), examined the design of information systems (Staggers, 1997; Zielstorff, 1998), or developed and evaluated NI models (Gassert, 1990, 1996a,b, 1997; Staggers & Park, 1993; Turley, 1996). Nursing informatics researchers also have investigated the decision-making processes of nurses (Fonteyn & Grobe, 1994; Thompson, 1997; Panniers & Walker, 1994). All of these examples support topics identified as research priorities for NI by the National Institute for Nursing Research at the National Institutes of Health (National Council on Nursing Research, 1993).

A third attribute needed for qualification as a specialty is to be represented by at least one professional body. Three major nursing organizations, the ANA, the National League for Nursing (NLN), and the American Organization of Nurse Executives, have established special interest groups that target NI. An interdisciplinary organization, the American Medical Informatics Association (AMIA), also has a nursing informatics working group (NIWG). At the international level, the International Medical Informatics Association (IMIA) has an NI special interest group with representation from member countries. There are also many regional NI organizations that promote information sharing among NI members. The formation and maintenance of NI special interest groups is extremely important in providing information exchange, mentoring, and educational experiences for nurses who are new to the field. With the support of so many organizations, NI has more than met the attribute of representation by a professional body.

The fourth attribute needed for recognition as a specialty is a mechanism for credentialing members of an interest area. The certification process for NI has been developed through the ANA and its affiliate, the American Nurses Credentialing Center (ANCC). Two separate task forces of nurses representing NI practice, education, and administration were appointed by the ANA to develop the scope of practice document and standards for NI practice. The ANA Council for Nursing Systems and Administration (formerly the Council of Computer Applications in Nursing) coordinated the task forces, and a certification examination for credentialing nurses as generalists in NI was developed under the direction of the ANCC. Although an NI specialist certification examination was originally planned, to date it has not been developed.

As a final attribute, a specialty must have educational programs to prepare nurses to practice within that field. Nursing informatics education will be discussed later in this chapter.

Nursing Informatics Practice

The scope of practice document outlines in detail what is and is not NI practice. In terms of educational preparation, it is important to note that although informatics nurses are expected to be competent in the use of information technology, NI practice should not be defined solely by the use of technology. The scope of practice document further describes the boundaries, core, intersections, and dimensions of NI. In essence, the document states that while the field focuses on the nursing perspective of data, information, and knowledge, NI also recognizes that collaboration within the larger umbrella of health informatics is requisite to developing integrated information tools that will benefit both providers and recipients of health care (ANA, 1994). Hence NI education should be interdisciplinary.

Authorizing legislation passed in 1992 prohibited further funding of nursing administration educational programs by the Division of Nursing, the federal agency charged with nursing work force preparation. This led to discussion of whether nursing informatics practice is clinical or administrative in nature (Simpson, 1993). Some have defined clinical NI and administrative NI as distinct entities, a distinction that seems artificial. Because NI activities have as a foundation the handling of clinical data and information, it seems best to describe all NI as a practice in which the informatics practitioner moves back and forth between a direct or indirect practice focus depending on patient and client needs. Handling individual patient data in the clinical setting would be considered direct informatics practice, whereas handling aggregate-level data for allocating resources would be indirect informatics practice. Educational programs in NI should provide students with knowledge and experience from both direct and indirect practice.

Nursing informatics is generally practiced in one of five arenas: healthcare agencies, consulting firms, vendor corporations, academic settings, and private business practices. As health care shifts its focus to nontraditional environments (such as outpatient and home care) and to the use of telehealth systems to deliver care, NI practice needs to move into these areas. Specific practice activities may vary from one setting to another, but the following list of activities generally describes NI practice:

- Developing applications, tools, processes, and structures that help nurses manage data
- Evaluating applications, tools, processes, and structures to determine their effectiveness for nursing
- Adapting existing information technologies to meet nurses' and clients' needs
- Managing systems selection, implementation, and evaluation
- Collaborating with other healthcare informatics professionals in developing solutions to previously identified information needs for nurses and clients
- Using informatics theories and principles to develop and test computerized educational systems, such as those delivered through the World Wide Web
- Developing and testing informatics models and theories pertaining to handling, communicating, or transforming nursing information
- Developing a taxonomy or naming system to describe and order nursing phenomena
- Conducting research to advance the knowledge base of nursing informatics
- Consulting with patients and clients about NI
- Teaching the theory and practice of NI

As the field of NI practice expands, different activities may be added to the list. With such a large scope of practice, it is not uncommon for informatics nurses to try to focus their practice in a way that allows for the development of one or two areas of expertise. Some informatics nurses have developed expertise in building taxonomies, while others have refined the processes associated with systems implementation. Increasingly, informatics nurses will need to share their expertise within interdisciplinary teams. Limited resources and the need to develop information technology solutions that are common to all clinicians are fostering interdisciplinary practice.

Informatics Nurse Specialist Role

According to the scope of practice document, nurses who practice in the field of NI are designated as either informatics nurses (IN) or informatics nurse specialists (INS), depending on whether they are prepared at the baccalaureate or graduate levels in nursing (ANA, 1994). This specification is consistent with ANA requirements that specialists have graduate education in nursing. Many INs have graduate preparation in fields that are outside of but support nursing informatics, such as business or computer science (Carty, 1994; Gassert, 1994). Regardless of their academic degree, almost all INs and INSs bring clinical practice experience to their roles.

Nurse specialists have traditionally described their roles by identifying different components or facets of their jobs. It seems appropriate, therefore, to describe INS roles in terms of the components of practice, consultation, research, marketing, education, and management. The practice component covers such activities as design, development, selection, testing, implementation, enhancement, and use of information technology. The consultation component includes advising and helping others to reach solutions related to information technology. The research component covers investigation of such problems as research methodology, symbolic representation of data, clinical decision making, ergonomics, usability issues, and information system impact. Marketing activities include selling both products and ideas related to information and information technology.

The educational role component includes training, presentation of both informal and formal programs in informatics, and development of learning technologies. Management, the final component, involves overseeing issues of change, quality, redesign, adoption and innovation, project planning, and cost. Just as the activities depend on the practice setting, the INS's primary role component may change with the setting or priorities of the employer. A discussion of competencies needed to practice in the field of NI follows.

Nursing Informatics Competencies

A competency is defined as "having sufficient knowledge, judgment, skill, or strength" (Grobe, 1988b, p. 4). Identifying competencies for a specialty and certifying nurses who meet those competencies promotes higher quality in specialty practice (Parker, 1994). IMIA's Work Group on Nursing

Informatics initially identified levels of informatics competencies (Peterson & Gerdin-Jelger, 1988). The statements of competency were intended to describe preparation of the general population of nurses relative to informatics as they accomplished their roles of clinician, nurse administrator, nurse educator, and nurse researcher (Grobe, 1989). The Work Group's designation of levels of preparation, however, has been used as the basis for organizing specialty programs in NI at the University of Maryland at Baltimore (UMB) (Gassert et al., 1992).

Nurses prepared with level 1 competencies are considered to be information technology users. These individuals know, understand, use, and interact with computer applications and healthcare information systems. These nurses must also be prepared to collect relevant data for patient care, access information needed for providing nursing services, and implement policies to ensure privacy, confidentiality, and security of data. Such preparation should take place in baccalaureate (basic) nursing programs. The scope of practice for NI states that these competencies are required for all nurses (ANA, 1994). Historically, nursing education programs have been slow to incorporate informatics competencies into the curriculum, and many practicing nurses still lack "user level" competencies.

Nurses with level 2 competencies are recognized as information technology modifiers, who analyze, manage, critique, develop, modify, and evaluate information technology for nursing. In addition to information technology skills, modifiers apply theoretical knowledge of nursing science, information science, computer science, and business to their practice. Modifiers' practices are focused in nursing informatics, and they are expected to conduct research to contribute to the body of knowledge. Modifiers are the INSs prepared at the master's level in graduate specialty programs in nursing informatics.

Nurses with level 3 competencies are identified as information technology innovators. These nurses design and develop research-based information technology for nursing, analyze and define the structure of nursing language, and explain the processing of information by nurses as they make both clinical and administrative decisions. Innovators are prepared at the doctoral level in nursing. With highly sophisticated preparation in research, nursing science, and information and computer science, innovators should contribute significantly to the body of NI knowledge and design information technology that truly supports nurses in delivering patient care.

Nursing Informatics Standards of Practice (ANA, 1995) defines the responsibilities for practice and professional performance for which generalist-level (initially competent) INs are held accountable. There are six standards that address the practice activities of INs. Eight standards speak to the professional performance of INs, and six additional standards delineate expectations for performance relative to the domain or field of NI. Informatics nurses are expected to meet each of the 20 standards but not every measurement criterion within each of the standards. The scope of practice document, competency lists, and standards should serve as the basis for developing educational programs in nursing informatics.

Nurse educators interested in NI programs should consider using lists of expected competencies requisite to developing the curriculum. Such lists are available in Peterson and Gerdin-Jelger's publication (1988) and in the ANA scope of practice document (1994). The standards are also distributed through the ANA (1995).

Nursing Informatics Education

Nurses frequently ask how they can learn more about informatics education. The NIWG of AMIA maintains a Web page that lists educational opportunities (Nursing Informatics Working Group, 1999). Generally, educational opportunities can be divided into six categories, as shown in Table 2.1.

Continuing Education in Nursing Informatics

Many professional development (continuing education) opportunities are available in NI through workshops and conferences sponsored by profes-

TABLE 2.1. Models of nursing informatics education.

Type	Programs
Continuing education and professional development	AMIA congresses NLN conferences HIMSS annual conference IMIA international NI meeting New York University NI conference Rutgers University international conference University of Maryland summer institute
Graduate programs with a specialty in NI	New York University Saint Louis University University of Maryland University of Utah
Post-master's certificate in NI	Duke University New York University Saint Louis University University of Arizona University of Iowa University of Maryland
Graduate programs with NI concentrations and minors	Northeastern University University of Arizona University of Iowa
Post-master's fellowships in NI	Partners HealthCare System Harvard Medical School and Deaconess Medical Center
Informatics courses	Graduate and undergraduate courses

sional nursing organizations, informatics organizations, and universities. The ANA has included NI educational sessions at its biennial convention. The NLN Council for Nursing Informatics (CNI), an active special interest group, has sponsored an annual conference focusing on NI. In 1998, the CNI implemented an exciting conference and membership meeting through a webcast (Nelson et al., 1999).

An interdisciplinary organization, Healthcare Information Management Systems Society (HIMSS), has conducted an annual informatics conference that includes informatics issues pertinent to nursing. The organization also invites nurses to learn about clinical information systems issues by joining an interdisciplinary special interest group.

AMIA, another interdisciplinary organization, has a very active NIWG that offers workshops, seminars, and other educational sessions in conjunction with spring and fall meetings. The NI Special Interest Group of IMIA sponsors an excellent international NI conference every three years. The 2000 meeting will be held in New Zealand, and Brazil will host the 2003 meeting. IMIA also sponsors MedInfo, an interdisciplinary international informatics conference, every three years.

Several universities have offered continuing education in NI. For more than 10 years, New York University (NYU) Medical Center conducted an NI conference each spring. NYU now offers a fall meeting through the nursing department. Rutgers University also has hosted a spring NI conference for 17 years.

While directing nursing informatics at the UMB School of Nursing, this author collaborated with the director of the campus Information Resources Division to develop a summer institute in 1991 (Gassert, 1994). The institute continues to focus on information technology and its effects on administrative and clinical nursing practice, information systems selection and evaluation, strategies for systems implementation, and informatics trends and issues from the nursing perspective.

Increased informatics educational opportunities are evidenced by the number of workshop and conference announcements distributed through traditional and electronic mail. Most conferences provide an excellent opportunity to learn about state-of-the-art technology and informatics issues, but some nurses, particularly those who enter informatics without academic preparation in the field, are looking for programs to help them learn how to perform their role. In addition, few conferences focus on the theories and concepts nurses need to practice NI as delineated by the standards.

Courses in Nursing Informatics

To prepare nurses in informatics, nursing schools are adding informatics to undergraduate and graduate curricula. For example, Travis and Brennan (1998) describe a series of courses that prepare undergraduate students to be sophisticated "users" of information and information technology. Earlier literature describes informatics courses that prepare practicing nurses and graduate students to be "users" of information technology (McGonigle & Eggers, 1991; Magnus et al., 1994). The Web lists NI courses offered by Lewis University, Loyola University, Georgia State University, Wichita State, and Hunter College (Nursing Informatics Working Group, 1999). Given the importance of appropriate information management in health care and the prevalence of using information technology to process information, one would expect all nursing schools to include informatics in the curriculum. Surprisingly, Carty and Rosenfeld (1998) found that less than one third of nursing schools in a stratified random sample of NLN-accredited schools included informatics in the curriculum.

Master's Specialization in Nursing Informatics

Not only is there a need for basic informatics preparation for nurses, but with the growing sophistication of information technology in nursing, there is also a need for specialized NI education. The purpose of graduate specialization in NI is to prepare INSs, individuals who can modify information management processes, data structures, and the technology needed to support information processing.

Master's specialty education in NI is built on several assumptions. First, one major area of coursework must be nursing science. Students must have baccalaureate preparation in nursing to allow them to increase their nursing knowledge at the graduate level. Increased theoretical understanding of nursing and nursing research facilitates the INS's ability to represent accurately nursing's view of informatics issues and solutions. Another assumption is that coursework must have an interdisciplinary focus on either information systems management or biomedical computing. This concentration of coursework builds students' knowledge base of technical and management issues related to information and information systems. Learning with another discipline also prepares the INS to work with other disciplines to identify problems and offer solutions from an interdisciplinary perspective. The result should be more representative and integrated information management solutions for all clinicians.

A third assumption is that state-of-the-art technology must be available to support students' technological growth. Not only must students have access to the latest technologies, they must also be able to use technologies from different technical environments. The INS must be flexible and able to move with advances in technology. Implied in the third assumption is that NI programs will have personnel available to support students (and faculty) technologically. The nursing informatics faculty can help with technological support, but additional personnel are needed.

The fourth assumption is that adequate numbers and a variety of practicum sites must be available to students. Sites in traditional and non-traditional healthcare agencies, vendor corporations, and consulting firms should be available. Having additional sites in organizations that set informatics policy, academic settings, and entrepreneurial NI practices would allow students to match career interests with available NI activities as they apply newly acquired knowledge during guided experiences.

The final assumption is that students must be prepared in basic computer competencies before starting NI specialty and interdisciplinary courses. The NI scope of practice document indicates that graduates of basic nursing programs should be able to use informatics applications that have been designed for the clinical practice of nursing (ANA, 1994). To expand on this thinking, if students decide to *specialize* in NI, which uses the computer as a tool, they should have basic microcomputer skills in word processing, spreadsheet applications, database manipulation, e-mail, World Wide Web, and presentation graphics. Furthermore, rather than being intimidated by computers, they should be inquisitive and self-directed in learning to use new applications and technologies.

This author developed the curriculum and implemented the first graduate specialization program in NI at UMB in 1988 (Gassert, 1989; Heller et al., 1989). The program was funded as a prototype for NI education within nursing administration. In 1990, the University of Utah was funded as a second model of NI education because of its focus on clinical nursing (Graves et al., 1995). These two programs received their start-up funding from the Division of Nursing, Health Resources and Services Administration. For several years, only UMB and Utah awarded master's degrees in NI (Carty, 1994), but additional NI specialty programs are now open. In 1998, NYU opened an NI specialty program at the graduate level. Saint Louis University also offers a specialty program in NI.

All four programs build on a master's core that emphasizes scientific inquiry, theoretical bases for advanced nursing practice, and healthcare delivery systems. Consistent with the philosophy of the informatics community, all of the programs emphasize the need for their students to understand interdisciplinary approaches to informatics solutions. All but the Utah program require NI students to take informatics courses in departments outside of nursing. Utah utilizes an interdisciplinary approach within the NI courses and encourages students to take elective courses outside of nursing.

The total number of credit hours of specialty courses varies among the four NI programs, but the content is similar. The UMB program requires 30 semester credit hours of coursework in informatics (Table 2.2). There are 15 credits allocated to the NI major and 15 credits of information science support. The total NI program requires 40 credits.

The master's specialization program at the University of Utah requires 25 to 26 semester credit hours of coursework in informatics (Table 2.3). Students take six credits of systems core courses and 19 to 20 credits of specialty area courses. Utah students also take six credits of a thesis or master's project focused in informatics. The NI program requires a total of 38 to 39 credits.

TABLE 2.2. University of Maryland at Baltimore nursing informatics courses.

Major courses
  Organizational Theories
  Managerial Health Finance
  Computer Applications in Nursing and Health Care
  Concepts in Nursing Informatics
  Practicum in Nursing Informatics
Support courses[1]
  Structured Systems Analysis and Design
  Project Management
  Database Program Development
  Data Communications and Networks
  Decision Support Systems

[1] Support courses could also focus on expert systems, neural networks, telehealth, or interface design.

The NI program at NYU requires students to complete 21 semester credit hours in the specialty. Courses are listed in Table 2.4.

The final NI specialty program to be covered is at Saint Louis University. It requires a total of 41 semester credits. Students in the program take 29 credit hours of informatics courses from the Schools of Nursing, Business and Administration, and Public Health (Table 2.5).

Some nurses who are master's prepared in other specialties have asked the academic community to allow them to attend informatics courses along with the NI specialty students. This has resulted in the development of post-master's certificate options in NI. Such options are available at schools of nursing at Duke University, Saint Louis University, NYU, University of Arizona, University of Iowa, and UMB.

TABLE 2.3. University of Utah nursing informatics courses.

Systems core courses
  Program Planning and Development
  Program Management and Evaluation
Required specialty area courses
  Introduction to Nursing Informatics
  Clinical Systems Analysis and Design
  Clinical Decision Support
  Clinical Database Design
  Clinical Systems Implementation
  Practicum in Nursing Informatics
  Master's Project or Thesis

TABLE 2.4. New York University nursing informatics courses.

Nursing Informatics: An Introduction
Assessment and Analysis of Clinical and Nursing Information Systems
Database Design and Decision Support in Clinical and Nursing Systems
Implementation, Management and Evaluation of Clinical and Nursing Systems
Nursing Informatics Internship

Master's Programs with Nursing Informatics Concentrations and Minors

Three programs indicate that their graduate curricula include courses in NI along with other requirements for other specialties in nursing (Nursing Informatics Working Group, 1999). Northeastern University requires their nursing administration majors to take three NI courses. The University of Arizona offers an MS degree with Role Development Option for Systems Management. Within this major, informatics is one of the emphasis areas. Finally, the University of Iowa offers a 20-semester credit hour certificate in informatics within the administration focus.

Doctoral Specialization in Nursing Informatics

The purpose of a doctoral program in NI is to prepare innovators or NI scientists. The NI scientist will be prepared to

- Conceptualize nursing information requirements for the future
- Design effective nursing information systems
- Create innovative information technology
- Conduct research regarding integration of technology with nursing practice, administration, education, and research
- Develop theoretical, practice, and evaluation models for NI
- Augment work to develop taxonomies and lexicons for atomic-level nursing data.

Given the expected activities, the NI scientist focuses on the role components of researcher and designer/developer. Employment opportunities

TABLE 2.5. Saint Louis University nursing informatics courses.

Health Information Systems
Program Development Techniques
Introduction to Object-Oriented Programming
Systems Analysis and Design
Nursing Informatics Concepts
Information Systems in Public Health
Database Management Systems
Administration of Care Systems I and II
Practicum in Nursing Informatics

could be available as appointments in academic institutions, directors of research and/or information systems in healthcare facilities, research and development for software companies, appointments to government agencies, and consultants in research for information systems.

Doctoral programs should be built on several assumptions. Because of the informatics activities expected from these innovators, the doctoral program should build on a master's degree in nursing informatics. Included in this assumption is a belief that students must have sophisticated information management and technology competencies before entering the doctoral program. Because the number of master's specialization programs is limited, students may need to be admitted without such a background, but they should take additional courses to build their knowledge base in NI.

A second assumption for a doctoral program is that an interdisciplinary approach must be maintained. Students should take doctoral-level courses required for information systems students with an emphasis on improving their capabilities in designing and developing information technology. A third assumption is that adequate state-of-the-art technology and technological support must be available to students, as discussed previously. In addition, the physical environment should allow doctoral students to be assigned to their own computer and working space to facilitate design and development efforts. The final assumption of doctoral study is that adequate informatics researchers must be available in the academic community to support student research activities.

As of this writing, only UMB offers a doctoral program with a prescribed curriculum in NI (Gassert et al., 1992). Many universities, however, provide an opportunity for doctoral students to develop a program of study in informatics. Examples are the University of Utah, University of Texas at Austin, University of California–San Francisco, University of Wisconsin–Madison, and University of Iowa.

Postgraduate Fellowships

Since 1993, a one-year fellowship in NI has been offered by the Massachusetts General Hospital (MGH) and, since the merger of MGH and Brigham and Women's Hospital, by Partners Health Care System. The fellowship, directed by Rita Zielstorff, is designed to promote the development of NI practitioners by allowing them to gain additional informatics experience of their choosing. Fellows are selected from qualified applicants. Admission preference is given to graduates of master's or doctoral programs in NI (Nursing Informatics Working Group, 1999). Fellows have included Mimi Hassett, RN, MS, from UMB, 1993–94; Emily Welebob, RN, MS, from UMB, 1995–96; Andrew Awoniyi, RN, ND, from University of Colorado Health Sciences Center, 1996–97; Beth Tomasek, RN, MS, from UMB, 1998; and Cheryl Reilly, RN, PhD, from University of California–San Francisco, 1999.

A second fellowship, the Douglas Porter Fellowship in Clinical Computing, is available to nurses through the Harvard Medical School and the Divisions of Medicine and Nursing at Beth Israel Deaconess Medical Center. This fellowship is three years in length and multidisciplinary in focus. Nurses who apply must have at least a master's degree, should have a strong clinical background, and should be interested in advancing the practice of nursing using technology and information science. Fellows have included Denise Goldsmith, RN, MS, and Heimar Marin, RN, PhD.

Nursing Informatics Education in the Future

This chapter has described NI education in the United States. In the past few years, more educational opportunities have become available in academic centers, and nurses now have choices about the type and location of NI programs they wish to enter. Federal legislation passed in 1998 allows the Division of Nursing to fund administration programs. Because most NI programs have been aligned with administration, we anticipate that more schools will apply for NI funding in the future. The National Advisory Council on Nurse Education and Practice (1997) has also recommended a national informatics agenda to the Secretary, Health and Human Services. These activities and the ubiquitous nature of technology are of increasing interest in NI.

With all these changes, it is interesting to ponder what the NI program of the future will look like. Will NI programs exist, or will all informatics professionals be educated through interdisciplinary programs? Will existing programs require students to take courses in the broad range of informatics topics available, or will specialization within the field be encouraged? Finally, will individual schools continue to spend precious resources on isolated programs, or will they collaboratively pool informatics resources from across the nation or across the world to develop new NI education models? The evolution of NI education over the next five to ten years will be fascinating to follow.

Summary

Nursing informatics has become well established as a specialty within nursing and health informatics. Development of scope of practice and standards documents and NI educational models has facilitated further curriculum development within the field. A mechanism for certification has added legitimacy to the specialty. Finally, NI educational opportunities include specialty programs, post-master's certificate programs, programs with a minor in NI, fellowships, continuing education, and individual courses.

Questions

1. Define nursing informatics.
2. How has nursing informatics qualified to be designated as a specialty practice by the ANA (what attributes are present)?
3. Discuss your beliefs as to whether NI is a clinical or an administrative practice.
4. List specific activities that reflect the practice of an NIS.
5. Compare and contrast the master's level specialty programs in NI presented in the chapter.
6. How does NI practice differ at the doctoral level from the master's level?

References

American Nurses Association. *Scope of Practice for Nursing Informatics.* Washington, DC: American Nurses Publishing, 1994.

American Nurses Association. *Nursing Informatics Standards of Practice.* Washington, DC: American Nurses Publishing, 1995.

Ball MJ, Hannah KJ. *Using Computers in Nursing.* Reston, VA: Reston Publishers, 1984.

Brennan PF. Improving health care by understanding patient preferences: the role of computer technology. *Journal of the American Medical Informatics Association* 1998;5(3):257–262.

Carty B. The protean nature of the nurse informaticist. *Nursing & Health Care* 1994;15(4):174–177.

Carty B, Rosenfeld P. From computer technology to information technology: findings from a national study of nursing education. *Computers in Nursing* 1998;16(5):259–265.

Fonteyn ME, Grobe SJ. Expert system development in nursing: implications for critical care nursing practices. *Heart & Lung* 1994;23(7):80–87.

Gassert CA. Opportunities to study nursing informatics. *Input/Output* 1989;5(2): 1–2.

Gassert CA. Structured analysis: a methodology for developing a model for defining nursing information system requirements. *Advances in Nursing Science* 1990;13(2):53–62.

Gassert CA. Summer institute: providing continued learning in nursing informatics. In: Grobe SJ, Pluyter-Wenting ESP, eds. *Nursing Informatics '94: an International Overview for Nursing in a Technological Era.* Amsterdam: Elsevier Science, 1994;536–539.

Gassert CA. Defining information requirements using holistic models: introduction to a case study. *Holistic Nursing Practice* 1996a;11(1):64–74.

Gassert CA. A model for defining information requirements. In: Mills ME, Romano CA, Heller BR, eds. *Information Management Nursing and Health Care.* Springhouse, PA: Springhouse Corp., 1996b;7–15.

Gassert CA. Using a revised model to identify information requirements for cardiac surgery patients operating mobile computing technology. In: Gerdin U, Tallberg M, Wainwright P, eds. *Nursing Informatics: the Impact of Knowledge on Health Care Informatics.* Amsterdam: IOS Press, 1997;172–175.

Gassert CA, Mills ME, Heller BR. Doctoral specialization in nursing informatics. In: Clayton PD, ed. *Proceedings of Fifteenth Annual Symposium on Computer Applications in Medical Care*. New York: McGraw-Hill, 1992;263–267.

Graves JR, Amos LK, Huether S, Lange LL, Thompson CB. Description of a graduate program in clinical nursing informatics. *Computers in Nursing* 1995; 13(2):60–70.

Graves JR, Corcoran S. The study of nursing informatics. *Image: Journal of Nursing Scholarship* 1989;21(4):227–231.

Grobe SJ. Nursing informatics competencies for nurse educators and researchers. In: Peterson HE, Gerdin-Jelger U, eds. *Preparing Nurses for Using Information Systems: Recommended Informatics Competencies*. New York: National League for Nursing, 1988a;25–33.

Grobe SJ. Introduction. In: Peterson HE, Gerdin-Jelger U, eds. *Preparing Nurses for Using Information Systems: Recommended Informatics Competencies*. New York: National League for Nursing, 1988b;4.

Grobe SJ. Nursing informatics competencies. *Methods of Information in Medicine* 1989;28(4):267–269.

Grobe SJ. The nursing intervention lexicon and taxonomy: implications for representing nursing care data in automated patient records. *Holistic Nursing Practice* 1996;11(1):48–63.

Hannah KJ. Current trends in nursing informatics: implications for curriculum planning. In: Hannah KJ, Guillemin EJ, Conklin DN, eds. *Nursing Uses of Computer and Information Science*. Amsterdam: Elsevier Science, 1985;181–187.

Heller BR, Romano CA, Moray LR, Gassert CA. Special follow-up report: the implementation of the first graduate program in nursing informatics. *Computers in Nursing* 1989;7(5):209–213.

Henry SB, Warren JJ, Lange L, Button P. Review of major nursing vocabularies and the extent to which they have the characteristics required for implementation in computer-based systems. *Journal of the American Medical Informatics Association* 1998;5(4):321–328.

Lange LL. Informatics nurse specialist: roles in health care organizations. *Nursing Administration Quarterly* 1997;21(3):1–10.

Magnus MM, Co MC, Derkach C. A first-level graduate studies experience in nursing informatics. *Computers in Nursing* 1994;12(4):189–192.

Martin KS, Norris J. The Omaha System: a model for describing practice. *Holistic Nursing Practice* 1996;11(1):75–83.

McCloskey JC, Bulechek GM, Donahue W. Nursing interventions core to specialty practice. *Nursing Outlook* 1998;46(2):67–76.

McGonigle D, Eggers R. Establishing a nursing informatics program. *Computers in Nursing* 1991;9(5):184–189.

Milholland DK. Congress says informatics is nursing specialty. *American Nurse* 1992;July/August:1.

National Advisory Council on Nurse Education and Practice. *A National Informatics Agenda for Nursing Education and Practice: A Report to the Secretary of the Department of Health and Human Services*. Rockville: Department of Health and Human Services, 1997.

National Council on Nursing Research (NCNR) Priority Expert Panel for Nursing Informatics. *Nursing Informatics: Enhancing Patient Care*. Bethesda, MD: National Institutes of Health, 1993.

Nelson R, Curran CE, McAfooes J, Thiele J. The NLN webcast: developing and implementing an online conference and business meeting. *Nursing and Health Care Perspectives* 1999;20(3):122–127.

Nursing Informatics Working Group, American Medical Informatics Association. *Education in Nursing Informatics.* http://amia-niwg.org, 1999 (October, 1999).

Ozbolt JG. From minimum data to maximum impact: using clinical data to strengthen patient care. *Advanced Practice Nursing Quarterly* 1996;1(4):62–69.

Panniers TL, Gassert CA. Standards of practice and preparation for certification. In: Mills ME, Romano CA, Heller BR, eds. *Information Management in Nursing and Health Care.* Springhouse, PA: Springhouse Corp., 1996;280–287.

Panniers TL, Walker EK. A decision-analytic approach to clinical nursing. *Nursing Research* 1994;43(4):245–249.

Parker J. Development of the American Board of Nursing Specialties (1991–1993). *Nursing Management* 1994;25(1):33–35.

Peterson HE, Gerdin-Jelger U. *Preparing Nursing for Using Information Systems: Recommended Informatics Competencies.* New York: National League for Nursing, 1988.

Saba VK. Why the home health care classification system is a recognized nursing nomenclature. *Computers in Nursing* 1997;15(Suppl 2):S69–S76.

Schwirian PM. The NI pyramid—a model for research in nursing informatics. *Computers in Nursing* 1986;4(3):134–136.

Simpson RL. Shifting perceptions: defining nursing informatics as clinical specialty. *Nursing Management* 1993;24(12):20–21.

Staggers N. Notes from a clinical information system program manager: a solid vision makes all the difference. *Computers in Nursing* 1997;15(5):232–233, 235.

Staggers N, Parks P. Description and initial applications of the Staggers & Parks nurse–computer interaction framework. *Computers in Nursing* 1993;11(6):282–290.

Thompson CB. Use of Iliad to improve diagnostic performance of nurse practitioner students. *Journal of Nursing Education* 1997;36(1):36–45.

Travis L, Brennan PF. Information science for the future: an innovative nursing informatics curriculum. *Journal of Nursing Education* 1998;37(4):162–168.

Turley JP. Toward a model for nursing informatics. *Image Journal of Nursing Scholarship* 1996;28(4):309–313.

Zielstorff RD. Online practice guidelines: issues, obstacles, and future prospects. *Journal of the American Medical Informatics Association* 1998;5(3):227–236.

3
An International Perspective on Nursing Informatics Education

Evelyn J.S. Hovenga

Nursing informatics evolved from the computing and information processing sciences introduced in the late 1960s to support medical practitioners, health service administrators, and governments. The field began as part of medical and nursing informatics during the 1970s. At that time, medical informatics education consisted of health professionals—mostly physicians and some nurses—undertaking computer or information science studies. Although nurses constitute the largest group of health professionals in any health system, the field of nursing informatics education has not been sufficiently addressed. It was not until 1992 that the American Nurses Association (ANA) officially recognized the discipline as a nursing specialty and defined its scope of practice.

Browsing through various contributions published in medical and nursing informatics conference proceedings, the yearbooks published by the International Medical Informatics Association (IMIA), and health-related informatics journals gives some insight into the global developments and foundations of the medical and nursing informatics disciplines. This plus a search of the World Wide Web illuminates the available associated educational programs and the pioneers who promoted the discipline in Europe and the United States.

In 1998, Morris and McCain reviewed the health-related informatics literature to elucidate the disciplinary nature and internal structure of this emergent interdisciplinary field, which draws upon and contributes to both the health and information sciences. Using intercitation network analysis, these authors concluded that a core literature exists, marking this as a separate discipline. Of the 29 journal titles identified, only three were nursing related, and two of these were removed from the final analysis because they had their own slant on informatics, one that was not evident for any other health profession. According to Morris and McCain (1998, p. 465), "nursing has sought more actively to differentiate its own unique and particular information needs."

Of course, several other nursing journals also include articles pertaining to nursing informatics literature. The way the literature has organized the topics included in our discipline may be a useful guide to curriculum development, although the discipline is still developing and changing. This may explain the potpourri of courses available and the difficulties associated with decisions about what to include during the program development phase.

Early medical informatics educational programs were not exclusively for medical students or medical practitioners, and a number of nurses successfully completed these. The "medical" in medical informatics denotes all of health care in other European languages, although it connotes "physicians" in English. Today, as a result, the term *health informatics* is gaining greater acceptance. Protti and Anglin (1992, p. 1066) noted that "this parallels a shift in public attitudes towards a new concept of health, i.e., one that not only includes the treatment and prevention of disease, but also the promotion of health and wellness and the concept of personal responsibility for it." Thus medical and nursing informatics become a subset of health informatics. It is clear that there exists a set of topics describing the discipline core that applies to each of these.

Nursing informatics education may be viewed from three different perspectives:

- It is about nurse academics using computers, information, and telecommunication technologies to support teaching and learning.
- It is about teaching nurses to use these technologies to support their practice.
- It is required to prepare nurse informaticians.

Each of these perspectives gives rise to distinctive educational programs. The mission for all nurse educators is to educate nurses to use health, medical, and nursing information together with telematics (informatics and telecommunication technologies) to enhance global health, health service delivery, and health system effectiveness.

Special Projects Promoting Nursing Informatics Education

The Center for Health Informatics and Multi-professional Education (CHIME) at University College London Medical School, England, maintains a public website with information and resources for education and training in medical, nursing, and dental informatics. The group at CHIME has compiled and classified 1,700 records and made them available via the Gateway to Health Informatics for Teaching (GHIFT) at www/chime.ucl.ac.uk. The database is divided into the following categories: acronyms, computer-assisted learning, events (courses and conferences), Internet resources, learning resources, organizations, people, and print resources.

The United Kingdom has established numerous Computers in Teaching Initiative Centers as part of their Teaching and Learning Technology Program. One such center, based at the University of Sheffield, is for Nursing and Midwifery. Created in 1995, the Center was scheduled to be reconfigured in late 1999. The center's website at www.shef.ac.uk/uni/ project/ctinm tracks developments, supports the use of computers in teaching and learning, and generally functions as a clearinghouse for nursing informatics.

The European Union has funded a number of special projects to improve health informatics education and training for health professionals. The Advanced Informatics in Medicine in Europe (AIM) initiative began in 1989. Under its auspices, the IT-EDUCTRA Concerted Action was established in 1992 and resulted in the development of general guidelines for European curricula in health informatics. These guidelines and the production of the ELITE PC-based program were designed to introduce healthcare professionals to information science and technology.

Other initiatives formed around that time were the interuniversity cooperation programs. The Erasmus Bureau of the European Commission, which implemented a master's program in health informatics, financed one. Another was financed via the TEMPUS-PHARE project, which provided assistance to central and eastern European countries. This joint European project involved 14 universities in providing education in medical informatics, statistics, and epidemiology at the Charles University in Prague (Hasman et al., 1995). These activities have contributed significantly to health and nursing informatics education in Europe.

In 1996, the Nightingale project was launched to provide curricula in nursing informatics for all levels of nursing education and training. These are now being implemented at various demonstration sites across Europe. Outcomes of the Nightingale project include a website at www.dn.uoa.gr/ nightingale, courseware, a CD-ROM with computer-based teaching software, and several publications by IOS Press. Mantas (1997) and Mantas and Malliotakis (1996) give excellent overviews of nursing informatics throughout Europe. The Nightingale project represents the first concerted effort to educate many nurses in the discipline.

Classification of Educational Outcomes

Historically, health and medical informatics education has had a strong orientation toward research and development, including software engineering at the postgraduate and postdoctoral levels (Hovenga, 1998b).

Graduates of such programs are highly trained individuals, categorized as level 3 professionals. This international reference point of an educational outcome was the result of work undertaken by the combined IMIA and International Federation of Information Processing (IFIP) at their first conference on education, held in Lyon, France, in 1973. This forerunner of today's IMIA Working Group 1 (WG1) on Education developed a schema with three levels:

- Level 1. General knowledge of computer and data processing beneficial to all health service users
- Level 2. Primary professional training complemented by skills facilitating cooperation with data processing and computer experts
- Level 3. Dual specialist qualification requiring detailed learning to professional standards in both medicine and computer science (Protti & Anglin, 1992)

This three-level schema was adapted by a task force formed by IMIA Working Group 8 on Nursing Informatics, which defined the levels as user, modifier, and innovator in the context of informatics competencies (Peterson & Gerdin-Jelger, 1988, p. 118). Ronald and Skiba (1987) referred to the informed user, the proficient user, and the developer to denote three different competency levels in nursing informatics. The schema has been retained by the newly developed Nightingale Nursing Informatics curriculum (Mantas & Malliotakis, 1996). This author believes that one more category should be included for graduates in computer science or informatics who have also acquired general knowledge of the health industry or one of the many associated disciplines like nursing informatics.

More recently, as discussed below, IMIA's WG1 has used a three-dimensional framework that includes type of professional in health care, type of specialization in health and medical informatics, and the stage of career progression for each.

Within the American Medical Informatics Association (AMIA), the nursing informatics expert panel identified four levels: beginning, experienced, informatics specialist, and informatics innovator. The AMIA panel is now describing more specific educational outcomes in the form of competency statements.

The ANA has developed competencies expected of a generalist nursing informatics nurse. These provide the foundation for the American Nurses Credentialing Center (ANCC) examination for nurse informaticians.

Competencies

Whether they are defined in terms of educational outcomes or educational levels, competencies vary according to role and function. Gonczi et al. (1993, p. 5) define professional competence as "having the attributes necessary for job performance to the appropriate standards." They note that a combination of such attributes as knowledge, skills, and attitudes is needed for successful professional performance. Defining successful professional performance requires analyzing the role and tasks performed by the target group and making judgments regarding what constitutes competent versus incompetent performance. To be reliable, this assessment process requires clearly defined performance criteria or competency standards. Gonczi et al. (1990, p. 10) had previously defined a competency-based standard as

... a level of achievement required for competence in some areas of professional practice. Specifying the standard involves stating the kinds of tasks and contexts in which the required level of achievement is to be exhibited. Performance at the required level of achievement is indicative of the presence of the underlying competencies, i.e. the appropriate combinations of knowledge, abilities, skills and attitudes. When this is done for a range of areas of practice within a profession, the result is a set of competency-based standards for the profession.

In Australia, nursing competencies first developed in 1989 are used as a basis for accreditation of university courses. According to Chapman (1999, p. 130), employer and university expectations in terms of educational outcomes converge on competence, although each may have different expectations. There is a tension between the need for vocational skills, highly valued by employers, and the universities' desire to produce lifelong learners.

The Nightingale curriculum guidelines, as well as the IMIA WG1 guidelines for health and medical education, essentially list topics to be covered by these curricula. They do not include a required set of competencies.

In contrast, a national expert panel convened by AMIA's nursing informatics working group has been reviewing and refining an existing set of competencies. They have established definitions for four levels of nurses: beginning, experienced, informatics specialist, and informatics innovator. They plan to have a list of competencies for each level validated by the expert panel and a larger Delphi study, and they are developing competencies that solely fit the doctorally prepared nurse. It has yet to be decided at what level and in what detail various concepts should be presented to undergraduates, postgraduate nursing students, and students in nursing informatics specialty programs.

Although clearly useful for curriculum developers, these standards may be too prescriptive and unsuitable outside the United States. Collectively, courses offered may not cover all aspects of this very broad discipline if each uses the same set of competencies. After all, it is impossible to include all of nursing and all of informatics in any one-degree course. Furthermore, individual nursing positions frequently require a unique range of skills and knowledge dependent on the technologies in use, the services provided, and the size and structure of the organization. Flexibility in curriculum design is essential.

Nonprescriptive guidelines such as those developed by IMIA WG1 permit individual courses to be designed to suit specific student populations and to meet the needs of the health industry in accordance with each country's educational system. These guidelines permit variations in the depth and breadth of the many topics covered. They use the European Credit Transfer System as the standard against which student workload may be measured (http://europa.eu.int/en/comm/dg22/socrates/ect.html). In essence, these features promote the use of a modular approach to curriculum design. This makes it well suited to student-led, customized course design and the use of flexible learning principles. Such an approach ensures diversity so that all aspects of the nursing informatics discipline, which is very broad indeed, can be covered. Each country is able to set the total credit points required for a degree of equivalent standing.

Nursing Informatics Educational Developments

Most efforts at the undergraduate level have focused on integrating informatics into the basic nursing curriculum, with varying levels of success. Many programs still do not include any informatics; others include very little.

A number of authors have tried to identify the content in these curricula (Vanderbeek & Beery, 1998; Arnold, 1996; Thede, 1998). A survey of European schools of nursing found that the inclusion of informatics into the curricula was not common. In 1986, the academic staff of only three percent of all nursing programs in the United States were prepared to integrate computer applications into their courses (Parks et al., 1986). By 1997, only 27 percent of undergraduate nursing programs had actually incorporated informatics in some way (Carty & Rosenfeld, 1998). Despite heavy use of computer technologies to support educational process and administration, the programs gave scant coverage of the development of nursing classification systems in patient care, the evolution of and research on nursing taxonomies and vocabulary, and the use of computers to store patient and nursing data.

According to Carty and Rosenfeld (1998), a majority of schools lacked a coordinated plan for technology implementation and were underfinanced for technology and related personnel. Furthermore, less than one third of the schools addressed nursing informatics in the curriculum. Only 19 U.S. nursing schools (10% of respondents) indicated that nursing informatics was offered as a separate course.

According to a 1990 study, the situation in Australia is better. Twenty-seven percent (10 of 37 respondents out of a total of 47 nursing programs) had more than five years' experience with teaching computing to nurses, and 73 percent (27) included computing within their nursing programs, often as a core unit. A more recent national survey conducted by this author indicates that little has changed.

Barnett observed in 1995 that after 20 years of effort by nursing informatics enthusiasts in the United Kingdom, only small proportions of the nursing and midwifery professions have become active in applying nursing informatics to their field of practice (Barnett, 1995). This appears to be true for Australia as well, judging by anecdotal evidence and this author's experiences in promoting nursing informatics to nurse academics. In the late 1980s there were more Australian nurses interested in nursing informatics than there are today, as is evidenced by the decline in nurse membership of our well-established national professional informatics organization.

Most nurse academics are struggling to learn the technology to support teaching and learning. All surveys to date, including a 1998 study in Finland by Saranto and Tallberg, point to a shortage of academic staff sufficiently experienced and comfortable with technology, despite widespread access to computers. The reluctance of nurse academics to embrace informatics may be explained by heavy teaching loads, compounded by the need to stay up to date clinically, and, for many, to upgrade their own educational qualifications. A 1999 survey by Sellers and Deans showed that 48 percent of all Australian nurse academics were themselves enrolled in a higher degree program, due in large part to the move of nursing education to the university level. The dearth of educational programs in nursing informatics is another contributing factor. In the absence of strong demand for such programs, however, universities do not regard them as financially viable and are reluctant to fund curriculum development.

Interestingly, as early as 1979, the Lincoln Institute of Health Sciences (now Latrobe University) gave nurses undertaking postregistration degrees the opportunity to include a computer studies course in their curricula. (This author undertook the course and was able to direct her career into nursing informatics.) In 1989, Central Queensland University introduced nurses to computers with its commitment to a Computer Assisted/Managed Learning project and the inclusion of basic computing studies in its curriculum. As from the year 2000, however, that will no longer be the case. Students are expected to have acquired the necessary computer skills prior to entry, and information literacy and nursing informatics will be fully integrated into the nursing program.

At the undergraduate level, nursing informatics is taught as part of a basic nursing bachelor's degree program. In countries where basic nurse education is not at this level, programs can be developed to offer registered nurses foundation degrees in nursing informatics. In Australia, all basic nurse education was transferred from hospital-based programs to the university sector's during the 1980s. Conversion courses allow registered and certificate nurses the opportunity to obtain academic qualifications—initially diplomas, and more recently, bachelor's degrees. With credit for prior learning, this typically takes one year on a full-time basis. Degreed nurses may take such courses for professional development or in preparation for higher degrees in nursing informatics. At least two programs now include a nursing informatics course. Although there are no nursing informatics programs in Australia, there are postgraduate health informatics programs, including doctoral-level studies.

In 1983, the University of Victoria, Canada, began to offer a four-year Bachelor of Science degree program in health information science, using a mandatory cooperative education model. Students are admitted after one year of university-based studies at a "better than pass" level. In addition to clinical, sociological, epidemiological, administrative, judicial, and economic perspectives of health information, the program includes a significant information technology component. Prior health professional qualifications are not required (Protti & Fisher, 1996).

Since the late 1980s, several schools in the United States have offered master's level programs in nursing informatics. There are only two programs at the doctoral level, which means that nurses wishing to specialize in nursing informatics at the doctoral level often do so within other specialties. South American countries, notably Brazil and Argentina, have just begun to introduce nursing informatics education. In Asia, Hong Kong, South Korea, and Japan are actively promoting the discipline.

Short courses, including preparation for the ANCC examination in the United States, and annual conferences complement formal degree programs. Professional nursing informatics groups are providing much of the nursing informatics education in the form of continuing education or staff development programs, seminars, and conferences.

Despite considerable progress, it appears that nurses as a group are strongly resisting the use of information technology to support their practice worldwide. This may well be gender based. Clearly, more needs to be done to promote the nursing informatics discipline and to motivate nurses to undertake studies in the discipline. Educational strategies must be sensitive to the special needs of nurses, but first we must convince those who educate nurses.

Curriculum Issues and Guideline Development

Nursing informatics education needs to address four issues:

- The scarcity of suitable educators
- The difficulty of adding new material to existing nursing curricula
- The variability among students in computing knowledge and skills
- The diversity of possible content due to the many combinations of foundation disciplines that, when combined and given a nursing information focus, make up the nursing informatics discipline

A review of the nursing informatics education literature and course materials makes it clear that every course is unique in structure and content. Each course depends on a number of factors: where within a university it originates, the mix of courses offered prior to the introduction of nursing informatics, the available expertise, and perceived or known market needs. Internet discussion groups have explored what constitutes the core content and what qualities or skills graduates of health informatics programs should have.

In 1991, the New Zealand Ministries of Health and Education introduced Guidelines for Teaching Nursing Informatics into their undergraduate nursing programs. The extent of implementation at any given school has depended on its resources: interested staff, hospitals with information systems to use as live examples, and classroom facilities with computer suites for teaching. In 1998, the University of Otago, in conjunction with Wellington Medical School, offered a diploma in health informatics for the first time.

Although the English National Board issued its framework for incorporating health informatics into the basic nursing curriculum in 1997, nursing informatics as a postgraduate specialist subject has yet to be recognized or developed by any of the schools of nursing. According to Barnett (1999), it is likely to be well into the next decade before all nurses have had the opportunity to learn more about informatics.

The Nightingale project has identified three distinct domains that make up their recommended nursing curriculum: building nursing knowledge; informatics and telematics; and people and organizational aspects. In the textbook written to support this curriculum, each of these domains was broken down further.

At the 6th International Conference on Health and Medical Informatics Education (Newcastle, Australia, August 1997), IMIA WG1 held a number of workshops on curricula. These resulted in recommendations for courses in health and medical education that would suit a number of different categories of health professionals. They were incorporated into one set of guidelines, with the following domains:

- Methodology and technology for the processing of data, information, and knowledge in medicine and health care
- Medicine, health and biosciences, health system organization
- Informatics, computer science, mathematics, biometry

These are broken down into greater detail, with separate specifications for specialists in computer/information management and health/medical informatics. In addition, the recommendations specify three levels of knowledge and skills for different health professions.

The guidelines were discussed by various groups and passed through iterative revisions. The national informatics societies that make up IMIA were invited to comment, and the framework was discussed during the 1999 AMIA spring congress, which was devoted to informatics education. A follow-up discussion was scheduled for the AMIA fall congress, when the IMIA board, its general assembly, WG1, and the Nursing Informatics special interest group also met. The final document is expected to be adopted by the IMIA general assembly in November 1999 and published in the *International Journal of Medical Informatics*. The document can be accessed at the IMIA WG1 website (www.imia.org/wg1).

Information Literacy

Information literacy among the general population has never been more important. In the twenty-first century, information literacy will include the abilities

- To use a variety of information and telecommunications technologies, information research skills, and higher order thinking skills
- To find, select, retrieve, decode, critically evaluate, and use information to create knowledge and insight
- To communicate this knowledge and insight to others through the use of a variety of technologies.

These abilities are crucial in the knowledge-intensive health industry. All teaching staff must accept this challenge and prepare health professionals for a lifetime of reskilling, redirection, and reorganization. A knowledge economy requires lifelong learners who communicate effectively and are capable of working both independently and in teams.

Nursing has always been an information- and knowledge-intensive profession, although it is not generally perceived as such. This is increasingly true. Nurses need inquiring minds and a sense of how nursing knowledge is created, including an understanding of the methodological and substantive limitations. Nurses must, wherever possible, base their practice on valid and reliable evidence obtained from studies on the effectiveness of nursing. They must have a sense of the interconnectedness of nursing relative to other health-related disciplines, and they must have a breadth of vision and be able to frame researchable questions.

As autonomous learners, nurses need to be aware of their own strengths and weaknesses, know their preferred learning styles, and be able to develop learning strategies (Tinkler et al., 1996, p. 77; Cheek & Doskatsch, 1998). The identification of these and related competencies are needed to guide curriculum and educational material development, as well as independent learning in nursing informatics.

Paradigm Shift in Education

With the use of new technologies to support education, delivery methods undergo change. Traditional classroom-based didactic lectures give way to problem-oriented and self-directed learning with a variety of flexible learning modes. Education faces a paradigm shift in every area. New technologies supportive of learning and teaching, such as CD-ROMs, the World Wide Web, and intranets and the Internet, are facilitating the shift from teacher-centered to student-centered learning. Indeed, "the rapid convergence of computing, audio-visual media and communications technologies is starting to have a profound transformative effect on how people work, learn and play" (Tinkler et al., 1996, p. 149). With the paradigm shift in healthcare education, open or flexible learning becomes the delivery method of choice for many.

Flexible learning encompasses distance education, which historically used print materials and correspondence. In Australia, this was often supplemented by short-wave radio, and later by audiotapes, videotapes, and teleconferencing. During the late 1980s, a host of electronic technologies came into use in distance education, ranging from facsimile machines to broadcast television and on to the World Wide Web. Technology entered the classroom too, where the white board replaced the blackboard, the document camera replaced the overhead projector, and the use of presentation software is becoming the norm for many.

The benefits of the convergence of these technologies are now coming to electronic classrooms, where the lecturer is able to control lights and microphone via motion sensors and touch screens. Electronic classrooms integrate networked and Internet-connected computers with document cameras, large high-resolution projection screens, and multipoint videoconferencing. They connect any number of classrooms at remotely located campuses.

Outside the classroom, students participate in Internet-based class mailing lists, communicate with lecturers via e-mail, and access study materials from class-based Web pages or CD-ROMs. Universities use intranets to provide multimedia resource materials, such as X-ray and pathology slides, to any number of clinical locations where medical and nursing students engage in problem-based learning. Students and staff have online access to library services from their desks at work or at home supplemented by any number of Web-based resources from around the world.

In short, distance education is converging with on-campus education to become open and flexible learning for everyone. To support this type of educational service delivery, universities and other institutions must change their traditional organizational structures and establish the infrastructures needed.

Central Queensland University (CQU) is a distance education provider with an international reputation in open and interactive learning and a well-developed infrastructure for the preparation of quality print and multimedia learning materials. During the early 1990s, CQU began to transform itself into an integrated multicampus regional university. Implementation of this mission began in 1994, and by early 1997, in time for the academic year, CQU's electronic classrooms were operational. All electronic facilities and support services are used extensively by all academics in all disciplines.

Changes in teaching practices generate the need to retrain academics in developing teaching materials that best suit the new technologies and support learning. Although material preparation time increases initially, effective use of the new technologies reduces the time and effort spent on some existing tasks. It can free up time for higher level tasks requiring teacher–student interaction if the infrastructure includes the right staff mix. This means less secretarial and administrative support and more technical support, both routine and skilled, including instructional designers and multimedia technicians. The teacher can no longer operate as an individual but rather must become a team leader and project manager who coordinates the skills needed to deliver the desired educational content.

The use of technologically mediated modes to deliver educational programs requires new skills and a high level of systemic support for teacher professional development. Teachers need to learn about the relationship between new technologies and pedagogy. They need to translate old skills and apply them in new environments, prioritizing and managing electronic resources, online communication, and team teaching. Teachers need to be competent in using new technologies and informatics applications in health and in producing multimedia teaching materials.

With these changes comes a shift in educational principles, from teacher-centered teaching to student-centered learning. Not only is this difficult for some teachers, it is also difficult for students who know how to be taught but not how best to learn. In university settings, the first task of teachers is to help students understand their learning styles and the delivery methods best suited to them. As learners, they also need to become independent and proactive, not dependent and reactive. With access to technology, control of access to learning can reside with the student rather than the distant instructor.

Proponents of flexible delivery tend to assume that students have the skills and access that allow them to use the required technologies, prefer these new modes of delivery, and have relatively uniform learning styles and preferences. This may not be the case. Assessment strategies may require changing from traditional examinations to project work, written assignments, or random computer-generated multiple choice questions to be answered anywhere and anytime. Because flexible learning must accommodate diverse student groups to be effective, there must be a range of instructional approaches from which students can choose, once they have been taught how to identify their particular learning styles and circumstances. Multimedia packages in particular should not be designed on a "one size fits all" basis.

Consistent with educational theories, Knowles (1990, p. 66) recommends the following strategies to facilitate learning:

- Foster interactivity, ensuring that the learner is active in the pursuit of new knowledge or acquiring new skills
- Reinforce through repetition and feedback
- Nurture ability to apply new knowledge and skills in new contexts through simulation

- Present problems so that the learner is provided with features that stimulate questioning
- Make use of the students' and others' experiences
- Organize and make easily available the widest possible range of resources for learning
- Nurture divergent and original thinking
- Organize knowledge, permitting learning to begin with simplified wholes and progressing to complex wholes to ensure that meaning and context are evident throughout the learning process
- Make learning goals explicit to enhance motivation to learn
- Allow for variations in progress among learners
- Create an environment that encourages learning and gives learner satisfaction
- Provide opportunities for the learner to test knowledge and skills in a safe environment
- Reduce frustrations when learners encounter difficulties, through the provision of adequate student support services

There are several forms of flexible learning. The first is a function of time (i.e., synchronous versus asynchronous modes of delivery). The second is a function of location, that is, fixed place versus anywhere. These, along with student and teacher access to and familiarity with technologies, determine how best to deliver education to a given student population. Mixed modes can be critical to accommodating variations in these prerequisites.

Telecommunication infrastructures around the world, including previously underdeveloped areas, are being developed and upgraded. These enable more people, communities, and organizations to use the Internet, videoconferencing, and other emerging technologies like video on demand for multiple purposes, including telehealth. As these technologies are used to deliver medical and nursing services via telehealth, all nurses—not just nurse academics—need to be familiar with them.

Globalization

As globalization and increasing international competition for market share continue, forward-looking universities will collaborate to establish educational multinationals capable of delivering high-quality flexible learning. Already a small number of academics are able to freelance, work from their chosen locations, and accept a predetermined number of students to mentor. In the future, these academics will provide assessment services, develop individual learning packages, or both.

Success will depend on market forces. Modular curriculum development will enable students to customize their own degrees to suit their career aspirations, educational opportunities, and capacity to pay. No longer will every university in the country offer all common courses. Credit transfers between universities will become more customary, and there will be a greater concentration on niche markets in education.

In health, medical, and nursing informatics education, IMIA WG1 has taken vital first steps, developing curriculum guidelines and establishing a database repository of courses currently offered by universities and other educational institutions (www.imia.org/wg1). This complements nursing informatics initiatives undertaken as part of the Nightingale project (curriculum) and by the AMIA nursing work group (competencies).

Educational collaboration of this type may lead to the establishment of a virtual Health Informatics University that draws on the collective expertise of academics. Such an approach is necessary if we are to

- Overcome the worldwide shortage of health and medical informatics educators
- Realize the economies of scale to justify the investment in quality educational products suited to multimedia technologies
- Prepare health professionals to work and function effectively in our emergent global knowledge economy and information society.

Summary

Nursing informatics is a distinct discipline for which a variety of educational programs are required. Much needs to be done to raise the awareness and skills of nurse academics so they can ensure that nurses, now and in the future, are adequately prepared to leverage new technologies. Despite the lack of consensus regarding the desired educational outcomes, progress has been made in developing generic curriculum guidelines, and initiatives have targeted the provision of new opportunities for nursing informatics education.

The increasing availability of new technologies is enabling the use of new educational delivery methods that promote student-led independent learning. This makes possible a more global approach to education, an approach that will help nursing informatics overcome the dearth of educational programs and make better use of available experts.

References

Arnold JM. Nursing informatics educational needs. *Computers in Nursing* 1996; 14(6):333–339.

Barnett DE. Informing the nursing professions about IT. In: Greenes RA, Peterson HE, Protti DJ, eds. *MedInfo '95. Proceedings of the Eighth World Congress on Medical Informatics*. Edmonton, Canada: International Medical Informatics Association and Healthcare Computing & Communications Canada, Inc, 1995; 2:1316–1320.

Barnett DE. Tomorrow is only a vision. *ITIN* 1999;11(1):8–11.

Carty B, Rosenfeld P. From computer technology to information technology: findings from a national study of nursing education. *Computers in Nursing* 1998;16(5):259–265.

Chapman H. Some important limitations of competency-based education with respect to nurse education: an Australian perspective. *Nurse Education Today* 1999;19:129–135.

Cheek J, Doskatsch I. Information literacy: a resource for nurses as lifelong learners. *Nurse Education Today* 1998;18:243–250.

Gomez A, Hager P, Oliver L. Establishing competency-based standards in the professions. Research Paper No. 1, Department of Employment, Education, and Training. AGPS Canberra, 1990.

Gomez A, Hager P, Athanasou J. The development of competency-based assessment strategies for the professions. Research Paper No. 8, Department of Employment, Education, and Training. AGPS Canberra, 1993.

Hasman A, Albert A, Wainwright P, Klar R, Sosa M, eds. Education and Training in Health Informatics in Europe. Amsterdam: IOS Press, 1995.

Hovenga EJS. Global Health Informatics Education. Keynote address at the Third European Conference on Health Telematics Education, June, Athens, Greece, 1998b.

Knowles M. *The Adult Learner, a Neglected Species*, 4th ed. Houston: Gulf Publishing Co., 1990.

Mantas J. The Nightingale project: an outline. In: Mantas J, ed. *Health Telematics Education*. Amsterdam: IOS Press, 1997.

Mantas J, Malliotakis J. European Commission project number HC 1109 Nursing Informatics: Generic High-level Training in Informatics for Nurses; General Applications for Learning and Education, Deliverable D5.1, December 1996.

Morris TA, McCain KW. The structure of medical informatics journal literature. *Journal of the American Medical Informatics Association* 1998;5:448–466.

Parks PL, Damrosch SP, Heller BR, Romano CA. Comparison of nursing faculty and student definitions of computer learning needs. In: Salamon R, Blum B, Jorgensen M, eds. *MedInfo '86. Proceedings of the Fifth Conference on Medical Informatics*. Amsterdam: North Holland, 1986.

Peterson HE, Gerdin-Jelger U, eds. *Preparing Nurses for Using Information Systems: Recommended Informatics Competencies*. New York: National League for Nursing, 1988.

Protti DJ, Anglin CR. The continuum of health informatics education: where do existing curricula fit? In: Lun KC, Degoulet P, Piemme TE, Rienhoff O, eds. *MedInfo '92. Proceedings of the Seventh Conference on Medical Informatics*. Amsterdam: North-Holland, 1992;1066.

Protti D, Fisher P. Health informatics at the University of Victoria. In: van Bemmel J, McCray AT, eds. *1996 Yearbook of Medical Informatics*. Stuttgart, Germany: Schattauer, 1996;135–139.

Ronald JS, Skiba DJ. *Guidelines for Basic Computer Education in Nursing*. New York: Natiional League for Nursing, 1987, April (41-2177):i–viii, 1–63.

Sellers ET, Deans C. Nurse education in Australian universities in a period of change: expectations of nurse academics for the year 2005. *Nurse Education Today* 1999;19:53–61.

Thede L. Undergraduate informatics: what should it include? Presentation at the 16th Annual Rutger's Informatics Conference, April 27, 1998. www.nursingcenter.com/treasures/rutgers/thede/uginform.html (October, 1998).

Tinkler D, Lepani B, Mitchell J. *Education and Technology Convergence. Commissioned Report No.43.* Canberra, Australia: National Board of Employment Education and Training, 1996.

Vanderbeek J, Beery A. A blueprint for an undergraduate healthcare informatics course. *Nurse Educator* 1998;23(1):15–19.

4
Using Computers in Basic Nursing Education, Continuing Education, and Patient Education

MARGARET J.A. EDWARDS AND R. MARJORIE DRURY

As the use of computers, information science, and the Internet in nursing practice, education, and administration expands, the need also increases for knowledgeable nurses to use and manage information technology in nursing environments. The task of nurse educators is changing. They now carry the responsibility of teaching students and colleagues to become discriminating users of information. To do this successfully, all nurses will need competence in the use of computer-based information systems in the healthcare organizations in which they are employed. They must use technology as a tool to practice their chosen profession rather than practicing their profession to suit the needs of technology.

In healthcare delivery, nurses traditionally have provided the interface between the client and the healthcare system. They are now called upon to fulfill this function in new ways in a technologically advanced environment. One obstacle they face is the fact that computer technology and Internet development have far outpaced the ability of educators and the health system to incorporate it. This chapter provides an overview of the opportunities and issues related to the use of computer-based multimedia and the Internet in formal nursing education (both undergraduate and graduate), continuing nursing education, and patient education.

Multimedia*

In the education of healthcare professionals, the traditional modes of learning are straining under the requirements of technological change. Although technology has created problems within the traditional educational system, it has also provided the solutions for resolving them. Computer-based multimedia can be used by educators to create order from confusion. Multimedia materials can be applied to the initial education of nursing students,

---

* This section is an edited extract from RS Hannah (1998). Used with permission.

staff development (continuing education), and patient education. With computer-based multimedia, education can move from an era of scarce resources into an era of abundance.

Computer-based multimedia aids in the knowledge and information transfer process, provides feedback to students about the efficiency of their learning processes, improves access to a vast warehouse of electronic data-bases, and enables students to problem solve and apply their learning. Ulti-mately, computer-based multimedia will free educators to concentrate on assisting students with their individual learning needs with emphasis on the "art" rather than the "science" of nursing.

What Is Multimedia?

In general, *multimedia* refers to computer-based technologies that integrate traditional forms of communication to allow seamless access or interaction by users. It also implies that computer-based technologies go beyond a single computer to include national and international networks like the Internet. Because the field is evolving so fast and includes many diverse interest groups, a more concise definition is not possible at this time.

The primary advantage of a multimedia approach is the freedom it allows for innovative expression of ideas and interactive student–teacher dialogue through one common tool, the computer. Multimedia technology provides for a flexible method of instructional delivery that attracts the learner's interest, maintains attention, and accommodates a variety of learning styles (Ribbons, 1998a). Many traditional modes of communication form the "pieces" comprising multimedia, including textual material, graphics, video (both still and motion), animation, and sound. Advances in technology will soon see virtual reality capabilities added to this list.

Just as there are many diverse tools that come together to make up a multimedia program, so there are many different ways in which multime-dia can be used. How well multimedia will be able to fulfill its potential remains to be seen. A major hurdle to overcome is clarification of the mul-tiplicity of related terms that abound in the literature. Although there are many ways to combine multimedia, there are only two basic types of appli-cations: information gathering programs, which provide the user with infor-mation and are controlled by the user; and learning activities programs, which generate learning and skill development through exercises controlled by the system.

Information Gathering Programs

- Hypermedia/hypertext programs use highlighted text or terms that the user selects to receive more information, such as a definition, graphics or animation about that term, or a link to another area or topic. The World Wide Web, for example, is an experimental hypermedia/hypertext system.

- Multimedia books are electronic versions of conventional textbooks. In addition to text and images, they contain video and audio clips and allow the reader to interact dynamically with the content.
- Multimedia databases are set up as records and fields like the familiar, conventional text-based databases, but they feature user-controlled access to all the "pieces" that comprise multimedia (e.g., graphics, video).

Learning Activities Programs

- Tutorials include classic computer-assisted instruction (CAI). Historically, users of CAI were presented with information, tested with an activity such as a question, and given appropriate feedback for a wrong response. Computer-assisted instruction has evolved so much over the years that some use the term to mean multimedia or refer to it as "multimedia CAI." The term CAI has, however, fallen into disfavor because of the negative connotation associated with it, which calls to mind merely the drill and practice format of early computers.

  A modern multimedia tutorial attempts to mimic a live lecture that guides users through a series of objectives, allowing them to undertake the operation at their own pace and providing the option of interactivity with the "teacher." This provokes thinking and motivation rather than a simple stimulus-response. Some national organizations, such as the National Council of State Boards of Nursing (1997) in the United States, are developing computerized testing programs to measure competence as a potential component of licensure examinations.
- Simulations in the health sciences usually feature nurse–patient situations. The simulation attempts to provide the user with the same type of experience that student pilots would have learning to fly using a flight simulator. Health-related examples are such programs as "Ethical Dilemmas in Nursing" by the *American Journal of Nursing*.
- Practice programs, which somewhat overlap simulation programs, allow the user to develop skills by using repetition.
- Problem-solving programs present the user with a problem, provide a number of resources to solve the problem, and expect users to independently arrive at the correct answer.

In summary, available programs are varied in content and presentation and typically use combinations of these categories. Several resources discuss the process of authoring and delivering multimedia material (Hannah, 1998; Jerram & Gosney, 1996; Kristof & Satran, 1995; Locatis, 1992; Lopuck, 1996).

Effectiveness of Multimedia

Many studies of learner achievement using classic CAI have been conducted in undergraduate nursing education. These studies consistently conclude that classic CAI is at least as effective as other teaching strategies in effecting behavioral changes in students (Nyamathi et al., 1989). Substantial reductions in the time spent learning subject matter have been shown in studies of classic CAI (Chang, 1986). Similarly, when classic CAI was compared with traditional strategies, significant cost benefit in favor of CAI was shown. These findings, regarding the effectiveness of nursing CAI with respect to learner achievement, time savings, and cost benefit, are consistent with findings in the health professions collectively and with findings in general education. The consensus among findings from a variety of disciplines lends support to the generalization that classic CAI is at least as effective as other means of teaching (Belfry & Winne, 1988; Gaston, 1988).

The development of multimedia computers and software and the resulting enhanced capabilities have led to yet another round of comparison studies (Ayoub et al., 1998). The time has come to finally accept that computers are now as effective as any other traditional teaching tool, no better or no worse. Several factors help determine the effectiveness of computer instruction: the quality of the programs, the environment of use (location and accessibility of computers), and the characteristics of the learner (anxiety, level of computer knowledge) (Khoiny, 1995). Future research should be aimed at developing tools for evaluating new programs and determining how students learn with computers. This way, existing programs and new programs can be improved rather than constantly compared with other teaching methods.

Limitations of Multimedia

Limitations that emerge from detailed studies of computer usage in nursing education include the following:

- Cost factors. The initial time investment in developing good programs is extensive. For example, to author one hour of effective, terminal-tested tutorials requires 120 to 150 hours. Once instructors become more adept at design strategies, the time required is reduced. However, extensive analyses of cost benefit and detailed studies of cost figures for the development and operation of nursing CAI programs are unavailable. Although the cost of the hardware may be dropping consistently, software development costs are not. Hopefully, in the future, institutions will enter into joint development projects in order to control costs.
- Content control. Unless more nurse educators become knowledgeable in the area of multimedia, there could be a tendency to abdicate the preparation of computer programs for nursing to educational computer software firms. Decisions about nursing and nursing education could slip out of nurses' hands. Nursing educators must monitor their own learning programs to ensure that decisions related to nursing remain in the hands of nursing content experts. Conversely, without a firm foundation, sophisti-

cated computerized nursing curricula will instead become patchwork coverage of course material.

- Altered professorial roles. Teachers who have felt secure in their role as dispensers of information may feel uncomfortable as they find their role changing to that of facilitators, moderators, and coordinators. In addition, active involvement by faculty members in computerized instruction requires a reward structure that places value on published instructional design efforts to the same extent that it values research and other publication activities.

- Technology. The dominance of the Windows and Macintosh personal computer operating systems, along with Internet access, has greatly facilitated the sharing of programs within and among institutions. However, many programs are still locked into a single computer language and hardware system. Translating an existing program from one computer operating system and language to another may require more programming time than was required to produce the original. This is an impediment to wider dissemination of nursing material. For this reason, there is probably a redundancy of lessons among nursing users.

  Large central computer systems place the nurse user at the whim of the individual or group controlling the system. The autonomy and control provided by personal computers has removed this limitation. Nursing multimedia is now dominated by the personal computer world. However, with the number of programs available on the Internet increasing at a dramatic rate, and with the huge potential of distance education via the Internet soon to be realized, nursing institutions must consider developing a balance between personal computers and large computer systems.

- Lack of formal communication among users. In North America, the vast majority of information about multimedia in nursing education is communicated at such annual conferences as the American Medical Informatics Association (AMIA) Annual Symposium, Association for the Development of Computer Based Instructional Systems, and the Annual Learning Resource Center Conference. International exchanges, such as MedInfo and the International Congress on Nursing Informatics, also permit formal and extensive exchange of information about the quality and quantity of available nursing programs.

The Internet

The Internet is a specialized example of the use of multimedia. Computer-based multimedia programs and applications can be run on the learning system of a faculty or on the personal computer of a student, nurse, or patient. The Internet allows for worldwide access to similar multimedia programs and applications. It can be viewed as both a delivery method for all types of health education and as a source of information.

Delivery Method

Distance education using Internet capabilities can provide learning experiences without regard to location or time. Students can access educational content at their convenience by using the Internet and course management software. Online conferences, student "chat rooms," e-mailed assignments, and materials including articles, video, and audio clips are all tools available for Internet-based educational offerings.

The Internet provides opportunity for both synchronous and asynchronous education. Synchronous or "live" education involves immediate communication between student and faculty. This approach requires all students to be "present" at a specific time. The alternate approach, asynchronous education, is becoming a more popular choice, as students and faculty are often in different time zones, if not different countries. Asynchronous education involves delayed interactions. Material is posted to the Internet by faculty and accessed at a time convenient to the student.

Information Source

The availability of the World Wide Web (or WWW) has brought about an expansion of resources for students. The increased quality of hard copy journal articles available through upgraded library capabilities is notable, especially when students, nurses, and/or patients can themselves scan through electronic databanks and choose which full-text articles they would like to download from journals originating from anywhere in the world. In addition, the speed of interlibrary transfer of documents electronically has removed the barriers to having the latest references available.

Additionally, there are the vast resources of the Internet that are not part of course offerings, but are available for individuals to access as they need. A search for virtually any health-related topic yields hundreds of sites with such material as articles, video clips, or support groups related to the topic. Newsgroups and listservs on a vast array of health topics allow students, nurses, patients, and the public to discuss problems and issues with others having similar interests.

Formal Nursing Education

Today, student learning needs in informatics are changing. With computer literacy almost a universal requirement for graduation from high school, an increasing number of students enter the nursing curriculum with advanced keyboarding skills and an understanding of computer terms, concepts, and history as well as computer applications in nursing. Often, they have outdistanced their nursing instructors in understanding and applying computer technology to the educational process.

Progress

The last decade has seen significant changes in the quality and availability of instructional software for nurses. The increasing use of computer-assisted interactive videodisc instruction (CAIVI) and the advent of PC-based CD-ROM and Internet technology have changed the face of educational computing. Nurse educators, many of whom were educated before computers became a mainstay of instructional strategies, have struggled in the past to keep up with this rapidly evolving technology. Faculty computer courses and the increased use of personal computers have helped to increase the confidence with which nurse educators now approach the solutions that computer technology can offer.

Self-Education

The need for faculty to not only keep up technologically but also lead the way in the utilization of these resources has never been greater. Fortunately, the means for self-education and upgrading have never been more accessible.

The accessibility of education via the Internet or through computer-mediated delivery has made education available to many nurses unable to travel or relocate for their education. Most nursing education institutions now use multimedia applications and computer delivery for some components of their program. Additionally, many programs for post-basic baccalaureate, master's, and doctoral degrees are now entirely available over the Internet (Connors et al., 1996; Milstead & Nelson, 1998).

Classroom Education

The amount of literature documenting nursing educational uses of computers and the Internet is growing exponentially. The studies cited below are meant to be illustrative but not exhaustive of the available literature. To manage the educational environment of both undergraduate and graduate nursing students, nurse educators are using the computer in many ways:

- To instruct (Clark, 1998; Gee et al., 1998; Goodman & Blake, 1996; Gravely & Fullerton, 1998; Ritt & Stewart, 1996; Thomson, 1998; Wright, 1995)
- To evaluate (Krothe et al., 1996; Kuehn, 1996; Kuehn & Hardin, 1999; Wong et al., 1992)
- To identify individual students' learning problems (Abbott, 1993; Lawless, 1993; McGonigle & Eggers, 1991; Wilson, 1991)
- To gather data on how learning takes place (Cust, 1995; Gonce-Winder et al., 1993; Hanson et al., 1994; Jonassen, 1995; Ribbons, 1998b)
- To manipulate data for research purposes (Napholz & McCanse, 1994)

- To facilitate meetings and group communication (O'Brien & Renner, 1998, 1999)

In the first edition of this book (Ball et al., 1988), a major concern was the lack of quality software. Nurse educators had often been sold hardware to "solve" their instructional problems, but many were unable to find either software to run on their particular configuration or the time and expertise to design their own software. The listing of software in the previous edition (Bolwell, 1988) cited over 600 nursing educational software packages from over 70 vendors, while the list in the second edition (Bolwell, 1995) cited over 300 packages from only 22 vendors. Expertise in software development is now concentrated within a small number of vendors producing high-quality software. Additionally, the advent of CD-ROM technology has resulted in a plethora of locally produced multimedia materials. The problem is no longer the availability of quality software, but the vision, understanding, and expertise of nurse educators in knowing how to use this technology to full advantage.

Future Requirements

Many nursing schools and faculties have developed computer laboratories for students' use. There will be an ongoing need to develop learning centers that provide appropriate hardware and software for their students (Drury, 1997). However, with the rise of PC technology and availability and CD-ROM capabilities supported by textbook publishers, students will have a wealth of materials directly available at their fingertips, without the need to be physically present at a learning center.

To make rational decisions about integrating informatics content into nursing curricula, nurse educators must accept the responsibility of learning about the use of computers in nursing practice and education. In the meantime, they can make use of the model curricula described in the literature (Saba & McCormick, 1995). They should also expect guidance and advice from such professional organizations as the International Medical Informatics Association (IMIA), Canadian Organization for Advancement of Computers in Health (COACH), the National League for Nursing, the American Nurses Association, the British Computer Society, and the Computer Applications in Nursing Special Interest Group of the Royal Australian Nursing Federation. All of these have active groups addressing the need for nursing informatics content in nursing education curricula. In addition, curriculum planners must locate instructional materials, evaluate their utility, and use them to support the teaching of nursing informatics. Finally, they must take an active role in shaping graduates who are discriminating users of information and technology.

Continuing Nursing Education

Information is being generated at explosive rates. Between 6,000 and 7,000 scientific papers are written each day, and knowledge is expected to double every 20 months in the decade ahead. Therefore, five years after a nursing student graduates from school, more than 50 percent of the acquired knowledge will be obsolete (McCormick, 1984). To make up for this loss, nursing management must take on such new responsibilities as staff development and continuous education.

Staff Development and Continuous Education

Staff development can be viewed as synonymous with continuing nursing education, which can be defined as all the learning activities that registered nurses undertake to enhance their nursing competence following basic nursing education. The main goal of this ongoing professional educational process is to maintain and improve the quality of health care by providing opportunities for the personal and professional growth of the individual nurse.

Staff development includes but is not limited to activities directed at orienting new staff to a facility, updating technical competency, progressing toward professional goals (including development of leadership potential and of decision-making and problem-solving skills), and enhancing professional roles and accountability.

Although the use of computerized instruction in nursing education has focused on basic nursing education in the past, many of the indications for using computer-based multimedia and the Internet in formal nursing education also apply to continuing education. In many areas, the focus in hospitals and community agencies has been on using computer technology to address administrative tasks, including bedside documentation. This focus has allowed many nurses to become familiar with specific uses of computers.

The use of computers in continuing education for nurses varies widely across North America, and the amount of literature related to computerized continuing education for nurses is growing. However, many articles are similar to those published 10 years ago about the use of computer-assisted instruction for nursing students. Site-specific programs that have been developed for local use are reported (Neafsey, 1998; Tronni & Prawlucki, 1998).

Our view of continuing education and computer use should not be limited to learning new systems applications or using software developed for specific content review. Instead, practicing nurses, regardless of specialty, can also be directed to Internet resources critical to their area of expertise. Continuing education departments can encourage nurses to make use of the

Internet to become more aware of professional development opportunities through the listing and promotion of conferences and activities. Opportunities for participation in listserv communication and newsgroups can facilitate the discussion of common practice concerns and sharing of resources.

Not only does the Internet offer institutions a variety of resources for use in providing continuing education opportunities, it also offers the nurse many opportunities for accredited continuing nursing education programs online (Plank, 1998) The following list of websites is illustrative of some available programs:

www.springnet.com
www.ajn.org or www.lrpub.com
www.helix.com
www.nurseweek.com
www.wholenurse.com
www.nursing.ab.umd.edu

Requirements and Benefits

There are a number of advantages to the nurse using Internet-based continuing education programs for credit. With Internet-based programs, there are no travel or lodging costs, no loss of personal or work time, no specified times for program attendance, and no last-minute cancellations of the program. Online programs vary in length and cost. Certificates can be issued immediately upon completion by submitting payment online using a credit card. Online learning offers a growing number of selections. Entire nursing journals are online, so access to articles is not an issue.

Nurse managers must familiarize themselves with the concepts of computer-assisted learning and the Internet as means of maximizing the resources available for staff development. These are important factors, considering that "training and education departments are frequently viewed as the most expendable units in an agency when budget cutbacks are necessary" (Porter, 1978). Nurse managers must acquire sufficient understanding of the technology to make rational decisions about staff development. With the use of computer-based multimedia and the Internet, the benefits include the availability of learning materials, productivity increases and savings resulting from reduced learning time and less time away from assigned duties, and improved staff morale associated with maintaining the commitment to staff development.

Patient Education

Computer assisted instruction has been identified as a unique ally for the nurse in delivering patient education (Campbell et al., 1994; Gustafson, 1994; McRoy et al., 1998; Weaver, 1995). The benefits of patient education are now universally accepted. However, lack of time, lack of adequate resources, varying degrees of subject knowledge, and a perception among nurses that time spent on patient teaching is not valued by management have led to inconsistent and sporadic delivery of health education to patients. Computer-based multimedia instruction and the Internet are ideal technologies to address many of these concerns.

Again, thinking about patient education should not be limited to software available to teach specific content. Instead, the available technology can be harnessed to provide a variety of online educational opportunities for patients. Nurses must be aware of the vast array of patient-focused articles, websites, and support groups that can be found on the Internet. Patients will benefit when the nurse is able to pass along these resources or help patients locate materials on their own.

The website www.healthtrans.org is an excellent example of the ability of Internet resources to address patient needs. This site makes health information concerning a large variety of topics available in 11 languages. With the growing need in urban centers for transcultural resources, the Internet can be utilized to make available patient education materials translated by health professionals to provide culture-sensitive information as well as understandable materials in the patient's own language.

Nurses also play a vital role in educating patients and the public about screening and critiquing health information they may find on the Internet. Patients are already using the Internet to do their own searches about health topics. Nurses can help them become discerning users of the health information available over the Internet.

Advantages and Limitations to Using Computers in Patient Education

Advantages to using computers in patient education documented by Sinclair (1985) and by Tibbles et al. (1992) include the following:

- Standardized content and delivery of educational material
- Individualization of both instruction and evaluation
- Privacy, decreasing anxiety and embarrassment associated with learning new material
- Time- and cost-efficiency, once developed
- Available outside of traditional instruction times

Although there are many benefits to using computers in patient education, one overriding factor has limited the use of this medium. There has been a significant lack of quality commercial courseware, and the cost associated with development is prohibitive to most agencies. The state of patient education software is similar to that of nursing education in the past. Small numbers of individual developers have produced site-specific software; however, the quality of these programs varies widely. The advent of the Internet has allowed for global distribution of previously local products, and it has increased the availability of health information exponentially.

Categories of Patient Education Resources

Three categories of patient education resources have been identified: (1) instruction on acute health problems, (2) teaching aimed at chronic health problems, and (3) wellness education (Sinclair, 1985). Examples of these categories of patient education courseware are meant to be illustrative and not exhaustive.

- Instruction on acute health problems. This category includes preoperative and postoperative teaching and cardiac rehabilitation topics (Masten & Conover, 1990; Tibbles et al., 1992).
- Teaching aimed at chronic health problems. Teaching self-management to young people with cystic fibrosis (Cooper, 1992) or nutrition to persons newly diagnosed with diabetes (McKiel, 1991) are examples of this strategy.
- Wellness education. The literature notes very few current examples of the use of computers in wellness education (Kahn, 1993; Vargo, 1991). However, although the professional community has not made significant progress in providing courseware for wellness education, commercial vendors have. While the reliability of some programs could be questioned, there is an abundance of courseware related to such topics as healthy eating, nutrition, and stress management that healthcare consumers can use on their home computers.

Influencing Factors

Societal trends have accelerated the need for health education delivered in a manner that is both time and cost efficient. The increase in life expectancy has also triggered an increase in the number of people with long-term illnesses and disabilities. Because no cure exists for many of these conditions, such as diabetes or arthritis, patients need ongoing education to make decisions related to the personal and medical management of their illnesses.

Increasing healthcare costs are compelling all healthcare providers to examine alternative ways of delivering their services. Often, in such an economic climate, concerted efforts at developing patient education materials or programs are abandoned in favor of the individual nurse "fitting in" patient teaching as time permits. With the increasing use of minimally trained auxiliary staff in healthcare institutions supervised by a nurse, the time available for that nurse to provide individualized patient teaching has decreased dramatically. Finally, the Internet has given the public access to health and medical resources never before easily available. Healthcare consumers are not only more knowledgeable about their health, but they also expect to continue to gain knowledge that applies to themselves and their illnesses.

Evaluating Educational Resources

Evaluating Software

As nurse educators and continuing education coordinators gain experience with educational software, they have become more sophisticated and selective in evaluating software before purchase. On the basis of previous experience, these nurses have often established personal criteria for evaluation of software. There remains, however, a large number of nurses who are responsible for purchasing educational software but have no prior knowledge or experience in this area. The next section is designed as a resource for those nurses without a personal framework for evaluating educational software. The principles apply to formal nursing education, continuing education for nurses, and patient education. Educational criteria, quality assessment, and cost analysis are discussed.

Educational Criteria

Nurse educators must make a conscious effort to acquire the necessary skills of software assessment. In choosing among alternative CAL software or between CAL and other teaching/learning strategies, nurse educators must compare alternatives on the basis of effectiveness, quality, and cost. These variables must be included in the evaluation of each alternative and the comparison among different alternatives. This will result in increasing pressure on the marketplace to improve the quality of their products.

The evaluation process must address a number of key considerations. To begin, the evaluation team must take into account the fact that not all content is taught equally well with different teaching methodologies. For example, group process terminology or concepts can be taught using instructional computing, but group process interaction skills cannot. At the present time, there are few criteria for discriminating among teaching strategies to identify the most appropriate for learning specific content.

The evaluation team must also make a concerted effort to determine the congruence between instructional objectives and the objectives of a particular CAL program. Although to some this may appear obvious, experience suggests that decisions to purchase instructional computing software are sometimes made without examining the objectives of that software and comparing them with the program, course, or learning unit objectives.

TABLE **4.1.** Criteria frequently used for evaluating instructional computing software for nursing education.

Content	Documentation style
Accurate	Scholarship
Relevant	Parsimony
Current	Use of humor
Format	Personalization
Frames	**Strategies**
Graphics	Predominant type
Ergonomics	Variety
Psychosocial	Remediation
Physical	

Quality/Utility Assessment

Numerous guides, checklists, and evaluation tools are available to assist the nurse in judging the worth of a particular CAL package for a specific instructional purpose (Ball et al., 1988; Bork, 1984; Caissy, 1984; Hannafin & Peck, 1988; Hudgings & Meehan, 1984; Komoski, 1984; Posel, 1993; Sawyer, 1984). Table 4.1 summarizes the most frequently used criteria in the evaluation of the quality and utility of instructional computing software.

Cost Analysis

In comparisons of commercial CAL software, often only the purchase price is considered because all other costs are considered to be equal. In many comparisons of commercially available CAL versus locally developed CAL, only direct rather than full costs are considered. Direct costs are those costs related specifically to the alternative under consideration. Full costs are all costs associated with an alternative, including direct costs and indirect overhead costs like utilities or administration. However, remember that direct costs of locally developed CAL materials must include design, development, and operation of the CAI software program.

Comparisons between CAL and other teaching/learning strategies involve more elaborate and sophisticated calculations than do comparisons between different CAL software programs. When comparing CAL with other teaching/learning strategies, the following categories of costs should be included:

- Personnel salaries and benefits
- Administration fees or salaries and benefits
- Services such as printing, postage, telephone, equipment rental
- Hardware
- Software
- Facilities

$$B_1 - C_1 \geq B_2 - C_2$$

FIGURE **4.1.** Cost-benefit analysis model.

The most useful method of comparison would permit comparison among alternatives using all of the variables identified above—that is, effectiveness, quality, and cost.

Cost-Benefit Analysis

Cost-benefit analysis involves the calculation of the monetary costs and the benefits of alternatives. The relative attractiveness of each alternative is then assessed by determining which has the lowest dollar cost and highest dollar benefit (Fig. 4.1, where B represents the benefits in dollars and C represents the costs in dollars).

Cost-benefit analysis provides for the use of quantitative objective data to compare two alternatives. Unfortunately, many benefits and costs in nursing education are not quantitative; rather, they are qualitative. Because this model does not consider measures of either effectiveness or quality variables, it is usually not useful for evaluating instructional computer software for nursing education.

Cost-Utility Analysis

Cost-utility analysis compares ratios between alternatives. First, the costs of an alternative are calculated, and second, the decision makers determine its usefulness. These two factors are then compared with the same factors for other alternatives under consideration (Fig. 4.2, where C represents costs in dollars and U represents the subjective judgment of a decision maker of the perceived utility of the software).

The cost-utility analysis method relies on a combination of quantitative and qualitative data, but unfortunately, only the quantitative data are objective. The utility (qualitative) data are based on the subjective judgment of the decision makers of their perception of the alternative's utility.

Cost-Effectiveness Analysis

Cost-effectiveness analysis also establishes a ratio. In this case, the ratio is between the measure of the extent to which an alternative is effective in achieving a predetermined goal and the cost of the alternative in dollars.

$$\frac{C_1}{U_1} \geq \frac{C_2}{U_2}$$

FIGURE **4.2.** Cost-utility analysis model.

$$\frac{GE_1}{C_1} \geq \frac{GE_2}{C_2}$$

FIGURE **4.3.** Cost-effectiveness analysis model.

Ratios for different alternatives are then compared (Fig. 4.3, where GE represents measures of goal effectiveness, and C represents costs in dollars).

In this method, both quantitative (costs) and qualitative (goal effectiveness) data are considered, and objective measures are gathered for both types of data. Finally, this method of comparison permits both effectiveness and quality variables to be considered goals. Thus, cost-effectiveness analysis is the superior method for choosing among instructional alternatives.

With a conscious effort to develop experience through practice, nurses will become more sophisticated in judging the quality of CAL software. This will translate into increasing pressure on developers and distributors of nursing CAL software to improve the quality of their products.

Evaluation of Internet–Based Materials

Evaluation of Internet-based materials differs somewhat. There is little or no peer review, editorial input, or preselection of general Internet-based materials. Search engines return large unstructured lists of information, and users of the Internet must screen information for correctness, currency, and appropriateness. Several tools have been developed to evaluate Internet resources (Brandt, 1996; Silberg et al., 1997). The online tool developed by Berry et al. (1998) to evaluate both the educational style of an Internet site and its user interface system for use in medical education provides a comprehensive example of considerations necessary to the evaluation of Internet resources (see http://wwww.leeds.ac.uk/medicine/lime/docs/sample_review.html). Clark (1998) has also developed a tool for evaluating Internet resources for use by nursing students. This tool can be found at http://personal.lig.bellsouth.net/~lclark7/ProfNsg/NUR211S.html.

Conclusion

Computer-based multimedia and the Internet are exciting additions to the repertoire of teaching strategies available for use by nurse educators. Success in exploiting these two powerful teaching and learning tools will be dictated by the imagination and creativity of nurse educators. Ignoring or underutilizing the potential of the information superhighway will seriously limit the nurse's ability to adapt and keep pace with the revolutionary changes occurring in health care.

Questions

1. Name the two basic types of multimedia applications. How do they differ? What are some examples of each?
2. What are the benefits of using multimedia technology in nursing education? What are some limitations?
3. What are some methods nurses can use to evaluate educational resources?
4. What is the difference between cost-benefit analysis, cost-utility analysis, and cost-effectiveness analysis?

References

Abbott K. Student nurses' conceptions of computer use in hospitals. *Computers in Nursing* 1993;11(2):78–87.

Ayoub J, Vanderboom C, Knight M, Walsh K, Briggs R, Grekin K. A study of the effectiveness of an interactive classroom. *Computers in Nursing* 1998;16(6):333–338.

Ball MJ, Hannah KJ, Gerdin Jelger U, Peterson H. *Nursing Informatics: Where Caring and Technology Meet*. New York: Springer-Verlag, 1988.

Belfry MJ, Winne P. A review of the effectiveness of computer assisted instruction in nursing education. *Computers in Nursing* 1988;6(2):77–85.

Berry E, Parker-Jones C, Jones R, Harkin PJ, Horsfall HO, Nicholls JA, Cook NJA. Systematic assessment of world wide web materials for medical education: online, cooperative review. *JAMIA* 1998;5(4):382–389.

Bolwell C. Index to computer-assisted instructional (CAI) software for nursing education. In: Ball MJ, Hannah KJ, Gerdin Jelger U, Peterson H, eds. *Nursing Informatics: Where Caring and Technology Meet*. New York: Springer-Verlag, 1988;371–391.

Bolwell C. CAI for nursing education. In: Ball MJ, Hannah KJ, Newbold S, Douglas J, eds. *Nursing Informatics: Where Caring and Technology Meet, 2nd ed*. New York: Springer-Verlag, 1995;392–405.

Bork A. Computers in education today—and some possible futures. *Phi Delta Kappan* 1984;65–66:239–243.

Brandt DS. Evaluating information on the Internet. *Computers in Libraries* 1996;16:44–47.

Caissy G. Evaluating educational software: a practitioner's guide. *Phi Delta Kappan* 1984;65–66:249–250.

Campbell MK, Devellis BM, Strecher VJ, Ammerman AS, Devellis RF, Sandler RS. Improving dietary behavior: the effectiveness of tailored messages in primary care settings. *American Journal of Public Health* 1994;84(5):783–787.

Chang B. Computer-aided instruction in nursing education. In: Werely HH, Fitzpatrick J, Traunton R, eds. *Annual Review of Nursing Research*. New York: Springer-Verlag, 1986;4:217–233.

Clark DJ. Course redesign: incorporating an Internet web site into an existing nursing class. *Computers in Nursing* 1998;16(4):219–222.

Connors HR, Smith C, DeCock T, Langer B. Kansas nurses surf Web for master's degrees. *Reflections* 1996;22(2):16–17.

Cooper M. Playing the game . . . computer games . . . to teach young people selfcare in cystic fibrosis. *Nursing Standard* 1992;6(21):22–23.

Cust J. Recent cognitive perspectives on learning: implications for nurse education. *Nurse Education Today* 1995;15:280–290.

Drury RM. Considerations in planning a computer learning lab for nursing students. *OJNI (Online Journal of Nursing Informatics)* 1997;1(2).

Gaston S. Knowledge, retention and attitude effects of computer-assisted instruction. *Journal of Nursing Education* 1988;27(l):30–34.

Gee PR, Peterson GM, Martin JLS, Reeve JF. Development and evaluation of a computer-assisted instruction package in clinical pharmacology for nursing students. *Computers in Nursing* 1998;16(1):37–44.

Goodman J, Blake J. Multimedia courseware: transforming the classroom. *Computers in Nursing* 1996;14:287–296.

Gonce-Winder C, Kidd RO, Lenz ER: Optimizing computer-based system use in health professions' education programs. *Computers in Nursing* 1993;11(4):197–202.

Gravely E, Fullerton JT. Incorporating electronic-based and computer-based strategies: graduate nursing courses in administration. *Journal of Nursing Education* 1998;37(4):186–188.

Gustafson DH, Hawkins RP, Boberg EW, Bricker E, Pingree S, Chan C. The use and impact of a computer-based support system for people living with AIDS and HIV infection. *Journal of the American Medical Informatics Association* 1994;1:604–608.

Hannafin MJ, Peck KL. *The Design, Development, and Evaluation of Instructional Software.* New York: MacMillan, 1988.

Hannah RS. Education applications. In: Hannah KJ, Ball MJ, Edwards MJA, eds. *Introduction to Nursing Informatics*, 2nd ed. New York: Springer-Verlag, 1998;146–158.

Hannah RS. *Designing Multimedia for Health Education.* New York: Springer-Verlag, 1999.

Hanson AC, Foster SM, Nasseh B, Hodson KE, Dillard N. Design and development of an expert system for student use in a school of nursing. *Computers in Nursing* 1994;12(1):29–34.

Hudgings C, Meehan N. Software evaluation for nursing educators. *Computers in Nursing* 1984;2:35–37.

Jerram P, Gosney M. *Multimedia Power Tools.* New York: Random House, 1996.

Jonassen DH. Computers as cognitive tools: learning with technology, not from technology. *Journal of Computing in Higher Education* 1995;6:40–73.

Kahn G. Computer-based patient education: a progress report. *MD Computing* 1993;10(2):93–99.

Khoiny FE. Factors that contribute to computer-assisted instruction effectiveness. *Computers in Nursing* 1995;13(4):165–168.

Komoski K. Educational computing: the burden of ensuring quality. *Phi Delta Kappan* 1984;65–66:244–248.

Kristof R, Satran A. *Interactivity by Design.* Mountain View, CA: Adobe Press, 1995.

Krothe JS, Pappas VC, Adair LP. Nursing student's use of collaborative computer technology to create family and community assessment instruments. *Computers in Nursing* 1996;14(2):101–107.

Kuehn A. Documentation of patient encounters using a database. *Proceedings, 1st International Nursing Conference*, June 17, 1996; Hamilton, Ontario, Canada.

Kuehn AF, Hardin LE. Development of a computerized database for evaluation of nurse practitioner student clinical experiences in primary health care: report of three pilot studies. *Computers in Nursing* 1999;17(1):16–26.

Lawless KA: Nursing informatics as a needed emphasis in graduate nursing administration education: the student perspective. *Computers in Nursing* 1993;11(6):263–268.

Locatis C, Ulmer E, Carr V, Banvard R, Lo R, Le Q, Williamson M. *Authoring Systems*. January 1992. http://wwwcgsb.nlm.nih.gov/monograp/author/. Last accessed January 28, 1998.

Lopuck L. *Designing Multimedia: a Visual Guide to Multimedia and Online Graphic Design*. Berkeley, CA: Peachpit Press, 1996.

Masten Y, Conover KP. Automated continuing education and patient education. *Computers in Nursing* 1990;8(4):144–150.

McCormick KA. Nursing in the computer revolution. *Computers in Nursing* 1984;2:4–30.

McGonigle D, Eggers R. Establishing a nursing informatics program. *Computers in Nursing* 1991;9(5):184–189.

McKiel E. Computer-assisted instruction: its efficacy for diabetes education. *Beta Release* 1991;15(3):85–87.

McRoy SW, Liu-Perez MS, Ali SS. Interactive computerized health care education. *Journal of the American Medical Informatics Association* 1998;5(4):347–356.

Milstead JA, Nelson R. Preparation for an online asynchronous university doctoral course: lessons learned. *Computers in Nursing* 1998;16(5):247–258.

Napholz L, McCanse R. Interactive video instruction increases efficiency in cognitive learning in a baccalaureate nursing education program. *Computers in Nursing* 1994;12(3):149–153.

Neafsey PJ. Immediate and enduring changes in knowledge and self-efficacy in APNs following computer-assisted home study of The Pharmacology of Alcohol. *The Journal of Continuing Education in Nursing* 1998;29(4):173–181.

Nyamathi A, Chang B, Sherman B, Grech M. Computer use and nursing research: CAI versus traditional learning. *Western Journal of Nursing Research* 1989; 11(4):498–501.

O'Brien BS, Renner AL. Opening minds: values clarification via electronic meetings. *Computers in Nursing* 1998;16(5):266–271.

O'Brien BS, Renner AL. Wired for thought: electronic meetings in nursing education. *Computers in Nursing* 1999;17(1):27–31.

Plank RK. Nursing on-line for continuing education credit. *The Journal of Continuing Education in Nursing* 1998;29(4):165–172.

Porter S. Application of computer-assisted instruction to continuing education in nursing: review of the literature. In: Zielstorff RD, ed. *Computers in Nursing*. Rockville, MD: Aspen, 1978.

Posel N. Guidelines for the evaluation of instructional software by hospital nursing departments. *Computers in Nursing* 1993;11(6):273–276.

Ribbons R. Guidelines for developing interactive multimedia: applications in nurse education. *Computers in Nursing* 1998a;16(2):109–114.

Ribbons R. The use of computers as cognitive tools to facilitate higher order thinking skills in nurse education. *Computers in Nursing* 1998b;16(4):223–238.

Ritt L, Stewart B. Innovative strategies for teaching anatomy and physiology. *Techtrends* 1996;41:41–42.

Saba V, McCormick K. *Essentials of Computers for Nurses.* New York: McGraw Hill, 1995:561.

Sawyer T. Human factors considerations in computer-assisted instruction. *Journal of Computer-Based Instruction* 1984;12:17–20.

Silberg WM, Lundberg GD, Musacchio RA. Assessing, controlling and assuring quality of medical information on the Internet. *JAMA* 1997;277(15):1244–1245.

Sinclair V. The computer as partner in health care instruction. *Computers in Nursing* 1985;3(5):212–216.

Tibbles L, Lewis C, Reisine S, Rippey R, Donald M. Computer-assisted instruction for preoperative and postoperative patient education in joint replacement surgery. *Computers in Nursing* 1992;10(5):208–212.

Thomson M. Multimedia anatomy and physiology lectures for nursing students. *Computers in Nursing* 1998;16(2):101–108.

Tronni C, Prawlucki P. Designing a computer-based clinical learning lab for staff nurses. *Computers in Nursing* 1998;16(3):147–149.

Vargo GS: Computer assisted patient education in the ambulatory care setting. *Computers in Nursing* 1991;9(5):168–169.

Weaver J. Patient education: an innovative computer approach. *Nursing Management* 1995;26(7):78–83.

Wilson BA. Computer anxiety in nursing students. *Journal of Nursing Education* 1991;30(2):52–56.

Wong J, Wong S, Richard J. Implementing computer simulations as a strategy for evaluating decision-making skills of nursing students. *Computers in Nursing* 1992;10(6):264–269.

Wright DJ. The use of multimedia computers and software in nurse education. *Health Informatics* 1995;1:101–107.

5
Butterflies, Bonsai, and Buonarotti: Images for the Nurse Analyst

Marina Douglas

The roles and responsibilities of nurse analysts have changed since the early 1980s, when their title was "nursing liaison" (Zielstorff, 1980) and their role specifically focused on the nursing components of a hospital information system (HIS). Although systems once were called *nursing information systems*, the term *clinical information systems* more fully describes what is used by nurses and clinicians in today's healthcare environment, where information required for patient care is collected from many sources. These sources may include laboratory, radiology, dietary, medical records, and financial systems internal to an organization. The external sources of community healthcare providers, federal agencies, and research and education databases may also be involved in the development and implementation of a patient's treatment plan.

The recognition of the multidimensional healthcare information needs has expanded the role of the nurse liaison to include active involvement in nontraditional nursing systems design, development, implementation, and research (e.g., radiology, laboratory, and quality assurance). It has also increased their involvement in all aspects of the more traditional nursing applications (plan of care, acuity, assessments) (Travis & Brennan, 1998). The term *nurse analyst* or *informatics nurse* is used here to denote the nurse working in the healthcare information arena as an analyst supporting all healthcare information needs. The work setting may be a hospital, a consulting service, or private industry.

In 1993, the American Nurses Association (ANA) recognized nursing informatics as a specialty area of nursing practice. The ANA (1994, p. 3) has defined the scope of practice for nursing informatics and is in the process of developing the practice standards for informatics nurses:

As a scientific discipline, nursing informatics serves the profession of nursing by supporting the information handling work of other nursing specialties. Nursing informatics is the specialty that integrates nursing science, computer science, and information science in identifying, collecting, processing, and managing data and information to support nursing practice, administration, education, research, and the expansion of nursing knowledge. It supports the practice of all nursing specialties, in all sites and settings of care, whether at the basic or advanced practice level. The practice of nursing informatics includes the development and evaluation of applications, tools, processes, and structures which assist nurses with the management of data in taking care of patients or in supporting the practice of nursing. It includes adapting, or customizing existing information technology to the requirements of nurses. It involves collaboration with other healthcare and informatics professionals in the development of informatics products and standards for nursing and healthcare informatics.

Nurses who practice in the field of nursing informatics are designated "informatics nurses." It recognizes that the person is both a nurse and an informaticist.

Through education, research, and experience, nurses have applied scientific principles, developed a body of knowledge, and made a significant contribution to the design and development of today's clinical information systems. The multidimensional healthcare information needs of patients and clinicians and the specialized requirements of professional nursing pose challenges for the continued design, development, and implementation of systems. To meet these challenges, the science of nursing and the nurse analyst must blend the technology of healthcare delivery and information systems with the patient's need for competent, compassionate care. The images of butterflies, bonsai gardening, and Michelangelo Buonarotti assist in describing the roles of the nurse analyst and the balance between the "high-tech" and "high-touch" phenomena.

Butterflies

The metamorphosis to butterfly occurs only after the caterpillar stage has been completed. For the nurse analyst, experience in the direct delivery of patient care is the essential starting point. Thoroughly schooled in the nursing process—to observe, assess, plan, implement, and evaluate—nurses utilize an analytic problem-solving approach to patient care. The nurse providing direct patient care continually assesses the status of the patient. The involvement of the patient and family in the delivery of care is fundamental. When the patient is unable to communicate or do for himself, the nurse provides care based on best judgment, experience, and knowledge. The everyday role of the nurse providing direct patient care, therefore, requires the abilities to

- Constantly observe and assess the patient and environment
- Participate in the development of the multi/interdisciplinary treatment plan based on assessed needs
- Translate the treatment plan into terms understood by patient and family
- Elicit the cooperation of the patient, family, and healthcare team, using listening and communication skills to implement the treatment plan

- Utilize knowledge of and experience with both normal and abnormal physiology and the desired and adverse reactions to treatment in monitoring the progress of the patient
- Evaluate the outcomes of care relative to the treatment goal and plan.

The skills developed in the role of direct care provider form the foundation for the nurse analyst. The knowledge base of the nurse analyst expands to include the technology of information systems in conjunction with the principles and processes employed in system analysis, development, and implementation. It is a widely held tenet that while nurses have successfully learned and applied information systems principles and technology, it has been much more difficult for those trained in computer science to identify the information needs and assimilate the principles and technology of medicine, nursing, and health care. The metamorphosis requires the analyst to experience the role of a nurse providing direct patient care.

Because of their expertise and training, informatics nurses are adept in bridging the needs of patient *care and technology* (Lange, 1997; Parker & Gassert, 1996). According to the ANA (1994), qualifications for informatics nurse specialists include a master's degree in nursing where a high level of clinical expertise has been demonstrated and graduate-level studies in information systems.

Bonsai

The practice of bonsai gardening began in Japan centuries ago. It is a living art form utilizing three horticultural practices—pruning, shaping, and containerization. The goal is to produce small three-dimensional forms of pleasing lines and aspects (Bailey & McDonald, 1972). Considerable care and commitment is required, as well as a long-term vision and patience.

During the pruning and shaping, small cuts are taken. The future lines and the overall look of the garden are determined by these actions. The container or garden space, determining factors for the size of the plantings, play an important part in the presentation of the garden. The visionary gardener plans the garden based on the desired effect of the plantings at maturity.

The nurse analyst often functions in an environment with similar constraints where nurturing and strong communication skills are essential. Managing the pruning and shaping of expectations during all phases of design, development, and implementation presents a considerable challenge. Fiscal limitations frequently impact the hardware and information system software selection process; it is a balance between the cost of the desired features and functions and the allocated funds. Development and implementation schedules will be dictated by the number and availability of resources to complete tasks.

While maintaining enthusiasm and a focused vision for the strategic goals of the institution and/or information system, the nurse analyst must shape the expectations of the project team to coincide with a realistic plan. Understanding the needs and interactions of multiple health care providers, balancing those needs against the fiscal and resource constraints of the institution, and delivering a functional system in a timely fashion are essential components of the nurse analyst role. The nurse analyst must focus on the data, information, and knowledge of health care and nursing, as well as the use of information technology, to support patient care and advance the discipline of nursing (Lange, 1997).

General Principles for Automated Systems

Just as the basic principles of health and nursing are taught and assimilated into the daily practice of nursing, the nurse analyst must learn and assimilate the general principles of automated systems. Yourdon (1989) describes four such principles.

First, "the more specialized a system is, the less able it is to adapt to different circumstances" (Yourdon, 1989, p. 34). Helping to define system requirements takes creativity. From a system designed with flexibility and considerations of future needs comes a system in which minimal programming changes result in maximum benefits for the end users and patient care. The nurse analyst encourages users to look toward the realistic future by reviewing their current practices and future trends.

The users will likely benefit from the nurse analyst's observation skills, knowledge of industry trends in health care, information systems and technology, and problem-solving skills. For example, care planning software designed strictly to meet the needs of nursing may no longer meet the multidisciplinary requirements of case management. Care planning software designed with flexibility to differentiate among the care providers and their needs and track variations between expected and actual completion dates may be adapted more easily to support the added requirements of the trend toward case management.

The second of Yourdon's automated systems principles (1989, p. 34) is "the larger the system is, the more of its resources that must be devoted to its everyday maintenance." The design and implementation of clinical systems must factor in system maintenance requirements. The development of policies and procedures for system operations considers the needs of patient care and the healthcare providers. Where nightly maintenance for an HIS once took four to six hours of processing, newer technologies have nearly eliminated this downtime. With greater emphasis on the extraction of information (rather than simply data), development of reports and online views must consider the overall performance impact on the central processing unit. The nurse analyst ensures that the end user's response time for routine processing will not be adversely affected by new projects, report generation, or procedures.

Yourdon's third principle (1989, p. 35) is that "Systems are always part of larger systems, and they can always be partitioned into smaller systems."

The nurse analyst has first-hand knowledge of the smaller systems that comprise the larger healthcare organization. The challenge is to find ways to automate the smaller systems for the benefit of the larger system. Efforts to reengineer and redesign workflow must occur concurrently with the development and implementation of new information systems. The nurse analyst facilitates the end users' review of "the way we always do it" with an eye toward gaining efficiencies. Personnel productivity can then be focused on patient care rather than paper management.

In other instances, there may be factions of users unwilling to accept the activation of a system that is anything less than the ultimate information system. Even though total information systems perfection has not been attained, groupings of available applications can achieve benefits for the organization in the near term. Romano (1990) points out that putting technology to practical use is innovation. The innovative nurse analyst assists in establishing development and/or implementation plans to maximize achievable benefits as soon as possible. This can be accomplished by thoughtful planning and segmenting the implementation of a total HIS into smaller activation groupings. This may include helping to evaluate the vendors' development schedule during the system selection process relative to the strategic goals of the organization and the desired implementation plan. In instances where the organization is responsible for the development of the new system, definition of the development plan provides benefits to the end user as soon as possible. In both instances, benefits can begin accruing while the vision of attaining the ideal information system is maintained.

The fourth of Yourdon's principles (1989, p. 35) is that systems grow. The use of clinical information systems will expand greatly as healthcare networks are implemented. Traditional smaller systems (order communications, medical records, intensive care systems) will require data integration with community health information networks. A study by the Institute of Medicine in early 1990 put forth the concept of a computerized patient record for healthcare delivery; it has become the goal for communities, hospitals, and software development (Dick et al., 1997).

The computerized patient record initiative will provide automated longitudinal clinical information for patients. Participation in the definition and use of standard nursing nomenclature in automation will be an important first step toward the computerized patient record. Ensuring clinical data integration among the disparate systems will be the challenge and responsibility of the nurse analyst.

Buonarotti

Michelangelo Buonarotti had both curiosity and the talent for creating beauty. Michelangelo began his formal art studies as an apprentice; his studies included both painting and sculpture. He studied the human form through traditional studio sessions as well as in a nontraditional manner—

assisting with autopsies. By peeling back the layers, dissection of the human form provided him with an understanding of the form, function, and limitations of the body. In this manner, Michelangelo learned art through the combination of internal structure and external appearance. His mentor, Lorenzo the Magnificent (Mariani, 1964), provided a milieu in which curiosity and creativity were encouraged.

The nurse analyst approaches the design and implementation of a system in much the same manner—understanding the form and function as well as the underlying anatomy. A history of actively providing direct patient care gives nurses a foundation of knowledge about the healthcare delivery system and the general needs of healthcare professionals. This involves dedicated preparation and study and many long hours of direct patient care responsibilities to meet the qualifications of a registered nurse.

Understanding the operational aspects of healthcare delivery assists in the design and evaluation of the system's end-user interface. Exposure to administrative duties in the acute care environment provides the nurse analyst with knowledge of the regulations and requirements that often dictate hospital policy and procedure. These regulatory requirements have a significant bearing on the development and implementation of a system. Just as Michelangelo studied human anatomy to better his painting and sculpting, the nurse analyst should know database structures, program logic, and processing requirements to better support both the end user and the programming resources of a system. Participation in systems analysis and development gives the nurse analyst a complete picture of a system. Development of a system requires the nurse analyst to dissect the requirements of the user, apply the rigors of systems analysis, and piece it all together in a cohesive manner that is both pleasing to the end user and programmatically efficient for the technical staff.

Systems Analysis and Development

Yourdon (1989, p. 1) defines systems analysis as the study of the "interactions of people, and disparate groups of people, and computers and organizations." For the nurse analyst, the disparate groups of people include patients, a cadre of healthcare providers, administrators, accreditation organizations, researchers, educators, insurers, payers, software programmers, and federal and state governments, with each group identifying its own set of information requirements. In addition to the skills outlined for the direct caregiver, the nurse analyst must possess the ability to think of systems in both the abstract and physical terms, possess computer skills, and survive the political battles found in every organization (Yourdon, 1989; Gause & Weinberg, 1989).

Participation in the analysis and development of systems is the major component of the nurse analyst's role. Nurses in the hospital, community, vendor, and consulting settings participate in the design and development

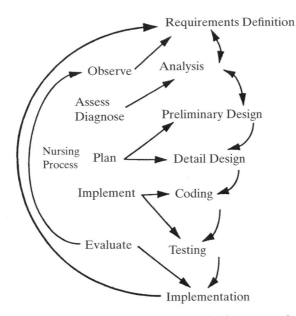

Figure 5.1. Comparison of nursing process and classic systems development life cycle.

of clinical information systems (Hersher, 1985). Figure 5.1 depicts the similarities between the nursing process and the system development life cycle. The comfort with which nurses utilize the nursing process for problem solving provides the foundation for assimilation of the systems analysis and development process. Active participation in systems analysis and development provides a detailed understanding of the needs of the end users, the information system's internal structure, and the system's limitations and potential.

The identification of system requirements is similar to the observation phase of the nursing process. At this stage, the requirements of the system's users are gathered. The nurse analyst gains insight into the requirements by observing the environment in which the system operates or will operate. The information needs of the users may not coincide with the current data collected because more data may have been collected than utilized. In other cases, insufficient data are collected.

Defining requirements helps bring clarity to the data issues and information needs. The nurse analyst may utilize a number of techniques to define requirements; the use of decision trees, mockups, prototypes, and/or data mapping assists in identifying the flow of information and data elements needed. While the nurse analyst must have the ability to conceptualize systems, these techniques allow for visualization of data requirements and information flow for the end users.

During the analysis phase of systems development, the nurse analyst works closely with the technical staff to determine the feasibility of the desired requirements. Hardware and communications technologies are evaluated relative to the desired goals, and financial and resource requirements are factored. The development/implementation plan is proposed. The nurse analyst communicates progress, seeks refined definition of requirements, and (when necessary) negotiates compromises.

Just as the nurse providing direct patient care continually communicates the patient's response to treatment to the patient, the healthcare team, and the family, the nurse analyst is the vital communications link between the users and programmers. The abilities to assess the political environment and mediate conflict resolution are required skills. Coordinating meetings, tracking task completion and programming progress, and maintaining frequent and effective communication are key to successful systems development.

The requirements definition and analysis phases of systems development are most critical to the success of a development project, yet they frequently have the least amount of time allotted. Gause and Weinberg (1989) note that fixing an error found when a project is in the requirements definition phase has a relative cost of one; in the analysis phase, the relative cost to fix an error is three to six times that of the analysis phase. The cost to fix an error increases dramatically as the project progresses, jumping to 40 to 1,000 times that of the analysis phase if found after the system is operational. The collecting, collating, reviewing, refining, evaluating, and documenting of the design are integral components of the success of a new system. Being open to new ideas, suggestions, and surprises is crucial as the design and implementation of the system is monitored. The direct patient care background provides the nurse analyst with a strong basis for understanding the information needs of smaller systems (e.g., in nursing, radiology, dietary, and laboratory), their relationship to the larger organization, and their potential impact on the new system.

The planning phase of the nursing process correlates with the development of the preliminary and detailed design phases of systems analysis and development. The nurse analyst assists by converting the desired requirements into formal specifications. The end-user interface—the "look and feel" of the system—is determined. The sequencing of screens and windows, data fields, and integration points is established and refined during these phases. The understanding gained from the requirements definition and analysis phases provides the nurse analyst with a strong sense of the desired sequencing and functioning of the system. The overall needs of the organization are considered as design and development of the smaller systems progress.

The coding and testing phases of systems development equate to the implementation phase of the nursing process. During these phases, the features and functions are programmed and tested. The nurse analyst seeks clarification from the end users on behalf of the programming staff. Communication during this phase is particularly important. Programmers rely on the nurse analyst for quick issue resolution, and the users are consulted on issue resolution and are kept apprised of the progress of the coding.

At least two levels of testing are recommended. The first level is functional testing, the level at which individual programs are tested to ensure that data are captured and processed within the individual function or application as specified. Responsibility for testing of individual programs as they are completed may be shared among the programming staff, nurse analyst, and end users. During functional testing, the nurse analyst develops testing scenarios or scripts that comprehensively test each feature.

The second testing phase for the newly developed programs or the implementation of a completed product is termed *integrated testing*. Coordinated by the nurse analyst, highly detailed testing scenarios are developed to mimic use of the functions in a production environment. Testing scripts and testing procedures are developed. The focus of integrated testing is on the points of integration with other applications and on the operational policies of both information systems and the end users. The testing scenarios should be executed as written, through-put followed closely, and thorough review of the output coordinated by the nurse analyst. The nurse analyst's evaluation of the success of the integrated test period has much bearing on the decision to implement the system in the production environment or to repeat testing.

The implementation of the new system equates to the evaluation phase of the nursing process. It is essentially the evaluation of the preceding analysis and development steps. The relative success of the implementation of a new system reflects the accuracy and in-depth understanding of the initial requirements and their translation into programs. As with the nursing process, the systems analysis and development life cycle will begin anew with the refining of previously defined requirements or the identification of new requirements.

The Nurse Analyst as Project Manager

Frequently, nurse analysts are called on to serve as design or software implementation project managers. The ability to rapidly apply a problem-solving approach (the nursing process) to situations, track the progress of multiple groups relative to the project's goal, gain consensus, and communicate issues and problems are skills the nurse analyst brings from the realm of direct patient care. The complex nature of the delivery of patient care affords the nurse analyst a solid background for assuming this role.

Summary

The role of the nurse analyst is complex and challenging. It requires observation skills with attention to detail, knowledge of healthcare delivery systems and trends, creativity in analytic problem solving, strong written and verbal communication skills, negotiation and mediation abilities, and the ability to conceptualize and communicate a vision for an information system. The nurse analyst builds these skills from the experience of providing direct patient care.

Expanding the skill set to include knowledge of information systems principles, technologies, systems analysis, and development begins the second level of requisite knowledge for the nurse analyst. Operating in a highly technical environment, the nurse analyst must balance the compassion of patient care needs with the coldness sometimes associated with technology to produce an accepted and utilized clinical information system.

As systems continue to grow, the needs of healthcare professionals will become more encompassing. The soft images of butterflies, bonsai, and Buonarotti provide important lessons for the role of the nurse analyst as the creation of clinical information systems progresses. The image of the butterfly's metamorphosis relates to the nurse analyst's prerequisite experience of providing direct patient care. Bonsai gardening teaches the need to work toward a vision fraught with constraints by using small prunings and shapings to accomplish a desired effect. Finally, Buonarotti's approach to the creation of art demonstrates the need to understand the internal structure of information systems as well as the outward appearance of the system.

Questions

1. Discuss Yourdon's four general principles of automated systems using examples from your own setting. Do they apply to your environment?
2. The author contends that a nurse is in a good position to take on the role of systems analyst for the design and implementation of an automated system. Do you agree or disagree with this statement, and why?

References

American Nurses Association. *The Scope of Practice for Nursing Informatics.* Washington, DC: American Nurses Publishing, 1994.

Bailey R, McDonald E. *The Good Housekeeping Illustrated Guide to Gardening,* vol 3. New York: Hearst Magazines, 1972;328.

Dick R, Steen E, Detmer D, eds. *The Computer-Based Patient Record: an Essential Technology for Health Care,* revised edition. Washington, DC: National Academy Press, 1997.

Gause D, Weinberg G. *Exploring Requirements: Quality before Design.* New York: Dorset House Publishing, 1989.

Hersher B. The job search and information systems opportunities for nurses. *Nursing Clinics of North America* 1985;20(3):585–594.

Lange L. Informatics nurse specialist: roles in health care organizations. *Nursing Administration Quarterly* 1997;21(3): 1–10.

Mariani V. *Michelangelo the Painter.* New York: Harry N. Abrams, 1964;13–33.

Parker CD, Gassert C. JCAHO management of information standards: the role of the informatics nurse specialist. *Journal of Nursing Administration* 1996;26(6): 13–15.

Romano C. Innovation: the promise and the perils for nursing and information technology. *Computers in Nursing* 1990;8(3):99–104.

Travis L, Brennan P. Information science for the future: an innovative nursing informatics curriculum. *Journal of Nursing Education* 1998;37(4):162–168.

Yourdon E. *Modern Structured Analysis.* Englewood Cliffs, NJ: Yourdon Press, 1989.

Zielstorff R. Preface. In: R Zielstorff, ed. *Computers in Nursing.* Gaithersburg, MD: Aspen Publications, 1980.

6
New Roles for Nurses in Healthcare Information Systems

Betsy Hersher

Opportunities for nurses entering the field of healthcare information systems are abundant. Now more than ever before, the opportunity for growth and advancement is unlimited in a dynamic, evolving, and challenging environment. Because of managed care, regulatory, and reporting issues, there is a general shift in systems direction to care management, clinical systems, clinical data repositories, care mapping, and outcomes measures.

These systems are vital to the success of every healthcare endeavor; in fact, in the last few years, they have become a major driver in care delivery. More physicians are entering information systems organizations to support these efforts. The increased number of clinicians (physicians and nurses) has increased the need for leadership. Nurses are a natural choice to lead these endeavors, as they are excellent managers. They are needed to define, develop, install, consult, and market these systems.

Technology has advanced rapidly. It has significantly facilitated complex interfaces, communication, and networking of diverse systems, not only across the continuum of care, but also across the complexities of integrated delivery networks and alliances. Data collected through sophisticated nursing systems are now available across the healthcare enterprise. The practice of nursing has evolved to take advantage of the technology and, in many cases, drive the technology.

We no longer need to make predictions regarding nurses' significance in healthcare information systems, as their roles have been securely established. Today, it is easier for nurses to move into these vital roles. In fact, nurses now have major roles in all aspects of the field. They are vital to the clinical success of any information systems endeavor and have attained important nonclinical leadership roles.

In addition to the explosion of clinical systems and the need for nursing leadership, one of the main factors in the establishment of nurses in clinical information systems roles has been the emphasis and preoccupation with Y2K over the last five years. Because of the resource demands for complete Y2K projects, clinical systems' leadership has been left to run autonomously. Those in charge have gained significant experience and exposure. Because of nurses' innate skills as project managers, they have been extremely successful—so successful that, in some instances, their projects have caused their managers to move them into nonclinical roles and further advance them to senior management within information systems.

Nurses are, by training and intuition, excellent managers and leaders. They are problem solvers and skilled jugglers of multiple priorities. Nurses also make excellent information systems candidates because they are adept at data gathering, documenting, viewing systems from a global perspective, setting priorities, managing all care, and understanding the need to access patient information. For those to whom implementation of information systems is an interest, this chapter describes how to combine skills, move into this field, and assume leadership roles.

The ability to learn on the job, communicate effectively, and exercise patience are important skills. Leaving the bedside to move into the development of patient care-related systems is a viable transition, but the prospective candidate must be comfortable leaving patient care. To make this transition, the nurse must also become a facilitator and user of resources without necessarily having control or authority over those resources.

Preparation: Requirements and Suggestions

Completion of a bachelor's degree is vital in all areas of nursing today, and many nurses continue their education to obtain a master's degree in clinical specialties. This helps them prepare for a leadership role in information systems. Consider a master's degree in business as an extra boost toward not only a future leadership role in information systems management, but also any executive role. It is much easier now for a nurse to move into the information systems field than it was five years ago.

One way to move into the field is to act as a user liaison on any information systems steering committees. Another way is to market new systems within the hospital and use the work experience to transition into a new career in information systems. The experience gained, combined with nursing expertise, can carry nurses into this field.

Volunteering for opportunities on information systems projects is also a smart way to gain experience and exposure. Get to know the chief information officer and other information systems mentors. Another valuable "nonactual job experience" is getting involved with vendors and user committees and attending national conferences.

Categories of Information Systems Jobs

Information systems jobs for nurses can be divided into many different categories and subcategories, as shown in Table 6.1.

TABLE 6.1. Information systems jobs for nurses.

Categories	Subcategories
Nursing divisions	Staffing
	Scheduling
	Acuity
	Care mapping/outcomes
	Quality
	Nursing informatics
	Research roles
Integrated delivery networks information systems organizations	Utilization review
	Outcomes measures and quality
	Client services
	Clinical systems
	Applications development
	User liaisons
	Chief information officers (CIOs)
	Associate CIOs
	Project management/installation management
Vendors	
Insurance companies	
Managed care	
Consulting firms	
Clinics	

User Liaison for the Hospital

When a clinical information system is installed in an integrated delivery network, it is necessary to coordinate the needs of the institution and staff with the capabilities of the system. Usually, a systems steering committee is formed. Participating in the steering committee is an excellent way to gain systems knowledge and exposure and to interact with hospital-wide users, vendors, consultants, and administrators. Duties of the steering committee also include needs analysis, participation in the selection of the systems, definition of the systems, and coordination of installation.

Becoming a steering committee member can help a nurse discover what level of interest this career holds. Members have an opportunity to conduct site visits, see a variety of systems, and attend training classes given by a chosen vendor. Active participation in the committee makes a nurse highly visible and the obvious first choice when the organization begins looking for a coordinator.

Nurses are naturals as user liaisons because of their training and background. There is order and organization in their profession, which includes teaching, accurate and complete documenting, and developing efficient and effective methods of patient care delivery with a step-by-step, problem-solving approach. Automation of patient care systems effectively helps nurses to analyze and handle problems.

Clinical Systems Installation/Vendor

There is a growing need for candidates qualified to install various components of medical information, order entry, communication, productivity, acuity, and staffing systems. An installation person is often on the market team during and after the sale of a software package. The main task of the installer is to train the users and help them over the rough spots during and after conversion to the new system. Many of the skills outlined above are imperative in this job. Additionally, the installer must be a negotiator and liaison, acting as the bridge between the user and the software vendor.

Working for the software vendor adds a new dimension. The job entails being an advocate of the user's position and needs while ensuring that the system is installed according to the design parameters. The vendor is paid as the various modules are installed. This position can sometimes require considerable juggling. In addition, leaving the nonprofit environment could be a large obstacle for a nurse to overcome.

These positions often require 50 percent or more traveling time, a solid understanding of how the components of an integrated delivery network operate, excellent communication and presentation skills, and a solid understanding of systems. A move into an installation role with a vendor can lead to a number of career possibilities, as this role also offers much visibility.

In-House Installation

The same skills required for vendor installers are needed for in-house installers. Additional skills in marketing the new system and user education are also vital.

Product Manager/Vendor

Product management is one of the most exciting professional moves that has become available in the last few years. The responsibilities of product management and production definition are loosely defined and can change from vendor to vendor. The duties often overlap into marketing. This is a position that is also beginning to develop on the integrated delivery network side.

A person in product management is responsible for constantly updating the current product and keeping abreast of all developments in the field. Product managers must be cognizant of the current and future needs of the clients and determine whether these needs can be or should be incorporated into the product. The people determining the product direction are the watchdogs of the product and the industry.

The characteristic role of product manager is the same in any industry. Product managers must interface with marketing staff, clients, technical staff, and management personnel to produce a usable and marketable product in a timely manner and at the best price. They must satisfy the needs of one client without compromising the needs of other clients or the capabilities of the technical staff. This position generally begins as a staff role requiring excellent communication and negotiation skills, as well as internal and external marketing expertise. Vendors and healthcare organizations are under pressure to define their current and future needs accurately, and this is an essential component. Success in this position can lead to high-level strategic planning positions with expanding responsibilities and compensation. Nurses are in high demand in the development of some new applications, including decision support systems, clinical ancillary systems, managed care, nurse staffing, outcomes and productivity, acuity systems, and bedside and hand-held terminals.

Marketing Support/Vendor

Market support is defined differently by various organizations. The classic definition involves technical sales support to the salespeople and additional explanations to the client. With so many patient care and ancillary systems in development, nurses are needed to assist in closing the sale.

To be a good marketer, it is important to listen closely to the needs of clients. Discovering the reasons why software products answer the needs of the clients is very important. Market support personnel must possess excellent written and oral communication skills and understand the marketing cycle. They must be able to identify the decision makers. On some occasions, it is necessary to act as a negotiator between the client and the salesperson.

The salesperson's role is to sell the product and close the sale. Market support personnel add the technical information, often demonstrate the product, and attempt to ensure that the client is not oversold or undersold. They play a significant role before, during, and after the sale.

During the sale cycle, market support staff will interface with the product management team, the technical staff of the hospital, the vendor, and salespeople. In many vendor situations, market support departments will answer requests for proposals and be involved in contract negotiations.

In a software vendor situation, the move from market support to sales rarely occurs because of the additional skills required. Notable exceptions are the patient care, ancillary, and alternative delivery systems. Additionally, medical personnel often move into sales for highly technical products, such as biomedical equipment.

The move into sales from marketing should not be taken lightly, as it is rare that an individual makes the transition successfully. A successful transition can, however, be quite rewarding. The skills required are negotiation, selling (sometimes more than is actually there), patience, and the ability to close a sale.

Consultant

All of the information systems consulting firms have nurses in senior roles and several as partners. The ideal candidate for a consulting firm has a master's degree, excellent written and oral communication skills, and a sound knowledge of systems. Consultants should be analytical problem solvers, independent, creative, and assertive. Additionally, an outgoing marketing personality is a plus and ensures growth. Listening and evaluative skills are essential in consulting.

Nurses make excellent consultants if they have the right personality. It is often necessary to make instant decisions based on analysis of fact. Generally speaking, nurses tend to have strong personalities, can take charge, and know how to establish their professional credibility. These are all traits that a consultant should possess.

Consulting is a high-pressure field. Assignments are usually carried out in project teams of more than two people. Projects can range from needs analysis and selection of vendors, to strategic planning, cost-benefit studies, and systems audits. These tasks fit well with nurses' abilities to manage teams.

Consulting stretches skills and abilities and offers excellent personal growth potential. One must operate independently and successfully, act as a liaison and expert, learn to lead projects, and be able to handle a variety of products. A career in consulting requires drive and the ambition to seek high levels of achievement. Consulting firms hire carefully and look for candidates who will be partner material.

One of the negatives of a consulting career is a heavy travel schedule. Another is that, although consultants get an opportunity for project management, they rarely manage large numbers. In many instances, consultants make recommendations but do not remain to implement them. Someone accustomed to following through might find it difficult to walk away before the entire task is completed.

Sales Representative/Vendor

Because of their keen ability to motivate, negotiate, and demonstrate credibility, nurses make excellent salespeople. A factor that adds to their credibility is the need to thoroughly understand a process (such as illness) and observe many signs simultaneously. Timing is a crucial skill in sales. If this skill is translated into sales, the nurse should be able to present the product from a sound base of understanding rather than a "smoke and mirrors" approach.

Because of training and experience, the nurse has the need to bring something to closure, an essential skill requirement in sales. A career in sales can be very rewarding financially, leading to sales management or operational management in a vendor environment. The downside is that it is a high-risk, high-frustration environment that requires a strong tolerance for rejection. Moving into sales can end up being the ultimate disconnect from the client (after the actual sale), which could clash with a nurse's gestalt.

Director of Quality Improvement

Directors of Quality Improvement deal with a combination of clinical and information technologies. Sophisticated organizations recognize how important the role of data is in process improvement. For this reason, there is increasing emphasis put on how to get the data necessary to measure outcomes and the effects of process improvement. Nurses with a solid understanding of informatics have a tremendous advantage in these positions. They understand the concepts of data mining and understand where to get the data necessary for clinicians to measure whether a process has been improved.

To be successful in the role of Director of Quality Improvement requires several clinical, personal, and technical skills. With regard to clinical skills, a well-rounded clinical background with an understanding of the importance of the continuum of care is desired. Quality improvement clearly involves process improvements that span across the continuum of care. Personal skills must also include a passion for excellence and the interpersonal skills to negotiate with caregivers. To be a change agent in process improvement requires the ability to work well with all kinds of caregivers and to sell them on the benefits of some of the necessary changes.

Finally, there are technical skills necessary in order to be successful. The Director of Quality Improvement must understand data and how to retrieve them. A sound knowledge of the existing systems and how they interface enables the director to identify where data can be found and to verify the reliability of those data. The frosting on the cake is to be technically sound enough to be able to use query language to obtain data from the existing systems.

Insurance Companies/Managed Care

More and more insurance companies and managed care organizations are paying attention to managing care, not just managing costs. They are looking to nurses to manage this "movement" with their focus concentrated on outcomes measures, quality, and utilization review (UR) systems, and nurses are rising to the occasion.

CIO/Deputy CIO

The CIO role has evolved quickly into a leader who manages technologists, facilitates change, and forces the use of data for all levels of decision making. The successful CIO is constantly developing key leaders within his or her organization for advancement. Because of all the pressures created by mergers, alliances, and the technology explosion, the CIO job has become a two or three person job.

Nurses have advanced significantly in information systems organizations due to their roles in major project management. They have an excellent opportunity to move into the CIO or deputy CIO role. In fact, nurses as information systems managers are no longer viewed as nurses, but as information systems executives and key project leaders.

If nurses are "regular" members of the team, the variety of jobs and growth potential is unlimited. More jobs open as information systems organizations become more complex. Also, due to recruitment and retention issues, there are a variety of opportunities available for internal transfers.

The number of nurses in the information systems field is rapidly increasing, and many are rising to the top. The progression of nurses in this field is evidenced by their occupation of CIO and deputy CIO roles.

Summary

The future of our industry lies in total healthcare systems that have expanded far beyond hospitals. Large non-healthcare corporations and business coalitions will have a strong influence. The management of care, sometimes called *care management*, has become as important as managed care and costs. Disease management systems and quality improvement and outcomes are essential factors in delivery of care. Because nurses lead these efforts, they must continually upgrade their skills and goals, examine career options, and be flexible. This is an ideal point in the growth of healthcare information systems for nurses to consider before becoming actively involved.

To be part of this growing and changing environment, nurses need to be proactive and visible, a goal that requires writing, speaking, and seeking out other ways to get involved. Many nurses have already attained key information systems positions and are willing to serve as mentors. There are jobs out there waiting for the right candidates, and with motivation and guidance, nurses can enter the rapidly expanding network of leaders.

Questions

1. What are the changes in the last five years that have led to new roles for nurses in healthcare information systems?
2. What learned and innate skills make nurses great managers and executives?
3. Given the explosion in technology and new applications, design three jobs in information systems for which you would like to apply.

Section 2
Enabling Technologies

Overview: Information Technology: Difference Engine of the New Millennium

Roy L. Simpson

The organizational buzzword for the last decade has been *total quality management* (TQM), or some variation on the theme. With managed care, however, the pursuit of quality became not only a competitive concern but also an economic dilemma. How could healthcare organizations provide better care for less cost and manage to stay in business? Over time, we have discovered the answer: by becoming a new type of organization. The key to building such an organization is information technology.

In the new millennium, consumerism, empowerment, and process flexibility will combine to create the world class organization, and information technology will be the foundation upon which it will be built. This overview explores several unique characteristics of the world class organization and how clinical information systems and information technology are evolving to support these characteristics. Issues for discussion include

- How patient-centered care and the interdisciplinary care team have engendered a new breed of clinical information systems
- How nursing's empowerment has created a need for systems and languages to measure and document nursing care and its outcomes
- How care across the continuum and rapid, constant change demand open systems that are scalable and interoperable

Defining the World Class Organization

The total quality organization of the 1990s is rapidly evolving into the world class organization of the new millennium. In many ways, they are similar. Both are focused on quality, and both operate on the principle that quality must be produced at a lower cost.

The difference between total quality and world class organizations is in how they achieve this cost-effective quality. While total quality organizations achieve quality by adhering to elaborate TQM standards and structures, world class organizations achieve it by focusing on customers, empowering their workforces, and implementing fluid, flexible processes and structures. Information technology (IT) makes this possible.

Information Technology: The Difference Engine

In 1822, the eccentric British mathematician and inventor Charles Babbage conceived the first device that might be considered a computer in the modern sense of the word. After seven years, he ran out of money and stopped building it. More than 150 years later, a team at London's Science Museum constructed the machine from Babbage's original drawings. It weighs seven tons, takes up an entire wing of the museum, runs on steam, and is slower than a $5 calculator. Still, it is a true digital computer that operates on binary code. Babbage called the machine his "Difference Engine." This precisely describes what IT is to health care—the engine built to make a difference.

Specifically, IT will support the world class organization's quest for quality by developing

- Scalable, interoperable new-breed clinical information systems that can support such new, quality-focused entities as patient-centered care, the interdisciplinary care team, and care across the continuum
- New systems and languages to measure and document nursing care and its outcomes.

The New Breed of Clinical Information Systems

When the original healthcare information systems were designed, the face of health care was entirely different—there was an acute-care focus, fee-for-service reimbursement, and caregiver autonomy. Managed care changed that. Today, outpatient and ancillary care is the focus, reimbursement is tied to outcomes, and success depends on managing care as opposed to simply providing it. As a result, the new model of care delivery is care across the continuum, and the new way to deliver it is via the care team.

This change makes caregivers responsible for controlling care quality and cost by way of their interaction with patients. To do this, they need access to sophisticated technology at the point of care. Paper-based documentation, with its inconsistencies, lack of accessibility, and potential for loss or damage, is almost useless for measuring or improving quality in the manner now required.

The new model of care demands new types of systems that can help caregivers identify best practices, coordinate team care, ensure compliance with established clinical protocols and referral guidelines, and get specialist feedback (Appleby, 1996). Legacy hospital information systems—which were predominantly financial, mainframe based, and written in proprietary operating systems—are giving way to systems that

- Integrate clinical and financial data
- Operate on almost all hardware platforms using predominantly "open" operating systems
- Place the patient at the center of the information-gathering process.

The result is better documentation that improves the quality of patient care by ensuring that the right information is collected and disseminated and that the best clinical practices are captured and translated into clinical care (Appleby, 1996).

Still, it is not enough that these new-breed clinical systems operate differently. They also have to operate with each other—and with other departmental systems, both old and new. Interoperability is critical. Systems must span the enterprise, integrating multiple care sites, multiple caregiver constituencies, and multiple episodes of care. This is particularly important in this era of consolidation, which calls for tying together disparate facilities, and in health care as an industry, which has a history of maintaining independent computer systems on a departmental or single-site basis.

The Empowered Nurse

In the world class organization, responsibility for improving quality rests squarely on the shoulders of caregivers. While this certainly makes them more accountable than ever for the care they provide, it also empowers them. Clearly, nursing is a discipline that can benefit from empowerment.

Empowerment provides a unique opportunity—and responsibility—for nurses to define and establish their contribution to the patient care process by

- Clarifying the value of advanced practitioners. Advanced practice nurses play a more critical and aggressive role in managing patient recovery and wellness. They bring superior clinical, academic, and practice experience that is directly reflected in higher quality care. They "cost" more, but world class organizations recognize that the higher price is justified by higher returns—improved quality of care and reduced patient care costs.
- Spearheading adoption of nursing minimum data sets. Traditionally, nurses have documented their care with medical data sets and nomenclatures. Unfortunately, the language of physicians is limited in its ability to reflect nursing care accurately. Without specific nomenclatures that can organize, classify, manage, and provide access to data about the context and support of direct healthcare delivery, nurses—and health care in general—can never compile the hard data needed to make today's difficult quality decisions (Simpson, 1997).
- Advocating and actively participating in the development of patient-based clinical systems. Over a decade has passed since people in health care began talking about the computerized patient record (CPR). The Institute of Medicine (IOM) endorses the CPR system and is calling for its widespread use by 2001. This is an unlikely goal, given the lack of standards, an industry-wide unwillingness to embrace new technologies, and overall confusion about what the CPR should be. Despite these obstacles, nursing can and should play a key role in furthering the development of the CPR, from adopting nursing minimum data sets to finding ways to apply its clinical expertise to the informatics arena.

Toward a New Organization

Without information technology, managed care would collapse, and the world class organization would be no more than a dream. With IT—health care's "Difference Engine"—the world class organization is a thrilling possibility. IT development cannot not happen in a vacuum, however, nor should its use be relegated to the elusive "somebody else." If caregivers are to be the new quality vanguard, then they should and must play an active role in the development of the technology that makes their empowerment possible.

References

Appleby C. The mouse that roared. *Hospitals & Health Networks*, 1996;70(4):30.
Simpson RL. What good are advanced practitioners if nobody at the top knows their value? *Nursing Administration Quarterly* 1997;21(4):91–92.

7
Usability Concepts and Clinical Computing

Nancy Staggers

A logical and often repeated mantra in healthcare computing is that applications must be easy for clinicians to use. What constitutes ease of use is, however, seldom articulated. What makes an application or system user friendly? How can decision-makers purchase systems that will be acceptable to clinicians as they use them in day-to-day operations? How can vendors design more usable applications? These questions address usability aspects of clinical information systems.

This chapter discusses the essentials of usability concepts: the existing problem of nonusable applications, definitions of usability and its broader concept, human–computer interaction, and components to consider in the usability of applications. Specific recommendations are outlined for incorporating usability concepts into the purchase and design of clinical information systems.

Usability Problems in Healthcare Computing

Many authors think that the key barrier to user acceptance of computers is the lack of user friendliness of current systems (Davis, 1993; Patel & Kushniruk, 1998; Staggers, 1995a; van Bemmel, 1988). In healthcare computing, evidence of usability problems is ubiquitous. We need usability concepts in healthcare computing because we still have systems fielded worldwide with screens like the one depicted in Fig. 7.1.

In the Department of Defense, for example, a text-based, dumb-terminal application predominates in ambulatory and inpatient care settings. To use this system, a variety of commands and menus must be memorized, a lengthy series of screens must be accessed to complete one simple action like creating a nursing intervention, and complex training and practice are required to become proficient with the system. Although there are plans to change to a more modern computer interface, migration away from this legacy system is slow and expensive. Inpatient applications are projected to continue with this interface for up to a decade or more into the future.

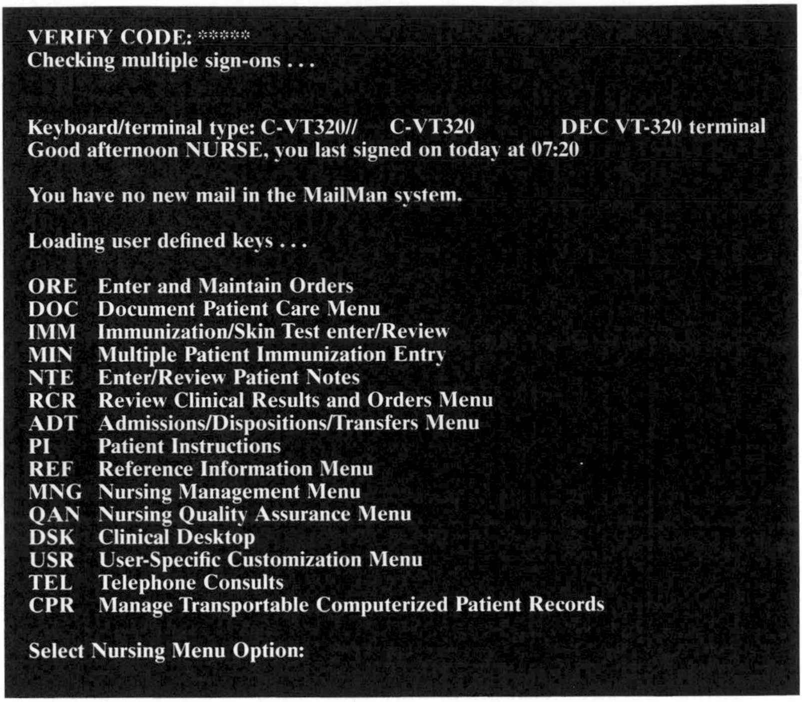

```
VERIFY CODE: *****
Checking multiple sign-ons . . .


Keyboard/terminal type: C-VT320//    C-VT320         DEC VT-320 terminal
Good afternoon NURSE, you last signed on today at 07:20

You have no new mail in the MailMan system.

Loading user defined keys . . .

ORE   Enter and Maintain Orders
DOC   Document Patient Care Menu
IMM   Immunization/Skin Test enter/Review
MIN   Multiple Patient Immunization Entry
NTE   Enter/Review Patient Notes
RCR   Review Clinical Results and Orders Menu
ADT   Admissions/Dispositions/Transfers Menu
PI    Patient Instructions
REF   Reference Information Menu
MNG   Nursing Management Menu
QAN   Nursing Quality Assurance Menu
DSK   Clinical Desktop
USR   User-Specific Customization Menu
TEL   Telephone Consults
CPR   Manage Transportable Computerized Patient Records

Select Nursing Menu Option:
```

FIGURE 7.1. Text-based computer screen.

Since its installation in 1988, this system has required an average of 40 hours of formal training for nurses. Even then, new users need a preceptor to help with system interactions during the first week or two. Another application installed in Defense, a clinical information system developed by CliniComp, International, requires only two to four hours of formal training for nurses to be proficient in using the application. The differences relate to the need to memorize commands and unusual language, nonintuitive interactions, and buried functions, all usability issues.

The general trend in computing has been to shift to graphical user interfaces (GUIs) (Head, 1997; Murphy, 1997). What would the impact be for nurse users if the system were redesigned into a GUI like the screen depicted in Fig. 7.2? More specifically, is there a positive impact on nurses' efficiency, effectiveness, and satisfaction with the introduction of a GUI? Or are users so adapted to the old system that the introduction of a GUI actually slows their productivity, creates more errors, and creates frustration? In fact, there is not yet an empirical study published about the impact of moving to GUIs for clinical applications, despite many institutions adopting these interfaces. In health care, we seldom assess these usability impacts before expensive changes from legacy systems are implemented, even if that assessment might prevent a strategic error.

On the personal computer (PC) side, informaticists have for years admonished our healthcare PC users to back up their files to avoid disaster. As Thimbleby (1990) noted many years ago, the blame was in the wrong direction. Usable systems ought to back up their own files. His admonition is still true today.

In another example, Windows 98 has a frequently seen and most uninterpretable error message: "Fatal exception OE has occurred at 0028:C678226B" followed by an entire blue screen filled with text. To whom or what is the error fatal? Can users prevent their system or themselves from dying? What is "OE?" What is "0028:C678226B?" For most users, the "blue screen of death" and its coded mystery message amounts to a large irritant. The usual action is to reboot the system with its potential loss of data and a long wait time. For this error message, the choice of language and lack of constructive guidance in correcting the error leave users frustrated and impatient to get on with their work.

A vivid usability example comes from a bewildering e-mail message sent to a new user of an existing hospital information system. The new user asked how to enter a patient problem list so that it displays on all pertinent screens/forms in the system. The response was:

The PROBLEM LIST is a Patient Text topic in Desktop. Place your cursor next to the patient you want to enter and press F9. This is a shortcut into Patient Text. Enter

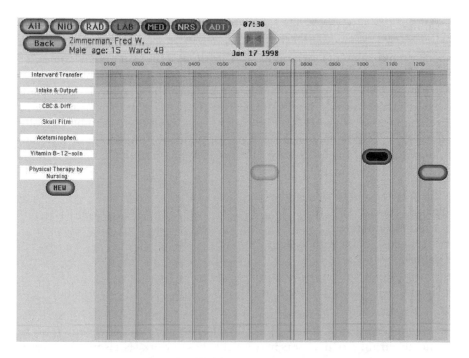

FIGURE 7.2. GUI-based computer screen.

the Patient Text topic as PROBLEM LIST (two words, all caps). Make the PROBLEM LIST "public." Enter the problem list as you like. The PROBLEM LIST automatically prints on the PBL and TXT options as with TEL. You could also set up a UDK.

The costs to individuals and organizations for poorly designed systems and usability issues range across these dimensions: decreases in productivity, extreme user frustration, underutilization or rejection of expensive systems, understated errors, extra personnel for help desks for cumbersome systems, open resistance to awkward applications, and millions of dollars for system redesign. Incorporating usability concepts can help defray these costs.

Many calls to action were issued to incorporate usability techniques into the design of healthcare systems (Lowrey & Martin, 1990; Staggers, 1991, 1995a,b; van Bemmel, 1988). In fact, some critics called the interaction between the provider and the computer interface an area in desperate need of attention. The first documented usability laboratory for health computing began operating at the Mayo Clinic in 1997, and one large clinical application vendor, Shared Medical Systems, recently began examining usability concepts in their Salt Lake City, Utah, office. Few others within health care, however, have integrated usability concepts into their design operations or their thinking about the purchase of systems.

What Is Usability?

Usability is a subset of the larger area of human–computer interaction (HCI), which concerns the interaction between people and computers in specific environments or contexts (Dix et al., 1998). Human–computer interaction blends psychology, applied work in computer science (Patel & Kushniruk, 1998), and information science into the design, development, or purchase of usable applications. The term *usability* is, at times, used interchangeably with HCI or human factors. However, usability usually addresses specific issues of human performance during computer interactions within a particular context (Rubin, 1994). Usability factors are multidimensional; they include

• Ease in learning
• Ease of use
• Ease to remember
• User satisfaction with system use
• Efficiency of use
• Error-free/error-forgiving interactions
• Seamless fit to the task(s) at hand.

All of these areas are necessary to consider when purchasing systems or creating clinical software. Usability begins with systems that require minimal learning so that users may quickly begin work (Nielsen, 1993). Ease of use implies easy navigation about the system, clear icons, and pertinent language for users. If systems are easy to remember, intermittent usage or returning after a lapse in use will not require relearning the entire system. Users should find interactions suitable, unobtrusive, and agreeable, facilitating desired tasks and leading to overall user satisfaction (Opaluch & Tsao, 1993). The system should be efficient for all levels of users, from naive to expert, by allowing high productivity and shortcuts for adapted users. Usability implies error-trapping to prevent catastrophic errors (Nielson, 1993) and the facility to undo actions where and when reasonable. The incorporation of usability concepts means the dyad of user and system is compatible in completing the task at hand. Most important, the task and user are central in computer interactions.

Typical usability assessments consist of three central goals: efficiency, effectiveness, and satisfaction. Efficiency concerns the speed with which users complete actions, effectiveness includes the quality of the interaction measured by the number and severity of errors, and user satisfaction is a subjective assessment of the application or system. These are not modest goals. If a system is designed well, the computer interface can effectively disappear, allowing users to focus only on the task at hand. This unobtrusiveness occurs not because the interface between humans and computer does not exist but because it blends seamlessly among user, task, system, and environment.

The Foundation of Usability: Users, Tasks, Systems, Contexts, and Their Interactions

Users

One of the most often repeated axioms of usability is to "know the user." But how do system designers or purchasers "know the users?" Knowing users involves understanding many characteristics of system users: ages, education levels, gender, computer experience, computer interaction experience (e.g., GUI, UNIX), work experience, general visual acuity, and language skills (Nielson, 1992; Rubin, 1994). More importantly, users' cognitive capabilities and limitations need to be understood (Patel & Kushrniruk, 1998). Other special considerations for clinicians, such as those listed below, are indispensable.

Shared Values

In the case of clinicians, knowing users also means understanding shared clinical values. Unlike informatics specialists, typical clinical system users are apt to view computers as tools, not captivating hobbies. Their first interest is patient care and expediting the care process. Although there are

pockets of computer enthusiasts in clinical settings, many outside informaticians do not have a penetrating interest in computers. Computers
merely facilitate work. More importantly, time is one of the most valued
assets for clinicians. Anything that wastes time is an anathema.

There are several implications from these observations. The problems
with systems that technicians view as interesting, clinicians will view as frustrating. Normal "bugs" in new software will not be seen as challenges (the
technician's view) but as impediments to work. Many clinical users have
little patience for system reliability problems, and they will quickly reject
slow systems. Therefore, sub-second screen changes are mandatory.

Interestingly, clinicians are reasonably tolerant of poor screen designs
and multiple screen changes as long as the system is blindingly quick. They
may, however, tolerate several-second delays if data such as complex
queries are being retrieved. Clinicians will use nearly any system if the perceived value of the product is more than the cost of using the system. That
is, clinicians may tolerate an inelegant results retrieval menu that takes
longer if the information they get in return is worth the extra time spent
navigating the system.

Most clinicians tend not to explore options in computers after the first
few days of learning a system. They search for "survival functions" based
upon what they need to complete their work. They quickly adapt to a familiar subset of options and expend little cognitive energy on system options
after that. Therefore, if good options are not readily apparent, many clinicians will miss opportunities to use them. Once users find options that they
value, they will employ them very quickly. In fact, many of our federal
system users know options so well that they do not look at screens as they
chart. They have long since memorized the key sequences. "Select 1, press
return 6 times," one user told this researcher about charting a function as
she stared at the keyboard, not the screen. When new releases change the
key sequence, users are dismayed.

Most clinical users want only essential, system survival training. Some of
the users will have competing time commitments and may not be able
to attend much training, especially new release training. Creative, clever
strategies are needed to accommodate everyday users like physicians and
intermittent users like per diem or agency nurses. Many users, including
clinical users, would rather not read user documentation. An informative
help desk, "superusers," or contextual online help may be better options.

Mental Models

An essential element of usability is the congruence between the way information is presented to users and the way clinicians cognitively process
information. These concepts concern users' mental models.

While interacting with almost any process, including those on systems,
users form internal representations or mental models of the processes at

hand (Allen, 1997). The idea of users' mental models is a widely accepted concept in the HCI literature, but other related terms need to be discussed. A target system is a particular system a user is learning or using. A design or conceptual model is invented by designers or educators as an accurate, consistent and complete representation of the target system. The system image is the impression the device portrays to users (Norman, 1983). The problem is that the conceptual model of the system may or may not be consistent with the system image. In fact, designers may not be cognizant of their models. Even if they are implicit, however, models are projected to users.

Mental models, on the other hand, are created by users as they interact with the target system and may or may not be equivalent to conceptual models. Mental models are "what people really have in their heads and guide their use of things" (Norman, 1983, p. 12). The basic dilemma between designers and users is summarized by Norman (1986, pp. 46–47):

> The problem is to design a system so that, first, it follows a consistent, coherent conceptualization—a design model and, second so that the user can develop a mental model of that system—a user model, consistent with the design model. . . . The user model is not formed from the design model: It results from the way the user interprets the system image. Thus, in many ways, the primary task of the designer is to construct an appropriate system image, realizing that everything the user interacts with helps to form that image. . . .

Mental models can range from fairly impoverished models to rich, visual images of systems and are important for system learning, performance, and design (Staggers & Norcio, 1993). Many authors propose that giving individuals a conceptual model of a system before instruction enhances user learning (Carroll & Mack, 1985). The model may then function as a knowledge organizer to promote understanding of the system. Mental models and user–system performance are intimately linked. Overall, even impoverished mental models assist users in system problem solving and allow more efficient and accurate user interactions. Therefore, designers must create a clear conceptual model and system image of a clinical workstation to allow users to create appropriate mental models.

User-Centered Design and Purchase

To ensure congruence between users' mental models, conceptual models, and target systems, an important usability concept concerns user-centered software design and purchase. As a software development method, user-centered design is used effectively outside our discipline but less within health care. Its decree is that users' needs are central to software design. Besides conceptually "knowing users," user-centered design is operationalized either by having end users as part of a project team through the entire developmental process or by having users as participants in an iterative software design process (Dix et al., 1998; Nielson, 1993; Opaluch & Tsao, 1993; Rubin, 1994).

User-centered design includes three principles (Rubin, 1994): (1) an early focus on users and tasks, (2) empirical measurement of a product usage, and (3) iterative design whereby a product is designed, modified, and tested repeatedly. User-centered design focuses on feedback from end users at every level of iterative product design. Users' comments about the product are then given utmost credence in redesign. Following on Rubin's principles, user-centered system purchase should include

- An early focus on user and task requirements
- Empirical measurement of candidate products or systems
- Iterative evaluations and discussions with end users as well as technicians before a purchase decision is reached.

Tasks

Many authors stress the importance of understanding tasks (Norman, 1990; Patel & Kushniruk, 1998; Rubin, 1994; Whitten & Bentley, 1998). According to Norman (1990), tasks should dominate, and the tool should become invisible. Both the user interface and the computer should be subservient to the task. Designers, then, must pay special attention to the tasks in order to understand how best the job can be done. Purchasers likewise need to clearly understand tasks central to clinical operations. Critical tasks can be outlined as requirements and used during testing of candidate systems. To determine the details of tasks, techniques in structured systems analysis (e.g., Whitten & Bentley, 1998) are useful. Focused interview questions might include

- What are the most frequently completed tasks to be done?
- What data/information do clinicians need?
- How is the task done now?
- How can the task be computerized for maximum efficacy?

Throughout the process, the fundamental question remains, "What does the user want to do?" (Laurel & Mountford, 1990).

Understanding tasks must include the concepts of cooperative group work. Work in clinical settings is frequently accomplished through a team approach. A team of nursing personnel may be organized for inpatient care. In medical centers, a separate team of physicians, from interns to attending staff, may care for patients. In other settings, an integrated team of providers may be organized around a clinical product line. Understanding tasks includes the analysis of the interactions within and between these team members. In addition to supporting integrated and separate views for the teams, information must be linked in unique methods to team members. For example, results retrieval information tasks must make laboratory results available to the entire team and notify the primary provider about abnormal results. If the primary provider is on vacation, the system must alert the covering provider about abnormal results.

Methods for Understanding Tasks

Clearly understanding clinical tasks is pivotal to purchasing and creating usable applications. A number of techniques are available to help with understanding tasks to include think-aloud protocols, cognitive walk-throughs, task analysis, ethnographic studies, semantic network representations (Patel & Kushniruk, 1998; Tang & Patel, 1994), focus groups, and more traditional techniques in structured systems analysis (Whitten & Bentley, 1998).

High-level task analysis was helpful in designing laboratory and radiology results retrieval for clinicians using a federal computer system. A team of software analysts, programmers, and clinicians analyzed the task by understanding the cognitive flow of information during manual processing of laboratory slips. Using the information processing model of Jonassen et al., (1989), a high-level task analysis was performed to understand how providers cognitively process paper laboratory slips. Analysts listened to clinicians describe getting a pile of inpatient/outpatient laboratory slips and sorting them into typical categories (more action required, discard, file). From that understanding, analysts created a computerized flow of information that was compatible with this model. All tests ordered by a particular provider were presented in a format allowing quick, visual identification of the set of results to be processed. Abnormal results were made visually distinct by highlighting. Quick access to the actual results was provided by circumventing the usual menu paths and allowing users to jump from the highlighted test name directly to the test results. An "action bar" allowed quick discarding or forwarding of listed results either individually or in groups. By understanding the task at hand, software was designed to complement that process.

Contexts

Considering user-centered design and tasks as embedded within clinical contexts is imperative. Clinicians, especially nurses, are information integrators. Information processing spans across sources—patients, medicine, nutrition, families, pharmacy, laboratory, radiology, social work, and occupational and physical therapy. However, this information processing is not independent of the context in which it occurs—from hospital ships to shock-trauma units to living rooms.

Many task and cognitive analysis methods do not emphasize the role of the environment or context (e.g., Dix et al., 1998; Patel & Kushniruk,

1998). However, the structured analysis techniques in Whitten and Bentley (1998) acknowledge context as "geography," and Lindgaard (1992) acknowledges the impact that systems have on the overall organization. According to Rubin (1994), the product's goals, tasks, and context are all from the user's viewpoint. As such, informaticists will analyze contextual information within user requirements and design precepts as well as perform usability within realistic contexts (or simulations of contexts) when possible.

Systems

Once the fundamental analyses of users, tasks, and contexts are completed, the knowledge gained can be used in iterative software design or solid evaluation of products for purchase. Iterative software design involves a series of system designs presented to users for evaluation. With each set of screens, designers assess user–system interactions and identify problems. These specific problems are the basis for software redesign and subsequent reassessment of user–system interaction. In this manner, designers effect steady refinements of the software. During iterative software design, systems are typically presented to users as prototypes rather than fully coded products. Severe design problems may then be corrected before the system is completely coded, a more economical technique than waiting until later in the software design cycle. Even small numbers of users, four or five, can uncover 80 percent of requirements or design flaws in an application (Patel & Kushniruk, 1998).

The principal precept of iterative software design includes user–task–system interaction evaluations. Both informal and formal methods are useful. Early in design, programmers may casually observe users as they interact with a particular design and ask their opinions about how the application functions.

More formal empirical testing includes traditional quantitative research methods and objective criteria such as online task metrics, capturing user keystrokes, or controlled user task performance measured in seconds with the numbers of errors committed per task. These data about efficiency, effectiveness, and satisfaction are useful in many instances for baseline usability data and determining optimal screen design methods (Staggers, 1993).

Designers must also ask focused questions about design preferences and explore the reasons underlying quicker interactions. Determining *why* one design or another is optimal is the key to effective design. The point is to determine where and why users trip in navigating systems, where language is inconsistent, where interactions are inconsistent, where functions are not intuitive, and where catastrophic errors occur. To capture these data, other research techniques may be useful for subjective but rich data: think-aloud protocols, videotaping interactions, and interviewing subjects. The prime notion in using any technique is that systematic methods are used to capture interaction information. The information is then fed directly into redesign, in this case clinical workstation design.

User Metaphor

User metaphor follows closely upon the concept of mental models. The purpose of a user metaphor is to provide users with a useful and easily recognizable model around which system functions are organized. This model is then portrayed as part of the system image. A good user metaphor will allow users to build a more complete mental model of the system in an efficient manner.

Typically, designers look for real-world objects or events that will allow users to relate to the system. For instance, current Windows user interface presentations use an office or desktop metaphor around which all user interactions proceed. The system has symbols and icons for file cabinets, folders, documents, and files. Users interact with familiar objects in a familiar order. More critically, users are able to predict the sequence of interactions by translating real-world experiences with the model into interactions with the system. This is the reason the office metaphor has been very successful for business applications. The same metaphor is useful for business transactions in patient care. However, the metaphor does not extend well into patient-centered clinical activities because the idea of an office, files, and documents does not depict realistic expectations of what happens with patient care processes.

Good metaphors are essential for ease of use in systems (Erickson, 1990). For patient care activities, finding a suitable metaphor is somewhat of a challenge. As Esterhay (1994) suggests, new metaphors are needed, and one metaphor may not be enough to encompass all clinical activities. Clinical workstations may have to use several metaphors to afford a comprehensive model of all activities.

Only a small amount of work has been done in this arena. Esterhay (1994) provides an excellent discussion of potential user metaphors for an oncologist's workstation. He suggests using flowsheets as a way of examining categories of patient data. For other activities, the use of rooms may be helpful in modeling users' work. Each room would contain tasks and interactive objects. Doors provide access to other rooms of activities.

Several current systems use a paper chart metaphor. There are tabs at the bottom or side of the chart much like dividers in the paper chart. Users interact with the system by clicking on the tabs and jumping to applications. This metaphor requires little training and is immediately familiar, but it ignores process redesign and leaves little room for growth into the future. Perhaps its best use is as a transitional model until better metaphors can be extrapolated and tested.

User–System Interactions

Usability Testing

An overview of usability testing was introduced earlier. For a detailed account of usability testing and how to plan, design, and construct effective usability tests, the reader is referred to Rubin (1994). His text is a practical guide for incorporating usability testing into the design of systems.

Usability laboratories provide a place to systematically study users as they interact with workstation hardware and software. Usability laboratories and usability testing have been used effectively by Xerox, Apple Computers, Bellcore (Bell Communications), Kodak, and Microsoft to ensure application usability. The use of these laboratories within health care is minimal, but these laboratories would be invaluable in creating usable clinical applications as well as other healthcare products.

Typically, usability laboratories provide a controlled setting for monitoring users' interactions with systems. The setting can be as informal as a personal computer in a quiet room with a trained observer and a user or as formal as a room with a one-way mirror, videotaping equipment, eye-movement tracking equipment, and a staff of trained analysts and researchers. A spectrum of research methods could be used. A laboratory might concentrate on a particular interest area, such as determining users' mental models for the clinical workstation or designing and testing applications for subspecialty system users. Other laboratories might focus on testing hardware for clinical personnel, for instance, whether portable technology, trackballs, or mice are preferable given scarce counter space in many settings.

Usability Testing for Clinical System Purchase

Usability goals are just as vital for application purchase as software design. Rubin (1994) suggests that usability goals be determined early in the system's life cycle. Thus, usability criteria should be a crucial part of purchase requirements. For example, an informaticist may determine that three common tasks for a new application are assessment, history, and vital signs. One portion of a product's usability assessment would include having end users interact with these three functions. Three outcomes would be determined: the amount of time it takes to complete the functions across products, the number of errors users make learning the functions, and a rating about their satisfaction using the application. Then, these objective data may be used to compare candidate applications and make the final purchase decision. Other usability assessments might include the ease with which users navigate from the progress notes to laboratory results retrieval functions or users' opinions about the adequacy of the user metaphor the vendor employs in an application.

For an anesthesia application purchase by the Department of Defense, nurse anesthetists and anesthesiologists used common tasks to evaluate two competing applications. They used a computerized mannequin to mimic clinical situations in anesthesia nursing and sent data to the interfaced application. Ease of use then included speed and accuracy of completion of realistic tasks as well as an assessment of the quickness and accuracy of the clinical data across the interface. The main point of usability testing is then to consider critical usability features of products early and systematically in the decision process when purchasing clinical systems.

Summary

Usability concepts must be imported from human-computer interaction literature and translated into healthcare operations. User-centered design, empirical measurement of user–system–context interactions, and iterative software design should be commonplace. Consideration of all four aspects of usability (users, tasks, systems, and context) as well as their interactions is imperative to achieve the goal of having usable applications in clinical computing.

Questions

1. Cite your own examples of usability problems in health care.
2. Compare and contrast the terms *usability* and *human–computer interaction*.
3. Determine how the three principles of usability (user-centered design, iterative prototyping, and empirical usability testing) have been used or not used in your agency. What are the consequences of having chosen to use or not use these principles?
4. Create a 15 minute presentation to convince your chief information officer that usability concepts need to be a part of your organization.

References

Allen RB. Mental models and user models. In: Helander M, Landauer T, Prablu P, eds. *Handbook of Human–Computer Interaction*, 2nd ed. Amsterdam: Elsevier, 1997;441–462.

Carroll JM, Mack RL. Metaphor, computing systems, and active learning. *International Journal of Man–Machine Studies* 1985;22(1):39–57.

Davis FD. User acceptance of information technology: system characteristics, user perceptions and behavioral impacts. *International Journal of Man–Machine Studies* 1993;38:475–487.

Dix A, Finlay J, Abowd G, Beale R. *Human–Computer Interaction*. London: Prentice Hall Europe, 1998;427–435.

Erickson TD. Creativity and design: introduction. In: Laurel B, ed. *The Art of Human–Computer Interface Design*. Reading, MA: Addison-Wesley Publishing Company, Inc., 1990;1–4.

Esterhay RJ. User metaphors of health care professional workstations. *International Journal of Bio-Medical Computing* 1994;34:95–113.

Head AJ. Question of interface design: How do online service GUIs measure up? *Online* 1997(May–June);20–29.

Jonassen DH, Hannum WH, Tessmer M. *Handbook of Task Analysis*. New York: Praeger, 1989.

Laurel B, Mountford SJ. Introduction. In: Laurel B, ed. *The Art of Human–Computer Interface Design*. Reading, MA: Addison-Wesley Publishing Company, Inc., 1990;xi–xvi.

Lindgaard G. Evaluating user interfaces in context: The ecological value of time-and-motion studies. *Applied Ergonomics* 1992;23(2):105–114.

Lowrey JC, Martin JB. Evaluation of healthcare software from a usability perspective. *Journal of Medical Systems* 1990;14(1):17–29.

Murphy T. Innovative interfaces: New GUIs help zero in on information. *Information Highways* 1997;4(4):20–23.

Nielson J. The usability engineering life cycle. *Computer* 1992;25(3):12–22.

Nielson J. Iterative user–interface design. *Computer* 1993;26(11):32–41.

Norman DA. Some observations on mental models. In: Gentner D, Stevens AL, eds. *Mental Models*. Hillsdale, NJ: Erlbaum, 1983;15–34.

Norman DA. Cognitive engineering. In: Norman DA, Draper SW, eds. *User Centered Systems Design*. Hillsdale, NJ: Erlbaum, 1986;31–61.

Norman DA. Why interfaces don't work. In: Laurel B, ed. *The Art of Human–Computer Interface Design*. Reading, MA: Addison-Wesley, 1990;209–219.

Opaluch RE, Tsao YC. Ten ways to improve usability engineering—designing user interfaces for ease of use. *AT&T Technical Journal* 1993;72(3):75–88.

Patel VL, Kushniruk AW. Interface design for health care environments: The role of cognitive science. In: Chute CG, ed. *AMIA '98: A Conference of the American Medical Informatics Association*. Philadephia: Hanley & Belfus, Inc., 1998;29–37.

Rubin J. *Handbook of Usability Testing: How to Plan, Design, and Conduct Effective Tests*. New York: John Wiley & Sons, Inc., 1994.

Staggers N. Human factors: the missing element in computer technology. *Computers in Nursing* 1991;9(2):47–49.

Staggers N. Impact of screen density on clinical nurses' computer task performance and subjective screen satisfaction. *International Journal of Man–Machine Studies* 1993;39:775–792.

Staggers N. Usability concepts for the clinical workstation. In: Ball M, Hannah K, Newbold S, Douglas J, eds. *Nursing Informatics: Where Caring and Technology Meet*, 2nd ed. New York: Springer-Verlag, 1995a;188–199.

Staggers N. Essential principles for evaluating the usability of clinical information systems. *Computers in Nursing* 1995b;13(5):207, 211–213.

Staggers N, Norcio A. Mental models: concepts for human–computer interaction research. *International Journal of Man–Machine Studies* 1993;38:587–605.

Tang PC, Patel VL. Major issues in user interface design for health professional workstations: summary and recommendations. *International Journal of Bio-Medical Computing* 1994;34(1):139–148.

Thimbleby H. *User Interface Design*. New York: ACM Press, 1990.

van Bemmel JH. Medical data, information, and knowledge. *Methods of Information in Medicine* 1988;27:109–110.

Whitten JL, Bentley LD. *Systems Analysis and Design*, 4th ed. Boston, MA: Irwin McGraw-Hill, 1998.

8
Solving the Vocabulary Problem

KATHLEEN A. McCORMICK

Without a language, nursing is invisible in healthcare systems and its value and importance go unrecognized and unrewarded. (International Council of Nursing, 1993)

There is no time like the present for the nursing profession to solve its vocabulary problem. The technology exists, the linking and mapping systems are available (Unified Medical Language System), and nursing is developing the International Classification of Nursing Project (ICNP). There is growing awareness and use of speech/voice technology in the healthcare environment. The reliability of content is becoming excellent, both in English and in up to 36 different languages. Natural language text processors, data mining algorithms for pattern analysis, and robust retrieval systems are tools being used commercially in robust applications requiring up to one billion documents to be read per day. The paperless environment is quickly approaching. The open system architecture that the Internet provides is offering additional solutions to the integration of vocabularies.

Vocabulary Needs in Health Care

Clinicians' reluctance to use a structured vocabulary may come from the training and skills that are developed through educational programs and reinforced in clinical practice. For example, nurses may use the terms *hypertension, high blood pressure, hypertensive*, and *elevated blood pressure* to mean the same thing. A nurse examining a child might look into the otiscope and describe the phenomenon as *glue ear, bulging eardrums, inflammation, reddening, infection, ear pain, earache*, or a number of other descriptions. Clinicians have not been trained to use structured vocabulary or to "talk like a computer" in the twentieth century. It is unlikely that any health professional in the new millennium, with the volume of information and the explosion in new diagnostic and treatment algorithms, will have time to learn all structured vocabularies in existence.

At the same time, networks like large academic practices, managed care plans, nurse practitioner organizations, and ambulatory/community care nursing networks often need a structured or fixed vocabulary to quantify the plan's major health issues and to describe group practice quality, outcomes, and major cost centers. For example, a network might have to define the variables from nursing care in ways summarized in Table 8.1.

The Health Care Financing Administration (HCFA) is the funding agency for health care of persons older than 65 (through Medicare) and the poor (through Medicaid). In this role, HCFA reimburses networks and individual practitioners based on a set of terms for reimbursement with codes from the International Classification of Diseases, Clinical Medicine, Version 9 (ICD-9CM codes). Soon HCFA will release the ICD-10CM, which has many significant improvements. The Current Procedural Terminology (CPT) coding scheme is also used by HCFA to reimburse procedures in health care. Together, these two classifications are used internationally to compare U.S. morbidity and mortality in health care and its management with that of other countries internationally.

McCormick and Jones (1998) described three healthcare needs in a framework: The clinician at the point of care needs an interface vocabulary to describe an individual patient or the practice, the network needs a fixed or structured vocabulary to manage group data or system policies, and the reimbursement or policy analysts need a universal vocabulary to manage populations and develop societal policies. The network vocabulary may also be called a *reference vocabulary*.

In their paper, McCormick and Jones (1998) also suggest that the multiple settings in which nurses work will also require unique point-of-care vocabularies to define the clinical practice for unique groups of patients. For example, nursing needs different vocabularies to describe patients,

---

TABLE 8.1. Network needs for structured or fixed vocabulary.

- Describe the number of infections
- Determine how many patients have pain
- Control the amount of antibiotics/medications being administered
- Justify costs in groups of patients
- Specify what procedures were used
- Specify what outcomes were achieved in individuals and groups
- Define if the symptom/condition is a recurrence
- Define if the symptom/condition is a complication of another condition or treatment
- Describe if procedure/symptom/or condition is occurring in a lateral body position (e.g., left eye, right eye)
- Describe if the condition/symptom is a comorbidity
- Define if the condition is a reportable condition
- Describe aggregate data on conditions and symptoms nurses are delivering in health care

consumers, or clients in school health, prison care, ambulatory care nursing, occupational health care, sub-acute care, inpatient acute care, primary care, and nursing homes. Likewise, there are many different kinds of networks that may require different fixed or structured vocabularies. Some of the networks may be integrated managed care organizations, large community networks, nursing homes, academic medical centers, and oncology special care facilities.

National Efforts Toward Vocabulary Solutions

Several national efforts in vocabulary have been focused on developing a linking vocabulary. In 1998, McCormick and Jones described the Unified Medical Language System (UMLS) of the National Library of Medicine (NLM) as a Rosetta Stone. This metaphor for classification and vocabulary solutions comes from the Egyptian stone that solved the riddle of three distinct and untranslatable languages in ancient Egypt: Hieroglyphs, Demotic, and Greek. The UMLS includes a metathesaurus to link and map vocabularies from different sources through a system of four knowledge sources. The UMLS includes about one-half million biomedical and nursing concepts and over one million different names. Information about the UMLS can be accessed at http://www.nlm.nih.gov/pubs/factsheets/umls.html. A license is required to use UMLS, but the application is obtained through the Internet.

The Unified Medical Language System

The UMLS is a long-term research and development effort that has been conducted through and coordinated by the NLM. It is designed to facilitate the retrieval and integration of vocabularies and information from multiple machine-readable biomedical sources(http://www.nlm.nih.gov/pubs/factsheets/umls.html). Information is retrieved from numerous sources for inclusion in the UMLS, including bibliographic material, clinical records, databanks, data repositories, knowledge-based systems, and directories. The UMLS electronically links vocabularies and classification systems developed by various groups of health professionals through a system of four knowledge sources: Metathesaurus, Semantic Network, Specialist Lexicon, and Information Sources Map. Lindberg et al., (1993) provide an in-depth discussion of these four knowledge sources and how they are used to aggregate and classify existing discipline-specific vocabulary systems.

All vocabularies and classifications for nursing that have been recognized by the American Nurses Association are incorporated into the UMLS. These include the North American Nursing Diagnosis Association, the Omaha System, Nursing Intervention Classification (NIC), Nursing Outcome Classification (NOC), the Georgetown Home Health Classification, and others. These nursing vocabularies and classifications included in UMLS offer the capability of extracting, synthesizing, and aggregating nursing phenomena to the universal level, the result of which would be the Unified Nursing Language System (UNLS) (McCormick et al., 1994). This UNLS has never been tested against large-scale nursing data repositories to determine if the new system represents such nursing vocabularies as are used in acute care, primary care, long-term care, outpatient, community, school health nursing, occupational health, and the many realms within which nursing care is delivered.

It is unknown how complete the UNLS within the UMLS is in relation to nursing phenomena.

Other National and International Efforts in Vocabulary

Other national and international efforts include the development of a national reference vocabulary as an outgrowth of the Systematized Nomenclature of Medicine (SNOMED) vocabulary. This vocabulary, started as a medical corollary of the Systematized Nomenclature of Pathology (SNOP) through the College of American Pathology (CAP), has matured to include most health conditions for humans and a veterinary vocabulary to classify animal conditions. Another type of reference vocabulary has been developed in the United Kingdom. This system, called *Clinical Terms v3*, was formerly called the *Read Codes* and is administered by the U.K. National Health Service. The Clinical Terms v3 are incorporated into the UMLS and are now being added to SNOMED. It is unknown if the addition of the nursing terms in SNOMED complement or contradict the U.S. vocabularies that have been accepted into the UMLS. Yet another reference type of vocabulary has been developed in Germany. It is called *Galen*, and it describes terms in detail.

In 1998, Dr. Chris Chute proposed a framework that was adopted by ANSI-HISB (Chute et al., 1998). This paper included a framework for comprehensive health terminology systems in the United States. The framework recommended four areas of consideration: (1) general basic characteristics, (2) structure of the terminology model, (3) maintenance, and (4) evaluation.

Other activities in medicine related to vocabulary structure and standards are beyond the scope of this chapter. However, these activities have included the Desiderata by Cimino (1998), the ToMeLo Architecture and Terminology by Rossi Mori (1998), and the concept of compositionality by Elkin et al. (1998).

International Nursing Efforts in Vocabulary

In an excellent review of the state of the European countries in nursing vocabulary, June Clark described the International Classification of Nursing Practice (Clark, 1998). She explains the logic behind the European countries' developing vocabularies that are culturally sensitive and linked to the model of healthcare delivery in respective countries. She notes that "by 1995, every major country in Europe was developing its own terminology and classifications" (Clark, 1998).

The ICNP Project, begun in 1990, was to develop a standard vocabulary and classification of nursing phenomena (diagnosis), interventions (actions), and outcomes. This came in response to a realization of nurses from member countries of the International Council of Nurses that "20 percent of what nurses do is recorded somewhere in a general health information system. However, that 20 percent is mostly of a technical nature (e.g. immunization, weighing, and dressings), and excludes much of the work that is often nursing's special responsibility e.g. teaching, counseling, community mobilization, family guidance training education, and supervision of other health workers."

All the member countries of the International Council of Nurses have been invited to Alpha test (1991) and now Beta test (1999) a cluster of phenomena (diagnoses), actions (interventions), and outcomes. The Beta version has become a multiaxial approach to the classification of phenomena. Table 8.2 includes the axes under development of ICNP Phenomena (Diagnoses).

In the Beta version, a classification of nursing phenomena has been put forward, as shown in Fig. 8.1. The Classification of Nursing Actions (interventions) in the Beta version are ordered by multiaxial axes of action types, objects, target or recipient, methods, and instrument. Table 8.3 includes examples of actions for those axes. The outcome is measured as a change or absence of a change in the nursing diagnosis. For example, if the nursing phenomenon were disturbed sleep, the outcome would be improved sleep.

TABLE 8.2. Multiaxial classification of phenomena (diagnoses) within the International Classification for Nursing Practice (ICNP), Beta version.

Focus of nursing practice	e.g., Sleep
Judgment	e.g., Disturbed
Degree	e.g., Extremely
Frequency	e.g., Daily
Chronicity	e.g., Chronic
Topography/laterality	Not appropriate
Body site	Not appropriate
Likelihood	Risk for

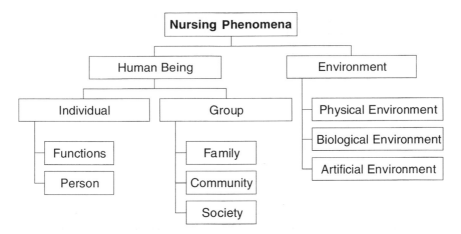

Figure 8.1. Classification of nursing phenomena in the International Classification of Nursing Practice (ICNP) Beta test version.

If the phenomenon were high risk of body nutrition deficit, the outcome would be improved nutrition.

The W.K. Kellogg Foundation has funded a three-year project to incorporate ICNP classification into computerized community-based practice and primary healthcare documentation systems. This study is ongoing and was scheduled to be reported at the June 1999 Centennial meeting of the International Council of Nurses (ICN). To keep up with the ICNP, there is a website: http://www.icn.ch/icnupdate.htm. It is the goal of ICN to have a dynamic vocabulary for nursing, one that will ultimately join the other classifications in the World Health Organization's ICD coding, probably among the "Other Health Related Classifications" category.

From Nursing Vocabulary into Computerized Documentation of Practice

Although medicine has taken the lead in defining the standards for vocabulary, nursing has defined the characteristics of nomenclature for an informatics environment. In 1998, Zielstorff described the characteristics of

Table 8.3. Examples of uses of action terms in the emerging Beta version of the International Classification for Nursing Practice (ICNP).

Action types	e.g., Alleviating	or Reducing	or Teaching
Objects	e.g., Pain	or Anxiety	or Nutrition
Target of Recipient	e.g., Individual	or Individual	or Family
Methods	e.g., Cold Pack	or Guided Imagery	or Instructional materials

TABLE 8.4. Characteristics of nursing nomenclature to be used in a computer environment.

Domain completeness
Granularity
Parsimony
Synonymy
Nonambiguity
Nonredundancy
Clinical utility
Multiple axes
Combinatorial

a nomenclature to be structured enough to capture data, sort, analyze, and report findings in a computer environment. These characteristics are incorporated into the concepts listed in Table 8.4. Each of these concepts and examples is described in a recent paper, available on-line at http://www.nursingworld.org/ojin/tpc7/tpc7_4.htm.

Solutions for the New Millennium

To receive speech from a clinician, the computer needs expert natural language processors to translate the natural language into a computer format. If the nurse is talking into a wireless microphone about reddening, inflammation, and bulging of a membrane, the computer needs to know that the ear is being assessed. Soon after the beginning of the new millennium, speech products will be in common use with home computers. When clinicians have these tools at home and in the office, they will ask those in nursing informatics where their applications are in their practice environments.

The clinician may also need feedback from the computer requesting that the practitioner describe more data elements; for example, in the above description, the practitioner may need to specify which ear, left or right, was assessed. If the computer is expecting input consistent with a guideline or protocol, the computer may suggest that the nurse describe whether this occurrence is a complication of another syndrome or a recurrence from a previous encounter. If it is a recurrence, the computer might prompt the clinician to document whether he or she has ordered a hearing test to determine if there is a five-decibel hearing loss since the last encounter.

With speech recognition and text processors or natural language processors, the nurse will be free of endless menus and lists of terms to select from, and coders will be free from endless drudgery. This should reduce the time of documentation because the vocabulary maps can be applied again and again to new data sets as they arise.

Friedman et al. (1999) have demonstrated that natural language processing can be used to create enriched documents from the patient reports, and that Extensible Markup Language (XML) tagging provides additional benefit by developing a document model that encodes structured clinical information while retaining the original contents using XML. The validity was 199 out of 200 patient records.

Extensible Markup Language is being used as an integrator of terms at the point of data convergence from multiple sources. Walsh (1998) describes what XML is on the Internet. It is markup language for documents that contain structured information. It is an extremely simple dialect of the Standard Generalized Markup Language (SGML) and Hyper Text Markup Language (HTML), both of which are languages of the Internet. Extensible Markup Language is intended for large-scale Web applications, for structured information that includes both content and some indication of what role the content plays. It is vendor neutral, and terms can be easily exchanged. The documents have more arbitrary structure. The specifications for making documents in the XML language are also available on the Internet.

Tags are still used in XML just like they are in SGML. The names of the tags and the rules for forming them are contained in the Document Type Definitions (DTD). To date, DTDs need to be described for each data element of nursing vocabulary. The DTDs describe the structure of the document and the name of the tags it contains. XML can be delivered without a DTD, but the structure must still have at least one tag pair, and all elements must be nested. United States organizations are currently trying to take patient-based record information and vocabulary structure and convert it into Health Level 7 (HL7) standards messages.

The backbone of the Web is the Document Object Model (DOM) (Dougherty, 1997). Because documents are becoming applications, developers have to set up documents as a user interface to information and to manage sets of interactions. Object-oriented technology is also advancing the way that vocabularies and classifications are converging from different sources. At the Internet level, XML and HTML are being fit into a DOM. The DOM is a platform- and language-neutral interface that allows programs and scripts to dynamically access and update content, structure, and style of all documents. The DOM provides a set of objects for representing HTML and XML documents, a standard model of how these objects can be combined, and a standard interface for accessing and manipulating them. Vendors can support the DOM as an interface with their proprietary data structures, thus increasing interoperability on the Web.

The Healthcare Domain Task Force (CORBAmed) is a committee working on the concept of object modeling and management within health. It advises the Domain Technical Committee (DTC) of the Object Management Group (OMG). The primary work of the CORBAmed group is to reach industry consensus on Interactive Data Language (IDL) interface specifications for health care. The task force recommends the adoption of these specifications to the DTC and the OMG member body as a whole.

One CORBAmed task force related to vocabulary, the Lexicon Query Service, has completed its work (Object Management Group, 1998). It described the set of interfaces that could be used to query and retrieve the contents of health terminology, vocabulary, and coding classifications. The interface specifications are partitioned in such a way that everything from a simple code value can pair with a total ontology.

Collectively, XML, Knowledge Discovery in Large Databases, (KDD), and the Object Models render content on the Web into a metadata syntax that fits within the framework of the World Wide Web. The XML has provided a mechanism for defining and documenting object classes. XML can be used for describing terms that are strictly syntactic, or for indicating concepts and relations among concepts with relational databases. Therefore, all vocabularies and classifications used at the point of care can be converged within networks, and converged yet again at the universal level. The universal level of taxonomy can be a convergence of many into a unicode or single taxonomy, or it can remain several taxonomies that are linked but not assembled at the universal level.

Summary

Times are changing for the needs of the nursing profession and its vocabulary, yet there remains little funding from industry or professional organizations for nursing to accomplish its work. The funding from the nursing government entities has not been sufficient to match the needs of vocabulary nationally and internationally. The message of this update is that one should be able to use vocabulary terms locally to map to networks of practice and to international classifications. New tools at our disposal that were not available in the past are the Internet, multilingual speech recognition tools, knowledge discovery solutions, text natural language processors with robust capabilities, and robust retrieval systems. When nursing's needs are joined with the tools, and when the market has sufficient reasons to fund these tasks, nursing will have all it needs to enhance clinical practice in any environment.

Questions

1. What new technologies are posing possible solutions to the vocabulary problems of the twentieth century?
2. Is one vocabulary needed to solve the vocabulary problems in health care?
3. What are an interface or point-of-care, a network, and a universal vocabulary?
4. What are five network needs of vocabulary?

5. What is the classification system that is used for reimbursement and classifying conditions internationally?
6. Why is the UMLS like a Rosetta Stone?
7. What is the theoretical framework of the ICNP for diagnoses and interventions?
8. How can XML and object-oriented technology advance the way vocabularies can be converged?
9. What are some consequences to the profession if nursing does not solve the vocabulary problem?
10. How will speech recognition change the current state of vocabulary needs in health care?

References

Chute CG, Cohn SP, Campbell JR. A framework for comprehensive health terminology systems in the United States: development guidelines, criteria for selection and public policy. *Journal of the American Medical Informatics Association* 1998;5(6):503–510.

Cimino JJ. Desiderata for controlled medical vocabularies in the twenty-first century (1998). *Methods of Information in Medicine* 1998;37(4–5):394–403.

Clark J. The International Classification for Nursing Practice Project. http://www.nursingworld.org/ojin/tpc7/tpc7_3.htm (October, 1999).

Dougherty D. The Document Object Model Explained. It's Not what Documents Say; It's What They Do. http://webreview.com/wr/pub/97/11/14/feature/concepts.html (October, 1999).

Elkin PL, Bailey KR, Chute CG. A randomized controlled trial of automated term composition. In: Chute CG, ed. *Proceedings of the AMIA '98 Annual Symposium*. New York: McGraw-Hill, 1998;765–769.

Elkin PL, Tuttle M, Keck K, Campbell K, Atkin G, Chute CG. The role of compositionality in standardized problem list generation. In: Cesnik B, McCray AT, Scherrer J-R, eds. *MedInfo '98, Proceedings of the Ninth World Congress on Medical Informatics*. Amsterdam: IOS Press, 1998.

Friedman C, Hripcsak G, Shagina L, Lie H. Representing information in patient records using natural language processing and extensible markup language. *Journal of the American Medical Informatics Association* 1999;6:76–87.

International Classification for Nursing Practice (INCP) Project. http://icn.ch/icnp.htm (October, 1999).

International Classification for Nursing Practice Emerging Beta Version. http://icn.ch/icnpupdate.htm (October, 1999).

International Council of Nurses. *Nursing's Next Advance: an International Classification of Nursing Practice (ICNP): A Working Paper*. Geneva, Switzerland: ICN, 1993.

Lindberg DA, Humphreys BL, McCray AT. The unified medical language system. *Methods of Information in Medicine* 1993;32:281–291.

McCormick KA, Jones CB. (1998) Is one taxonomy needed for health care vocabularies and classifications? *Online Journal of Nursing Research*. http://www.nursingworld.org/ojin/tpc7/tpc7_2.htm, September 30, 1998.

McCormick KA, Lang N, Zielstorff R, Millholland DK, Saba V, Jacox A. Toward standard classification schemes for nursing language. *Journal of the American Medical Informaties Association* 1994;Nov.–Dec.;1(6):421–427.

Object Management Group (OMG).
ftp://ftp.omg.org/pub/docs/corbamed/98-03-22.doc, 1998.

Rossi Mori A, Consorti F. Exploiting the terminological approach from CEN/TC251 and GALEN to support semantic interoperability of healthcare record systems. *International Journal of Medical Informatics* 1998;48(1–3):111–124.

Rossi Mori A, Consorti F, Galeazzi E. Standards to support development of terminological systems for healthcare telematics. *Methods of Information in Medicine* 1998;37(4–5)551–563.

Walsh N. What is XML? http://xml.com/xml/pub/98/10/guide1.html (October, 1999).

9
Determining Essential Nursing Information: Nursing Terms, Concept Representation, and Data Elements

KATHRYN J. HANNAH

This chapter explores international efforts to develop minimum health data sets, identify essential nursing data elements, and converge on standards for controlled clinical vocabulary in nursing. All of these efforts are essential underpinnings for the effective use of nursing information. Factors related to the role of the nurse in information management and obstacles to effective nursing management of information have been detailed elsewhere in this book. The issues for all nurses relate to information and information management, the salient concerns being the acceptance of core nursing data elements and the establishment of nursing data standards (controlled clinical vocabularies) for use within those data elements.

Nurses must be able to manage and process nursing data, information, and knowledge to support patient care delivery in diverse care delivery settings (Graves & Corcoran, 1989). Ozbolt (1999) maintains that

Standard terms and codes are needed to record as structured data the problems and issues that nurses and other caregivers address; the actions they take to prevent, ameliorate, or resolve the problems; and the results of their care. Such data could be used to increase the effectiveness of care and control costs in the following ways:

- Care plans or pathways for upcoming shifts, constructed of coded "building blocks" of known complexity and time requirements, could be used to project clinical workload requirements, so that managers could make appropriate staffing decisions. This would replace expensive patient classification or acuity systems that require a separate, redundant data collection and that are imperfectly related to the care the patient actually receives.
- Relevant decision support and supplementary information could be linked to statements of patient problems, care actions, and goals to provide assistance integrated into the workflow at the moment of need. For example, nurses could point and click for detailed instructions on how to carry out an unfamiliar procedure. Or the diagnosis of one problem, such as impaired mobility, could be linked to related problems, such as risk of falls, to assure that all relevant problems were included in the plan of care.
- Patient care data could be stored in relational or object-oriented databases for subsequent aggregation and analysis. It would become relatively easy (and much cheaper than by manual record audits) to discover patterns of variances from

expected care or outcomes and to identify places where corrective action was needed. It would also be possible to discover real best practices: not merely the cheapest, but those that produce the best balance of goal achievement and cost.

- The government and other regulators and purchasers of health care would have more sensitive measures of quality and effectiveness to consider in addition to cost when making purchasing decisions, establishing regulations, and mandating or refusing to authorize certain services.

To accomplish the goal of achieving standard nursing terms and concepts, nurses must attend to the data contained in local, regional, national, and international information systems. For some time, the technological aspect of information management has distracted nurses at the expense of ignoring the data. In fact, the initial systems for gathering minimum uniform health data can be traced back to systems devised by Florence Nightingale over a century ago (Verney, 1970). Despite Nightingale's early attempts to develop a nursing database, nurses in most countries have yet to define the minimum set of data elements essential to describing the practice of nursing, let alone achieve consensus on the standardization of terms and concepts within those essential data elements.

At the time of this writing, nursing data elements are not being regularly, comprehensively, or systematically collected and stored in any jurisdiction, either regionally or nationally, for use in research or decision-making related to either health policy or resource allocation. Ozbolt (1999) deplores

... the complete absence of standard terms and codes for documenting the care of nurses and other non-physician caregivers. The provision of care by nurses and other non-physician health professionals is the *raison d'etre* of hospitals, nursing homes, and home care services. The economic and clinical importance of this care would suggest that standard terminology to represent clinical events would have been established long ago.

The patient discharge abstracts prepared by medical records departments across Canada and the United States currently contain no nursing care delivery information. The abstracts, therefore, fail to acknowledge the contribution of nursing during the patient's stay in the hospital. This omission is important because the abstracts are used by many agencies for a variety of purposes, including

- Validation and authorization of payment for services
- Outcome measurement in terms of the quality, effectiveness, and cost-effectiveness of services
- Resource allocation
- Research
- Policy making.

We are losing much of the information needed to determine the costs of hospitalization and the effectiveness of nursing care in achieving appropriate patient outcomes. Given the current status, anyone looking back 500 years from now at today's national health databases would never know that nursing even took place in North America during the twentieth century!

Fortunately, these data gaps have been recognized, and nurses have developed a heightened awareness of the importance of collecting, storing, and retrieving nursing data. Attention is now being directed at developing the processes and means by which the nursing profession will begin to address the essential data needs of nurses in all practice settings. This activity is coinciding with an increasing international thrust for healthcare reform and restructuring, which has generated an increased awareness of the need to develop national health databases as a foundation for rational decision-making about national health policy and resource allocation. A minimum number of essential nursing elements must be included in such databases.

The nursing profession must provide leadership in defining appropriate nursing data elements to be included in national health databases—specifically, through patient discharge abstracts or summaries. There is an emerging international consensus that the unique nursing data elements to be included in health data sets are

- Nursing diagnosis (also known in some countries as *client status* or *nursing problem*)
- Nursing intervention
- Patient/client outcome
- Nursing intensity.

In Canada, these nursing data elements are beginning to be called the *Nursing Components of Health Information* (HI:NC). In the United States, the unique nursing elements are included in the current Nursing Minimum Data Set. The purposes of the Nursing Minimum Data Set are "to establish comparability of nursing data across clinical populations, settings, geographic areas, and time; to describe the nursing care of patients and their families in both inpatient and outpatient settings; to show or project trends regarding nursing care needs and allocation of nursing resources according to nursing diagnoses; and to simulate nursing research" (Werley et al., 1988, p. 1652). Such data are essential because they facilitate description of the health status of individuals, groups, and populations in terms of nursing care needs; establish outcome measures related to nursing care; and investigate the use and cost of nursing resources.

Besides the identification of nursing data elements, the other salient issue in information management for nurses is the establishment of appropriate nursing data standards for use within those data elements. Resolution and convergence on these two topics is essential for collection and storage of nursing data in national health databases. Data elements and their associated nursing data standards must reflect data that nurses use to build the information that provides the foundation for clinical judgment and management decision-making in any setting in which nursing is practiced.

Contextual Factors Influencing Development of Health Information

There are several factors influencing the drive toward unique nursing data elements of health information. These include

- Initiatives to facilitate the evolution of national systems for health information built on essential and comparable data
- Increasing costs of health services driven by rising drug costs, new technologies, and treatment modalities
- Changing demographics as a result of an aging population
- Growth of alternative approaches to managing hospitals and an associated drive to find alternative funding mechanisms
- A trend toward patient-specific costing of health services
- Analysis of health services in terms of patient outcomes
- A shifting paradigm in terms of the value and emphasis placed on community-based practice as opposed to acute care hospital-based practice
- Examination of the roles of health care providers and organizations to eliminate duplication of services and functions
- The trend toward consumerism.

We must identify ways and means by which nurses can become more efficient and effective and maximize the quality of care available to patients within available resources. To facilitate the use of ever-diminishing resources, we also need to identify strategies that will enable enhanced information management.

In addition to the preceding factors, the information revolution has prompted health care organizations to develop or acquire automated information systems focused on the use of data for resource allocation, patient-specific costing, and outcomes of services. The information revolution has also been a driving force in the evolution of national systems for health information.

Most healthcare providers still document client care in natural language narrative text (Toews, 1995). Although clinicians use a clinical vocabulary in client records, there is considerable variety of expression for similar concepts. Because natural language generates inherent inconsistencies in clinical data, retrieval of information in client records is very difficult. Computers can rapidly manipulate, analyze, and retrieve large amounts of data; however, they have limited capability to retrieve and aggregate information from natural language. A number of controlled clinical vocabularies have been developed to address the problem of standardized textual data in the computerized client record.

Current data aggregation usually begins with the coding of medical records abstracts in hospitals and of billing diagnosis and service encounter data in office practice. Coders usually extract data from paper-based clinical records and apply standardized codes for clinical data. Because the healthcare system of the future will permit sharing of electronic health records among health professionals independent of discipline, location, time, or sector of the health system, data must be entered in a standardized way, using standardized terminologies. It is impractical for caregivers to do the coding of data elements in the course of delivering care because the process of coding accurately (anyone can code inaccurately if forced to code what is irrelevant to them) is time consuming, and it interferes with the usual clinical work processes and procedures. Simply stated, the only data that will be accurate at the point of service are those that are crucial to the provision of care by the clinician. Therefore, reliable data for management can come only from an aggregation of this clinical information.

The terminologies used in health care need to serve different uses and users. Clinicians need specificity at the same time that they need usability, whereas managers need classification of clinical data into categories for analysis. Broad classifications, therefore, are to be preferred for health management, but rich terminologies are needed at the point of care. However, the size of the terminology necessary to achieve the richness required for clinical utility is a barrier to its usability, thereby creating a conundrum.

Information and information management will become increasingly important in the future. Nurses must demonstrate that nursing makes a difference in patient outcomes, and they must provide quantitative evidence to support this claim. We need nursing information to facilitate the articulation of our professional scope of practice and of our authority and responsibility within the healthcare system. We must determine the essential data elements required for inclusion in national, multidisciplinary patient-focused health data sets.

Current Status: Nursing Elements of National Health Data Sets

A national health data set containing a minimum number of elements with uniform definitions and classifications was first developed in the United States in 1969 (Murnaghan & White, 1970). Similar health data sets have been developed and implemented in the United Kingdom, Canada, and other countries. The historical background of the development and implementation of minimum health data sets has been described elsewhere (Anderson & Hannah, 1993). These data sets include almost no nursing data. The author is aware of only one health data set that focuses on nursing data: the Nursing Minimum Data Set, developed by Werley and colleagues in the United States.

A Nursing Minimum Data Set is defined by Werley (1988, p. 7) as a "minimum set of items of information with uniform definitions and categories concerning the specific dimensions of professional nursing, which meets the information needs of multiple data users in the healthcare system." (This data set consists of such nursing care elements as

- Nursing diagnosis, nursing intervention, nursing outcome, and intensity
- Patient demographic elements like personal identification, date of birth, sex, race, ethnicity, and residence
- Service elements like health record number, principal nurse provider identification, admission date, discharge date, disposition of the patient, expected principal source of payment, and facility number.

The absence of nursing data elements in national health information sets has been recognized by nurses in many countries, as evidenced by the ongoing activities in countries outside the United States. European nurses have also recognized that their health systems need to include nursing data elements that are significant in the nursing decision-making process. The seminal European research initiative in this area was launched in 1991. This project, entitled "A Concerted Action on European Classification for Nursing Practice with special regard to Patient Problems/Nursing Diagnosis, Nursing Intervention, and Outcomes," was known as TELENURSING. The objectives of TELENURSING were

- To create a network of nurses interested in classification of patient problems/nursing diagnosis, nursing interventions, and nursing outcomes
- To create minimum data sets and healthcare informatics
- To raise the awareness among nurses of standardization efforts in healthcare informatics
- To link the technical approach of national groups and the professional approach of international groups with regard to development of classifications of health care.

The TELENURSING group established an interest in developing data standards and a nursing minimum data set. The next step is to promote standardization of definition, classification, and coding of data as initial work that may contribute to the development of internationally comparable nursing minimum data sets (Mortensen et al., 1994).

Australian nurses also recognized and supported the need for integration and standardization of data from all disciplines involved in the provision of health care. To this end, they participated in the development of a National Health Care Data Dictionary of standard definitions and the nursing data element identification and classifications based on these standard definitions. Australian nurses also established and pilot-tested a National Minimum Data Set for Community Nurses, based on the work of Werley and colleagues in the United States (Foster & Conrick, 1994).

In Canada, many nurses recognized the need to identify the HI:NC to facilitate the development of a national health information system during the restructuring of provincial health information systems. To get nursing data incorporated into a national health information system, nurses took a proactive stance and mobilized resources to ensure the identification of those data elements that are essential to nurses in all practice settings in Canada.

In the closing decade of the twentieth century, the Canadian Nurses Association responded to a resolution calling for a national consensus conference "to develop in Canada a standardized format (Nursing Minimum Data Set) for purposes of ensuring entry, accessibility, and retrievability of nursing data" (Canadian Nurses Association, 1990). Direction was set at The Nursing Minimum Data Set (NMDS) Conference, held in Edmonton, Canada in October 1992. At the provincial level, the Alberta Association of Registered Nurses (AARN) provided national leadership in promoting the HI:NC: client status, nursing interventions, client outcomes, nursing intensity, and a unique provider number.

These examples clearly illustrate that internationally, there is an emerging consensus among nurses that the unique nursing data elements to be included in national health data sets are nursing diagnosis (also known in some countries as *client status* or *nursing problem*), nursing intervention, patient/client outcome, and nursing intensity.

Data Standards

Exchange of data among health professionals and institutions occurs with great regularity; however, common interpretation and understanding of those data does not. A common language through which health information can be shared does not exist. Accessing the valuable information contained in clinical records is more often a problem of linguistics than of technology (Toews, 1995). There is no consistency in the use of terms to identify client health status, interventions, or outcomes within a particular health profession, among the various health professions, or across the continuum of care.

Documenting care in a consistent and retrievable way requires the use of structured clinical vocabularies. Interpretability is one of the greatest challenges regarding useful information exchange—technology is no longer a barrier. Standardizing the terminologies used in communicating health data is essential to improving the quality of shared information, especially in electronic format. It is estimated that more than 150 health-related classification and code systems exist in the world today. Hence, there is a real problem with communicating effectively and producing integrated individual health records and health databases.

Effective standard "languages" for creating intelligible data, coupled with the tools for effective and secure data exchange, are essential for health information sharing, retrieval, analysis, and use. Creating standardized vocabularies for health care not only allows different health professionals and organizations to "speak" to one another, but it may also facilitate more efficient and effective data capturing. Ideally, data entry should be a by-product of clinical activity, captured as close to the (first-person) source as possible. Such entries could support data availability much closer to "real time" and allow information sharing among different and dispersed potential users. Also, the ability to consistently interpret health concepts enables their consistent retrieval and the further categorization of data for knowledge base searches (e.g., literature) or statistical analysis at group and population levels (e.g., for resource management, planning, outcomes measurement, and evaluation).

At the point of service, healthcare workers use their own natural languages. Healthcare managers, however, need accurate aggregate data. There is a necessary trade-off between natural language and structured languages. The less structured the language, the less likely that aggregated data will be accurate, valid, or reliable. Source data capture may be more accurate and efficient than deferred data capture; the more structured the language, the less likely the clinician is to find the language usable in haste at the point of service.

There are three main categories of language, which differ in freedom of expression. All three can be, and have been, used in electronic data and health information systems. Definitions and relative advantages and disadvantages of each are as follows:

- Natural language (or free text). Natural language is the way in which people "naturally" speak everyday language. Natural language is the least inhibited type of language and includes a multitude of ambiguities that require contextual understanding for correct interpretation. Although it is the easiest language to deal with "at the source," it is the most difficult for the next reader to precisely interpret or translate into different languages and conceptual classification structures.

  Unfortunately, natural language (or free text) does not allow for the reuse or systematic interpretation of data within electronic records. Only in codes can clinical data be transmitted in shared care and analyzed systematically.

- Controlled language (or controlled vocabulary). A controlled language is a subset of a natural language. In controlled languages, data are coded and possibly organized into one or more hierarchies. Coding places explicit restrictions on terminology, grammatical rules, and/or description formats. These restrictions result in fewer ambiguous statements, greater assurance of information reliability, and an increased potential for shared

understanding. On the other hand, controlled languages necessarily restrict the richness of clinical detail, and they require that the person using the language be skilled in its use.
• Formal language. In formal language, such as computer programming language, all terms and relations between terms are strictly and explicitly predefined. Although it is the most reliable type of language, it is the least flexible and the most difficult to learn and use.

Types of Controlled Languages

Nomenclature

A nomenclature is a list of all approved terms for describing and recording observations. A more precise definition of a nomenclature is a collection of terms relevant to a domain, or knowledge area, with no explicit hierarchic structure (Ingerf, 1995). The terms used to document the planning and delivery of care would be part of a nomenclature of health care. A nomenclature is simply an agreed-upon naming convention. The purpose of a nomenclature in nursing, for instance, is to have a dictionary of approved nursing terms so that all data are recorded in a standardized way. A nomenclature of health care would contain all the terms relevant to health care, including but not limited to

• Client status, demographics, needs, risks, and problems
• Diagnostic examination, physical findings, and symptoms
• Reason for encounter
• Treatment, interventions, and therapeutic procedures
• Treatment objectives and treatment endpoints
• Outcome measures
• Functional/health status
• Laboratory tests and results.

Classification System

A classification system is a means of giving order to a group of disconnected facts by assigning them to predesignated classes on the basis of perceived common characteristics. Ideally, a classification should be characterized by

• Naturalness—the classes correspond to the nature of the thing being classified
• Exhaustiveness—every member of the group will fit into one (and only one) class in the system
• Constructability—the set of classes can be constructed by a demonstrably systematic procedure.

Although some classifications aim to cover aspects of care broadly (e.g., the Systematized Nomenclature of Medicine [SNOMED]), many focus on specific areas—for example, the Home Health Care Classification (HHCC) is designed for home health and ambulatory nursing care. Classification systems are not meant to fully describe the health and health service needs of an individual; rather, they are more often intended to drive the statistical analysis of the health and health service needs of a population. For this reason, classification categories are not ambiguous. The determinants of each "class" must be mutually exclusive to enable statistical analysis. The trade-off for this lack of ambiguity, however, is a lessening of the clinical specificity of each record or concept represented.

Thus, by definition, a nomenclature of health care is the vocabulary (used to describe patients, problems, events, etc.) employed in the everyday practice of health care. A classification system is the grouping of terms from this vocabulary on the basis of characteristics shared by the terms. For example, "angina," "coronary artery disease," and "myocardial infarction" may be grouped together in the category "coronary heart disease. (Ontario Family/General Practice Data Standards Project, Process and Data Modelling Project Report, no date)

Controlled Clinical Vocabulary or Controlled Clinical Terminology

A structured and limited dictionary of clinical terms used at the point-of-service, a controlled clinical terminology (CCT) is intended to overcome the difficulty of term selection, the lack of reliable classification when using large nomenclatures, and the clinicians' aversion to the "formalistic and arcane nature of disease classifications." (COACH, 1998)

Controlled clinical vocabularies are standardized sets of encoded terms that allow clinical data to be captured "the source" (i.e., entered directly into an electronic record by a health service practitioner). (CIHI, 1997)

Unlike classifications, the detail represented in CCTs is meant to be comparable with that which is currently included in clinical records (e.g., textual summaries, reports, and progress notes). Controlled clinical terminologies seek to represent concepts in as much detail as is commonly useful for clinicians and other health professionals in describing health-related concepts. These concepts include both specific attributes (of the client and the service being provided) and modifiers or qualifiers of those attributes. Modifiers indicate degree, time, stage, and so forth of a condition or characteristic. Qualifiers indicate negation or uncertainty in a detail or condition.

Some level of categorization may occur internally in controlled vocabulary systems in order to group terms that are clinically related, usually in hierarchies according to concept and level of detail. These hierarchies are useful as a means to structure or conceptually frame the knowledge represented in the clinical domain for presentation, maintenance, and updating.

They are also useful in automated implementations as the basis for data structure that enables intelligent prompting or alerts the user to clinical events and that facilitates database searching and relating. Ideally, CCTs should balance the needs of natural language in individual documentation with the needs of shared interpretation (i.e., with less ambiguity than natural language).

Thesaurus

A thesaurus is a type of controlled vocabulary arranged so that relationships among terms are displayed clearly and identified by standardized relationship indicators. Synonym identification may also be included. The Unified Medical Language System (UMLS) is the best known medical thesaurus. The primary purposes of a thesaurus are

- Translation: a means for translating the natural language of authors, indexers, and users into a controlled vocabulary used for indexing and retrieval
- Consistency: to promote consistency in the assignment of index terms
- Indication of relationships: to indicate semantic relationships among terms
- Retrieval: to serve as a searching aid in retrieval of documents (American National Standards Institute, 1994).

Some experts suggest thesauri are not suitable for clinical purposes.

There is often confusion among controlled clinical vocabularies, nomenclatures, and classification systems. A specific, controlled clinical vocabulary will be called a *nomenclature* in one paper and a *classification* in another. This confusion is likely due to the fact that all three encode health information and also tend to involve some amount of concept representation. The fundamental difference, however, lies in the types of concepts being represented and categorized (CIHI, 1997).

Both CCTs and nomenclatures standardize the terms to describe health and health service-related concepts. The purpose is to create a shared "language of health" to enable the exchange of basic clinical data among different individuals, agencies, and institutions. Ideally, both should be easy to use at the point-of-service, and the data they create should be easily and reliably interpreted. Such data, although primarily designed to support clinical decision-making, should also support the aggregation of basic clinical data for research and administrative purposes.

The distinction between nomenclatures, controlled clinical vocabularies and classifications can be conceptualized as points along a continuum of increasing aggregation and decreasing richness: natural language → nomenclature → controlled clinical vocabularies → classification.

Nursing Data Standards

Although considerable work has been invested in identifying and achieving consensus on essential nursing data elements for inclusion in national health data sets, the linkages to international health data sets are only beginning to be explored. In addition to efforts to develop uniform definitions for the data elements, there has been considerable effort invested in developing nursing data standards (Delaney et al., 1994; Vanden Boer & Sermeus, 1994; Werley & Lang, 1988). Research has been directed at the development of standardized nomenclatures for nursing diagnosis, interventions, and outcomes to be used in describing the nursing care elements in a data set (Bulechek & McCloskey, 1990; Grobe, 1990; Jenny, 1989; Lang & Marek, 1990; McCloskey et al., 1990; McLane, 1987; North American Nursing Diagnosis Association, 1989; Ozbolt, 1999). The American Nurses Association has launched major initiatives to develop a Uniform Language for nursing. In addition, the national nursing associations have worked with the International Council of Nurses to develop and promote an international CCT that describes nursing care, the International Classification of Nursing Practice (McCormick et al., 1994; Zielstorff et al., 1995).

In the United States, the American Nurses Association has recognized seven terminologies as appropriate to support clinical practice. These are

1. Home Health Care Classification: developed by Dr. Virginia Saba
2. NANDA: developed by North American Nursing Diagnosis Association
3. Nursing Interventions Classification: developed by Dr. Joanne McCloskey and Dr. Gloria Bulechek
4. Nursing Interventions Lexicon and Taxonomy: developed by Dr. Susan Grobe
5. Nursing Outcomes Classification: developed by Dr. Marion Johnson
6. Omaha System: developed by Omaha Visiting Nurses Association
7. Patient Care Data Set: developed by Dr. Judy Ozbolt.

These seven terminologies differ in purpose, scope, form, content, and process of development. Some are nomenclatures, some are controlled nursing languages, and some are classifications (Fig. 9.1). None of these has emerged as a de facto standard, and together they do not constitute a standard or even a unified language. These nursing terminology sets have been criticized as lacking comprehensiveness, granularity, and rules for combining atomic-level concepts into more complex concepts.

The International Council of Nurses (ICN) undertook an initiative to compare and analyze existing nursing taxonomies. After extensive effort, the ICN developed the International Classification of Nursing Practice (ICNP). This controlled clinical vocabulary has been widely tested in Europe, the Asia Pacific region, and in Latin America.

In Canada, the AARN Ad Hoc Committee on HI:NC undertook comparison and analysis of the existing classification systems for data within

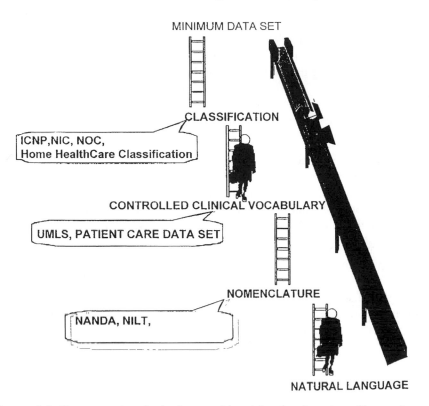

MINIMUM DATA SET

CLASSIFICATION

ICNP,NIC, NOC,
Home HealthCare Classification

CONTROLLED CLINICAL VOCABULARY

UMLS, PATIENT CARE DATA SET

NOMENCLATURE

NANDA, NILT,

NATURAL LANGUAGE

FIGURE 9.1. The seven terminologies considered by the American Nurses Association to be appropriate for clinical practice.

each of the HI:NC data elements (Alberta Association of Registered Nurses, 1994). The conclusion reached simultaneously and independently was the same as the one reached in the United States and at the International Council of Nurses: None of the classification systems was sufficiently comprehensive or granular to meet the needs of nursing in all practice settings. Ultimately, the AARN endorsed the ICNP for testing.

Issues

The first issue is the need to further develop and utilize existing controlled clinical vocabularies in nursing and work toward convergence rather than repeatedly starting all over again. Nursing must go forward, build on previous work, and avoid "reinventing the wheel." The second issue is the need to ensure integration of all unique nursing elements of national health data sets. Additionally, with the emphasis on a multidisciplinary approach to client care, the overlapping of professional boundaries with respect to interventions must be acknowledged.

Several issues germane to the development and use of minimum data sets emerge, including data integrity and the scope of data to include in a minimum data set (i.e., what does "minimum" really mean?). Other technical issues of relevance relate to aspects of data linkage. Once the unique nursing data elements of health information are developed, three more issues emerge:

- Promoting the concept to ensure consensus and widespread use among nurses and all other users of health information
- Educating nurses to ensure the quality of the data that are collected
- Establishing mechanisms for ongoing review and revision of the controlled clinical vocabularies to ensure their currency and relevance

There is much work to be done on the development of an international classification system(s) and controlled clinical vocabularies for nursing data. Nurses in all countries must raise their awareness of this important work. Linkages must be created among national and international initiatives to identify and resolve issues related to the development and use of these standardized nursing data. It is imperative that efforts not be duplicated.

Implications of Nursing Data

In the absence of a system for collecting, storing, and retrieving nursing data, it is evident that much valuable information is being lost. This information is important to demonstrate the cost-effectiveness of nursing care and the contribution nursing makes to the care of patients (Werley et al., 1988, 1991). The trend in health care is away from discipline-specific models of patient care delivery and toward patient-focused models that emphasize collaboration of disciplines, multiskilling of healthcare providers, standardization of care, and streamlining of documentation through charting by exception.

In this environment, it is imperative that nurses be able to articulate what is and is not nursing's role. Furthermore, nurses will be asked to demonstrate nursing's contribution to patient care in terms of objective and measurable outcome measures. Nurses require nursing data to identify their field's contribution to the outcomes of care, defend the allocation of resources to nursing, and justify new roles for nursing in the healthcare delivery system. Similarly, nurses need to understand and value nursing data so that, during the selection and implementation of information systems, they insist that nurses play a major role and that nursing data needs are incorporated into the selection and implementation criteria. For greater detail on the selection and implementation of information systems, see Hannah et al. (1999).

Although nursing must preserve its professional identity, this objective must be balanced against professional compartmentalization. Collection and storage of essential nursing data elements that are not integrated as components of national health data sets will serve to "ghettoize" nursing. This is dangerous at a time when significant emphasis is being placed on multidisciplinary collaboration, patient-focused care, and patient outcomes. In view of priorities such as these in health care, the need for integration of data elements could not be clearer.

Nurse clinicians need to know what nursing elements are essential for archival purposes so that nursing documentation includes data related to these elements. With the move toward standardization of care through the use of care maps, it is essential that outcomes of nursing care are determined and included. As healthcare organizations embrace the concept of charting by exception in an effort to decrease the valuable hours healthcare workers spend in documentation, nurses must be sure that the tools outlining the patient care delivered are not devoid of nursing's contributions and data. If there are no data that reflect nursing activities, there will be no archival record of what nurses do, what difference nursing care makes, or why nurses are required. In times of fiscal restraint, such objective nursing data are necessary to substantiate the role of nurses and the nurse–patient ratios required in the clinical setting.

Nurse researchers need a database composed of essential data elements to facilitate the identification of trends related to the data elements for specific patient groups, institutions, or regions and to assess variables on multiple levels, including institutional, local, regional, and national (Werley et al., 1988). Collection and storage of essential nursing data elements will facilitate the advancement of nursing as a research-based discipline (Werley & Zorn, 1988). Nurse educators need these essential nursing data to develop nursing knowledge for use in educating nurses and to help define the scope of nursing practice (McCloskey, 1988).

Finally, nursing elements of health information and CCTs for nursing must be defined if they are to influence health policy decision-making. Historically, health policy has been created in the absence of nursing data. At a time of profound international healthcare reform, it is essential that nurses demonstrate the central role of nursing services in the restructuring of the healthcare delivery system.

Clearly, a priority for nursing is the identification of the nursing components of health information—those essential nursing data elements that must be collected, stored, and retrieved from a national health information database. There is much work to be done to ensure that nursing data elements are included in these databases and to achieve consensus and convergence on a common controlled clinical vocabulary for nursing. The challenge for all nurses is to identify their role in helping to define the nursing elements essential for inclusion in such a database and to achieve international consensus and convergence on a common controlled clinical vocabulary for nursing. The time to respond to this challenge is now. If we do not, the essential nursing data elements and a common controlled clinical vocabulary for nursing will be defined by somebody else, or they will remain absent from national health databases.

Questions

1. Why is it important for nursing data elements to be collected and stored?
2. Briefly discuss some of the worldwide initiatives in nursing that are working toward the development of nursing data elements. Consider work from the countries of Australia, Canada, or the United States. How do the initiatives differ? How are they similar?

References

Alberta Association of Registered Nurses (AARN). *Client Status, Nursing Intervention and Client Outcome Taxonomies: A Background Paper.* Alberta: AARN, 1994.

American National Standards Institute ANSI/NISO Z39.19-1993. Bethesda, MD:NISO Press, 1994.

Anderson BJ, Hannah KJ. A Canadian nursing minimum data set: a major priority. *Canadian Journal of Nursing Administration* 1993;6(2):7–13.

Bulechek GM, McCloskey JC. Nursing interventions: taxonomy development. In: McCloskey JC, Grace HK, eds. *Current Issues in Nursing*, 3rd ed. St. Louis: Mosby, 1990;23–38.

Canadian Nurses Association (CNA). *Report of the Resolutions Committee.* Unpublished report, June 1990.

Canadian Institute for Health Information (CIHI). *Controlled Clinical Vocabularies: Background Document.* Ottawa, Ontario, 1997.

COACH. *Something Old, Something New, Something Borrowed.* A Review of Standardized Data Collection in Primary Care. COACH Conference 23, 1998 Scientific Program Proceedings, *www.coah.org*, 1998.

Delaney C, Mehmert M, Prophet C, Crossley J. Establishment of the research value of nursing minimum data sets. In: Grobe SJ, Pluyter-Wenting ESP, eds. *Nursing Informatics: An International Overview for Nursing in a Technological Era.* Amsterdam: Elsevier Science, 1994;169–173.

Foster J, Conrick M. Nursing minimum data sets: historical perspective and Australian development. In: Grobe SJ, Pluyter-Wenting ESP, eds. *Nursing Informatics: an International Overview for Nursing in a Technological Era.* Amsterdam: Elsevier Science, 1994;150–154.

Graves JR, Corcoran S. The study of nursing informatics. *Image: Journal of Nursing Scholarship* 1989;21(4):227–231.

Grobe SJ. Nursing intervention lexicon and taxonomy study: language and classification methods. *Advances in Nursing Science* 1990;13:22–33.

Hannah KJ, Ball MJ, Edwards MJ. *Introduction to Nursing Informatics*, 2nd ed. New York: Springer-Verlag, 1999.

Ingerf J. Taxonomic vocabularies in medicine: the intention of usage determines different established structures. In: Greenes RA, Protti D, eds. *MedInfo '95. Pro-*

ceedings of the 8th World Congress Medical Informatics. Amsterdam: North Holland, 1995;136–139.

Jenny J. Classifying nursing diagnoses: A self care approach. *Nursing and Health Care,* 1989;10(2):82–88.

Lang NM, Marek KD. The classification of patient outcomes. *Journal of Professional Nursing,* 1990;6:158–163.

McCloskey JC. The nursing minimum data set: benefits and implications for nurse educators. In: National League for Nursing, *Perspectives in Nursing 1987–1989.* New York: National League for Nursing, 1988;119–126.

McCloskey JC, Bulechek GM, Cohen MZ, Craft MJ, Crossley JD, Denehy JA, Glick OJ, Kruckeberg T, Mass M, Prophet CM, Tripp-Reimer T. Classifications of nursing interventions. *Journal of Professional Nursing* 1990;6:151–157.

McCormick KA, Lang N, Zielstorff R, Milholland DK, Saba V, Jacox A. Toward standard classification schemes for nursing language: recommendations of the American Nurses Association steering committee on databases to support clinical nursing practice. *Journal of the American Medical Informatics Association* 1994;1(6):421–427.

McLane AM. Measurement and validation of diagnostic concepts: a decade of progress. *Heart & Lung* 1987;16(Pt 1):616–624.

Mortensen R, Mantas J, Manuela M, Sermeus W, Nielson GH, McAvinue E. Telematics for health care in the European union. In: Grobe SJ, Pluyter-Wenting ESP, eds. *Nursing Informatics: An International Overview for Nursing in a Technological Era.* Amsterdam: Elsevier, 1994;750–752.

Murnaghan JH, White KL. Hospital discharge data: report of the conference on hospital discharge abstracts systems. *Medical Care* 1970;8(Suppl):1–215.

North American Nursing Diagnosis Association (NANDA). *North American Nursing Diagnosis Association: Taxonomy I: Revised 1989.* St. Louis: NANDA, 1989.

Ontario Family/General Practice Data Standards Project, Process and Data Modelling Project Report. Ontario, Canada. No date.

Ozbolt JG. Testimony to the National Committee on Vital and Health Statistics (NCVHS). Hearings on Medical Terminology and Code Development. May 17–18, 1999.

Toews, L. An evaluation methodology for clinical vocabularies and evaluation of the Read Codes. www.ualberta.ca/dept/slis/cais/toews.htm, 1995 October, 1999, (last accessed).

Vanden Boer G, Sermeus W. Linkage of NMDS-information and patient classification systems. In: Grobe SJ, Pluyter-Wenting ESP, eds. *Nursing Informatics: An International Overview for Nursing in a Technological Era.* Amsterdam: Elsevier Science, 1994;158–163.

Verney H. *Florence Nightingale at Harley Street.* London: Dent & Sons, 1970.

Werley HH. Introduction to the nursing minimum data set and its development. In: Werley HH, Lang NM, eds. *Identification of the Nursing Minimum Data Set.* New York: Springer, 1988;1–15.

Werley HH, Devine EC, Zorn CR. Nursing needs its own minimum data set. *American Journal of Nursing* 1988;88:1651–1653.

Werley HH, Devine EC, Zorn CR, Ryan P, Westlake BL. The nursing minimum data set: abstraction tool for standardized, comparable, essential data. *American Journal of Public Health* 1991;81:421–426.

Werley HH, Lang NM. The consensually derived nursing minimum data set: elements and definitions. In: Werley HH, Lang NM, eds. *Identification of the Nursing Minimum Data Set*. New York: Springer, 1988;402–411.

Werley HH, Zorn CR. The nursing minimum data set: benefits and implications. In: National League for Nursing, *Perspectives in Nursing 1987–1989*. New York: National League for Nursing, 1988;105–114.

Zielstorff RD, Lang NM, Saba VK, McCormick KA, Milholland DK. Toward a uniform language for nursing in the US: work of the American Nurses Association steering committee on databases to support clinical practice. In: Greenes RA, Peterson H, Protti D, eds. *Proceedings of MedInfo '95. Proceedings of the Eighth World Congress on Medical Informatics*. Edmonton: International Medical Informatics Association, 1995;1362–1366.

10
Knowledge Discovery in Large Data Sets: A Primer for Data Mining Applications in Health Care

Patricia A. Abbott

It is often said that not all things that count can be measured, and not all things that are measured count. This saying brings us face-to-face with pressing issues in informatics today: determining what data need to be collected and how to collect them, using information to enhance the efficiency of care, and providing knowledge-based support for the improvement of patient outcomes. It has become glaringly apparent that these issues cannot be addressed in the absence of focused, available, and integrated information.

The migration toward integrated enterprise-wide information systems that incorporate clinical, resource, and cost data is a result of the movement to achieve outcomes and effectiveness goals in health care. However, this headlong rush into automated systems has generated collections of data that are unwieldy for purposes of management and analysis, at least from a traditional methodologic standpoint. In the face of ever-expanding health-care data warehouses, questions are frequently raised:

- Now that we have the data, what do we do with them?
- Why did we opt to collect all these variables?
- What should we be collecting?
- Do we know the elements that contribute to outcome X?

It seems that health care is facing another engineering conundrum: how to manage what is being measured, as well as how to capture what is missing.

The management of what is being measured is challenging; massive warehouses of data are being captured and generated as a normal by-product of health services. Electronic data gathering devices, physiological monitoring equipment, digitized imaging, genetic coding, and enterprise-wide data warehousing efforts have led to gigabytes, terabytes, and petabytes of data. Often, this glut of data is referred to as "data smog," a rather negative representation of a seemingly fuzzy, unpleasant, and unmanageable phenomenon. On the contrary, the massive collections of data are increasingly valuable resources.

It is important to note that healthcare data are not like wine—generally, they do not improve with age. In reality, much of the data collected in health care lie moldering in data silos, with consequential decay in currency and value. Tremendous resources are being spent to capture data, yet the industry is slow in leveraging the value of the information gold mine. The failure to act can be called the "paralysis of analysis," most often due in this situation to the limitations of traditional methods of management and analysis.

Traditional approaches to data analysis, which are based primarily on humans dealing directly with the data, are generally unable to scale up to working with "big data." Instead, we must look to alternative approaches to data management, requiring adoption of methods that are unfamiliar and, for some, uncomfortable. Traditional use of fixed equations and numbers as ways of describing phenomena is often not suited to the adaptive and ever-changing biological events found in health care. The complexity of human data requires adaptive and evolving approaches to analysis and management.

One may suppose that working with highly dimensional patient data is best suited to specialized statistical analysts. In reality, many of the biggest benefits of understanding complex healthcare data are afforded to those in clinical practice, where decisions that directly impact resource utilization and patient outcomes are made. The issue at hand is how to assist clinicians in analyzing, leveraging, and understanding these huge bodies of information or, in other words, how to filter the "essence from the bulk."

In health care, clinical decision-makers are deluged with overwhelming sensory inputs. Patient presentations, beeping monitors, laboratory printouts, scientific studies, reports, consultations, business plans, insurance regulations, budgets, personnel . . . the list goes on. Ultimately, providers are responsible for assimilating the torrents of incoming data to make high-quality decisions. The capacity of the human processor is limited, however, and inputs are often purposefully and consciously limited. This limiting phenomenon may be due to high levels of experience, where the pieces of data necessary to come to a decision are "known" a priori (based on experience or bias) by the decision-maker. At the other end of the spectrum, inexperienced practitioners may find themselves at a data-overload point and make critical decisions in an information-poor environment.

There are many variables that impact a patient condition or clinical decision, some known and some not. Often, these data points are not available at the moment of need or are unknown by even the most skilled practitioner. Eckhardt (1981), in discussing the uncertainty inherent in the decision-making process, asserts that knowledge is relative to the "knower and the world being known." This statement illustrates that humans often make decisions in situations where much of the knowledge could be unknown or biased. Pauker et al. (1976) assert that clinicians make clinical decisions on "guesses" of initial hypotheses that are based on minimal amounts of data. Therefore, one might expect that increased amounts of data available for decision-making would enhance the quality of the decision. This is not the case, however. Classic work by Miller (1956) demonstrated that the human mind can only process a specific amount of information when it is viewed within definite and specifically sized "chunks." Simoudis (1996) asserts that the size of the data is not necessarily the culprit for overload, citing instead the impact of the presentation of disparate information.

All of these issues contribute to the peril and promise of working with large amounts of data and create new challenges for informaticists who are working to leverage the value of integrated healthcare data. How can the torrents of captured data be analyzed and presented to the decision-maker in a form that is comprehensive (yet not overwhelming) and situation specific (yet based on pooled population data sets)?

Converting massive collections of data into usable knowledge requires two new approaches to analysis and management: Knowledge Discovery in Large Databases (KDD) and data mining. Although differences between the two approaches are clarified later in this chapter, these terms will be used interchangeably throughout.

KDD Primer

What is KDD, and how does it differ from traditional statistical approaches to management and analysis of data? As defined by Abbott (1999), KDD is the melding of human expertise with statistical and machine learning techniques to identify features, patterns, and underlying rules in large collections of healthcare data. This fusion of approaches leads to the detection of nonintuitive, previously undiscovered relationships in the data.

KDD is defined by Fayyad et al. (1996, p. 6) as a "non-trivial process of identifying valid, novel, potentially useful, and ultimately understandable patterns in data". Fayyad et al. (1996) also refer to KDD as the process of deriving high-level knowledge from low-level data. This high-level knowledge is used to support knowledge-based decision-making.

It is critically important to understand that the tools of KDD are totally independent from the data on which they operate. Therefore, KDD utility is domain independent and can be used in any large collection of data. It has been noted that the value of KDD as an approach is often confused with the character of the data, which in health care have a tendency to be "noisy" or dirty. One should never confuse the validity of the tools and approaches of KDD with the characteristics of the data.

Ultimately, KDD or data mining is used to "discover" previously unknown patterns or nonintuitive relationships in the data. The use of the word "unknown" or "nonintuitive" reveals the value of the approach. In traditional approaches to statistical analysis, the researcher or investigator has an a priori hypothesis and structures the analysis session based on the hypothesis. An a priori approach to analysis is considered a "verification"-based approach in which the goal of analysis is to verify the hypothesis.

KDD, on the other hand, is a "discovery"-based approach that uses an exploratory analysis instead of an a priori hypothesis.

It is important to note, however, that KDD can be used to both verify and discover. In the experience of this researcher, the output of KDD has verified what was suspected and illuminated what was not. For example, Abbott (1999) used KDD to determine the major predictors of admission from a long-term care facility to an acute care facility. It was expected that such predictors as a broken hip, dyspnea, heart failure, and sepsis would emerge as predictors of admission. This was verified in the analysis. Many variables that were not expected, however, added true value to the output. In all, 23 major predictors of admission emerged, some expected and some discovered.

KDD has many semantic flavors. Titles such as data archaeology, data pattern processing, knowledge extraction, and information discovery can be found in the literature. As mentioned earlier, data mining and KDD are different. KDD generally refers to a several-step process of knowledge discovery, while the term *data mining* refers singularly to the use of algorithms to extract patterns. Data mining is a single step in the KDD process, which is discussed later in this chapter. The term *KDD* is most commonly used in the Artificial Intelligence (AI) and machine learning communities, while the term *data mining* is most often used by Management Information Systems (MIS) personnel.

The Process of Data Mining

The work of Fayyad et al. (1996) indicates that data mining is not a process in and of itself. Rather, it is only one step in the process of KDD. As a step in the KDD process, however, the semantic argument can be made that to effectively discover the nuggets of information in large, disparate data sets, the data sets must be quarried for nuggets of information. This extraction takes place through data mining. The process of KDD consists of five basic steps (see Fig. 10.1 for an illustration):

- Problem identification
- Data extraction
- Data preprocessing
- Data mining
- Pattern interpretation and presentation

These five steps include subprocedures, which in reality bring the number of steps in the KDD process to eight. Each step and substep build on each other, which attests to the criticality of expert involvement. Errors of ignorance can be easily propagated through the KDD process. Without all five steps working in concert, an incorrect data mining methodology may be applied. Blind application of data mining methods can lead to discovering

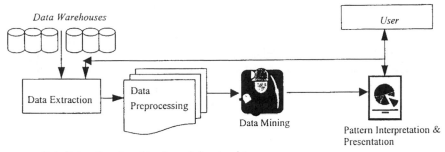

Data Warehouses

User

Data Extraction

Data Preprocessing

Data Mining

Pattern Interpretation & Presentation

Data Extraction: Searching for and choosing data

Data Preprocessing: Choosing variables, dealing with noise and multidimensionality

Data Mining: Analysis of data using association, clustering, modeling, classification, etc.

Pattern Interpretation & Presentation: Interpretation, evaluation, and presentation of patterns

FIGURE 10.1. Knowledge Discovery in Large Databases: the KDD process.

meaningless data patterns, or what is known as "data dredging" (Fayyad et al., 1996). Failure to include domain experts in the KDD process may result in improper discovery of erroneous patterns and consequent presentation without understanding the spurious nature of the results.

Broad outlines of the KDD steps are presented here, based on the work of Fayyad et al. (1996) and as originally published by Abbott (1999). This practical overview demonstrates the interactive and iterative nature of the KDD process.

The initial step of KDD involves obtaining an in-depth understanding of the application domain via experience and examination of prior knowledge generated in the domain. This is where the problem is identified, prior work in the area is examined, and the decision is made in relation to the need for further investigation. It also involves in-depth work with the end user to obtain an understanding of the needs and/or goals of the persons that the application of KDD will serve. Brachman and Anand (1996, p. 40) believe that for the development of successful KDD applications, it is critical that the developer "understands the exact nature of the interactions between humans and data that leads to the discovery of knowledge."

The secondary step involves creating a target data set, which involves selecting the warehouse or data set upon which KDD is to be tested. At this point, the data subselection process has not begun. This can be likened to mining for a commodity such as natural gas. A large oil company does not arbitrarily set up a drilling operation in the middle of a field. Instead, the underlying geology is studied, previous success in finding natural gas is considered, land forms are mapped, property rights are investigated, and so forth. A drilling experiment is guided by science and intuition. Data mining operates on similar principles. One does not pick a random warehouse and mine for a specific phenomenon, just as an oil company would not set up a drilling rig in Central Park. An understanding of both the domain and the data is critical in selecting an environment for KDD to be effective.

The third step involves subselection, preprocessing, and cleaning of the data to examine the impact of outliers and noise on the data set. It is during this step that decisions related to missing or "dirty" data are made. Wreden (1997, p. 47) refers to this step as "Purgatory before Nirvana." Brachman and Anand (1996) make the point that caution in "scrubbing" away anomalies in the data is warranted, as these could be crucial indicators of interesting domain phenomena. There are several approaches to dealing with missing or noisy data. These approaches range from advanced automated algorithmic data cleaning to simply dropping cases that are erroneous to statistical leveling.

The fourth step involves feature or dimension reduction. As is often the case, the number of variables that are gleaned in the second step are highly dimensional, and frequently there are certain dimensions that can be used to identify the factor structure and then model for the set of variables (Stephens, 1996). The use of dimensionality reduction or transformation methods is applied in this phase. Brachman and Anand (1996) labels this "parameter restriction" and suggests it as a way to deal with massively overwhelming amounts of data. These authors state that not all variables will have utility in an analysis, and they believe that parameter shrinkage makes a model more robust. For example, it would be unnecessary to include "gender" in a mining experiment focused on pregnancy. A common approach used for dimensionality reduction is a principal components analysis (PCA).

The fifth step involves choosing the data mining task. The selection of the data mining approach is based on the goal of the KDD process, such as summarization, dependency modeling, classification, association, and regression. (Fayyad et al., 1996) Each of these approaches has strengths and weaknesses, and the decision of what method to use depends on the task at hand and the inclination of the modeler. Brachman and Anand (1996) assert that the choice of approach can be determined as data sets are being investigated, a point that emphasizes the intertwining of data analysis and model creation in the KDD approach. These authors frame the model selection process in a "human-centered" approach, asserting that when completing the knowledge engineering that is required for model selection, "background knowledge of the domain expert is crucial." (Brachman & Anand, 1996, p. 47) Considerations of end user needs are also included here, for example, determining if the system is to be used to explain the patterns or to use the patterns for prediction purposes.

Classification is a commonly used data mining approach, where the goal of the analysis is to classify people into groups, such as those who survive and those who do not, or those who are admitted and those who are not. For example, classification is frequently used in the finance or banking industry as a way to classify people into good credit risks and bad credit risks. A mining approach is used on retrospective data for which the outcome (repayment or default) of the loan is already known. The classifier then determines the combination and degree of contribution that each variable makes to the outcome. Using the model built on this sort of analysis, the classifier is used prospectively (as a real-time decision support tool) to determine who runs a higher risk of default. This enables finance companies to approve or reject loans within minutes, many times while applicants are on still on the telephone.

Association, used to look for factors that cluster together, is another frequently used mining approach. In the business world, this is similar to an approach called *market basket* analysis. Customer buying patterns are examined for certain purchases that are associated with each other. One particularly humorous example appeared in a recent mining study that looked at association buying in convenience stores. One may expect that a purchase of diapers would be associated with a purchase of baby food or formula. To the surprise of the investigators, this analysis revealed that the purchase of diapers was closely associated with the purchase of a six pack of an alcoholic beverage. The interpretation of this phenomenon was interesting. It was decided that fathers who are sent to the local convenience store for diapers were not thinking of formula or baby food.

How does this all relate to health care? It is not hard to imagine how association and classification of symptoms, presentations, emergency room use, insurance buying habits, risk factors, and the like would have tremendous utility in health care. Knowing the probabilities of occurrence and then being able to predict the phenomenon has tremendous implications for health management and resource utilization.

The sixth step involves the actual data mining, which is the active investigation of the transformed data set for interesting patterns, frequently via the use of neural networks (NN), classification and regression trees (CARTS), or decision trees. Readers are referred to the literature for in-depth discussions of these techniques. Abbott (1999) describes neural network classification systems in detail.

There are a variety of software packages that enable this portion of the data mining process, and most are relatively easy to use. Connectionist machine learning techniques, NN, were used by Abbott (1999) via a software package called NeuralWare Professional II Plus. Neural networks have been shown to solve complex problems with high accuracy and fewer constraints associated with traditional statistical methods. Neural networks may constitute reasonable alternatives to current regression models in health care (Ohno-Machado & Musen, 1995; Penny & Frost, 1996) because they are particularly well suited to noisy, multidimensional, and explosive problems. Assumptions of normality and distribution are not as stringent as regression approaches, and the number of variables that can enter into the equation far exceed the limitations of traditional approaches. Each of these considerations is particularly apropos to healthcare data that are dirty, complex, and intensively multidimensional, with no assumptions of normality guaranteed.

The final two steps involve interpreting the output of the data mining and incorporating and/or disseminating the knowledge to the users. Interpretation is a critical step—again, the role of the domain expert cannot be overemphasized. Generally, output involves the analysis of results and can be represented in many different formats, such as reports of goodness of fit, outliers, scatterplots, graphical representations, and alarming (or monitoring) functions. The type of output and dissemination is once again based on the needs of the user and the type of problem. The final step also involves reconciling new findings with previously known facts, a point of particular importance in clinical situations.

These steps are iterative, adaptable, and a combination of manual, statistical, and machine learning techniques. Although some software packages purport to offer a single solution to all aspects of the KDD process, it is believed that a certain degree of knowledge of underlying statistics and domain expertise is required. As with many research projects, one of the most important things to implement is the assembly of a team of experts who specialize in these different steps of KDD. For example, a team may consist of the domain expert, a statistician, and a programmer. The programmer may assist with the merging of data sets, file transporting, software management, and standardization. The statistician can be responsible for dealing with missing or erroneous data, handling the dimensionality reduction, and assisting in interpretation and analysis. The domain expert is involved throughout the entire process. There are also industry firms that offer services in data mining; these can be found readily on the Internet. Although not a method to be approached casually, data mining is within the realm of "do-ability." KDD projects should be initiated and directed by those they will eventually serve. Instead of waiting for technology to deliver that service, these initiators must be proactive in driving the development of information systems in health care.

Application of Knowledge Discovery in Large Data Sets

A research project completed by Abbott (1999) used KDD and machine learning techniques to aggregate and sift through large federal databases, examining the web of causality related to admission from long-term care (LTC) facilities to acute care facilities. Admission from a LTC to an acute care facility is often a negative outcome, associated with increased morbidity and mortality as well as considerable financial outlay. This experiment resulted in the development of a model of admission risk, which can be used to prospectively determine the probability of a resident being admitted to an acute care facility and to reveal the variables that are contributing to the level of risk. The model was designed for incorporation into LTC Minimum Data Set (MDS) assessment tools as a method of decision support. It is anticipated that the inclusion of risk probabilities into a knowledge-based LTC assessment tool will help detect negative patterns and alert providers to increasing levels of risk, resulting in a positive impact on the process of care in LTC.

The initial sample size for the experiment was approximately 44,000 records from the Health Care Financing Administration, generated from three disparate warehouses: the OSCAR state survey files, Medicare inpatient claims files, and the MDS. Each record contained a potential of 1,095 variables. Preprocessing and statistical manipulation resulted in an experimental set of approximately 14,000 records for this research. Dimensionality reduction reduced the number of input variables to 135.

A neural network (NN) was utilized to classify patients into distinct groups based on the outcome of admission versus nonadmission. The trained model demonstrated an overall classification accuracy rate of approximately 94 percent, with a resulting sensitivity average of 88 percent and a 99 percent average specificity. A dithering function was used to counter the criticism of the NN "black box" phenomenon as a way to explain the derived output. Twenty-three variables emerged from the dithering as major predictors of admission, some that were expected (validation) and many that were discovered.

When one considers the size of this data set (albeit very limited) and the fact that the data came from three separate and totally unlinked databases, it is not hard to imagine that some discoveries were novel. Dealing with the distribution, fragmentation, complexity, and noise inherent in healthcare sets such as these were very challenging. However, it is important to realize that the growth of enterprise-wide data is expanding and the technology and infrastructure to connect disparate data collections is increasing in sophistication. The future may hold such innovations as intelligent agent architectures, highly advanced structures, and KDD mechanisms that will make data mining a common practice in large set management.

Conclusion

As health care moves into an increasingly automated future in which massive data warehouses are the norm, innovative discovery-based approaches will become more and more important. This will require adoption of techniques different from the traditional statistical approaches that are common to data analysis in health care today. Health care may find itself in a position similar to other industries, where the importance of prediction may begin to exceed that of explanation. Experiments are a first step in leveraging some of those innovative and challenging methods both to examine large data sets and to ensure that the patient and the clinician, who make up the absolute core of the domain, are the primary beneficiaries of information system solutions.

Questions

1. What is KDD? How does it differ from traditional statistical approaches to data management/analysis?
2. Name the five basic steps of KDD.
3. Name and describe two commonly used data mining approaches.

References

Abbott P. *Predicting Long-Term Care Admissions: A Connectionist Approach to Knowledge Discovery in the Minimum Data Set.* Doctoral dissertation, University of Maryland, Baltimore, 1999. Dissertation Abstracts International, in press.

Brachman R, Anand T. The process of knowledge discovery in databases. In: Fayyad U, Piatetesky-Shapiro G, Smyth P, eds. *Advances in Knowledge Discovery and Data Mining.* Cambridge, MA: MIT Press, 1996;37–57.

Eckhardt W. Limits to knowledge. *Knowledge: Creation, Diffusion, Utilization.* 1981;3:1.

Fayyad U, Piatetesky-Shapiro G, Smyth P. From data mining to knowledge discovery. In: Fayyad U, Piatetesky-Shapiro G, Smyth P, eds. *Advances in Knowledge Discovery and Data Mining.* Cambridge, MA: MIT Press, 1996;1–36.

Miller G. The magical number seven, plus or minus two: some limits on our capacity for processing information. *Psychological Review* 1956;63(2):81–97.

Ohno-Machado L, Musen M. A comparison of two computer-based prognostic systems for AIDS. *Proceedings of the Nineteenth Annual Symposium on Computer Applications in Medical Care.* Philadelphia: Hanley & Belfus, 1995;737–741.

Pauker S, Gorry G, Kassier J, Schwartz W. (1976) Towards the simulation of clinical cognition: taking a present illness by computer. *The American Journal of Medicine* 1976;60:981–996.

Penny W, Frost D. Neural networks in clinical medicine. *Medical Decision Making* 1996;16:386–398.

Simoudis E. Reality check for data mining. *IEEE Expert* 1996;11(5):20–25.

Stevens J. *Applied Multivariate Statistics for the Social Sciences,* 3rd ed. Mahwah, NJ: Lawrence Erlbaum Associates, 1996.

Wreden N. The mother lode: data mining digs deep for business intelligence. *Communications Week* 1997(February 17);43–47.

11
Electronic Imaging: Concept Overview and Application to Nursing

L INDA F ISCHETTI

Electronic imaging, a relatively recent technological development, has received broad and increasing acceptance in healthcare environments. This technology was first used extensively in the field of radiology. Later, it was adopted by the disciplines of gastroenterology, dentistry, dermatology, and other specialities. As electronic imaging begins to play a role in nursing practice, nurses can expect to see it become a major component of a fully developed patient's electronic medical record (EMR). Such a record will seamlessly integrate images obtained from radiology, consulting services, clinical pathology, nursing, and other patient care environments. The entire EMR will be instantaneously available for viewing throughout the healthcare delivery system without requiring access to a physical record. Integrating electronic images into the medical record can facilitate interprofessional communication and improve the quality and continuity of health care as a patient moves from one treatment environment to another.

The advent of electronic imaging technology in the nursing environment provides special opportunities for—and places special demands upon—nursing informaticists. They must develop clinical tools and clinical applications that allow this technology to be effectively and safely implemented in daily patient care routines. To ensure that the applications developed will support rather than hinder nursing practice, the nurse informaticist must have a basic understanding of electronic imaging concepts as well as patient care processes. Thus, the nurse informaticist is challenged not only to understand technical concepts and nursing processes but also to acquire knowledge of rapidly evolving technologies and their capabilities. The nurse informaticist who designs and implements an imaging program must constantly evaluate new concepts and products and adapt them for practical application.

Basics of Electronic Imaging

Image quality is influenced by the technical characteristics and handling of images through the processes of acquisition/capture, storage, and display. Image quality is of concern in all imaging systems; the higher the image quality, the greater the amount of potentially useful information that is captured and made available to an image user. To facilitate the expanding role of imaging in the healthcare environment, a basic understanding of image acquisition/capture, storage, and display is necessary. Additionally, electronic image handling in the healthcare environment adds unique conditions related to security and editing. Images, whether they are from the visible light spectrum (e.g., a picture of something that can be seen by the human eye) or gray scale (e.g., an X-ray), have the same stages of flow through an information system.

Image Types

In the healthcare field, most images are classified into two types, depending on the original image generation process. Images that are obtained by visible light, such as pictures taken by a camera or camcorder, are called *visible light images*. The purpose of such images is to provide an observer with the same image an individual could have seen when the image was first captured, except at a later time or a different location.

Images originally produced by means other than reflection of visible light are usually classified as *gray scale images*. Typical methods of producing such images are ultrasound, X-rays, CAT, MRI, PET, and SPECT. Although such images are not produced with visible light, they must be displayed by visible light to allow the information to be accessed by human beings. It should be noted that the nomenclature, although standard, is somewhat misleading. Visible light images can be captured, stored, transmitted, and displayed as gray scale images. This would be the case if black and white film were used in an ordinary camera, for example. Also, gray scale images are sometimes converted to pseudo-color images through an intensity/wavelength transformation performed by a computer.

Image Acquisition

When working with images, the terms *acquisition* and *capture* are used interchangeably to refer to the process of generating a representation of what the clinician wants to evaluate or record. This can be done directly from a device that saves all images in a digital file format, or it can be done with the use of a scanner that will digitize traditional films or photographs.

Images can be stored and transmitted digitally only after they have been broken into a large number of small elements called *pixels*. These are almost always arranged as a rectangular array, and the total number of pixels is equal to the number of rows times the number of columns. For each pixel, intensity and/or color is uniform throughout and is given by a digital code. The higher the number of pixels, the better the resolution and appearance of the reconstructed image.

The maximum resolution at the time of capture is determined by the capability of the capture device, but it may be set lower by the user of the device. The higher the number, the larger the digital file. If the image is in color, more bits per pixel are needed to include color information. For example, an image described as $1,024 \times 768 \times 24$ bit has its picture elements arranged in a matrix consisting of 1,024 horizontal rows and 768 vertical columns. Each pixel is capable of recording color information to a depth of 8 bits for each of the three primary light colors, red, green, and blue.

This modest example of pixel rating is already outdated in the consumer marketplace; it is used here because the low numbers are easily comprehensible. Advancing technology is quickly escalating pixel counts. With the increasing resolution comes an increased demand on storage and transmission media. The example of a $1,024 \times 768 \times 24$ bit image requires 2.36 megabytes of storage.

As the fully electronic patient medical record continues to incorporate images and maintain them on-line, there are escalating requirements for storage and display capabilities. The storage and transmission media demands can be reduced by resorting to image compression. This technology exploits the fact that in many portions of most images, large numbers of nearby pixels have very nearly the same brightness or color. Compression algorithms use this similarity to reduce the number of bits needed to store an image.

When a digital file is created, a specific file format must be used. All file types have different methods of organizing and storing the data contained within the file. One of the main considerations for selection of file format is whether the data compression algorithm used is "lossless" or "lossy." The final use or destination of the image also affects the choice of file format.

Image Storage

Storage and archiving of an image is the act of recording the image to a permanent storage media. Frequently, an image is stored in as many as three different places at the same time to meet the demand for database linkage to the EMR, both for clinician viewing and for back-up. For example, the image is stored within an optical jukebox for permanent association with the patient's EMR. It is then placed on a server for short-term storage, which will provide instantaneous delivery of the image in response to user requests, and it is stored within a tape storage system used for back-up and archival purposes.

Image Display

Display of an image involves presenting the image itself, the associated reports, and other patient information to the clinical area where the image is required for patient care. The quality of the image that is produced for the clinician is not solely dependent on the acquisition/capture and storage processes. The actual display device (e.g., a monitor or a printer) where the image will be presented for viewing must be carefully selected to ensure image quality. The display device must be able to reproduce accurately the information that has been captured. If it cannot, crucial information may be lost. For example, if a computer video monitor can display only a 640 × 480 resolution image, capturing the image at a higher resolution will not result in a better image. In this example, not all of the captured data are used in the display process, and the image is degraded. Such degraded views of images may have unintended negative impact in clinical practice by failing to display fine details that might affect diagnosis and evaluation of a condition.

Acquisition/Capture, Storage, and Display Infrastructure

The hardware and software infrastructure for electronic imaging capture, storage, and display most commonly used today is a Picture Archiving and Communication System (PACS). This infrastructure includes an information processing unit, image capture stations, a database for management of images with associated text, storage capabilities, and the ability to display images (Dwyer, 1996). Optimally, healthcare providers can access images stored on the PACS along with a patient's electronic chart from a clinical workstation within their office. When images are available for the patient, the clinician initiates a request for the image that begins a Hospital Information System conversation with the PACS. This is a Digital Imaging and Communications (DICOM) conversation, which requests retrieval of patient images for display at the clinician's workstation (Horii, 1996). Part of this conversation is the translation between the Health Level 7 (Hospital Information System) and the DICOM (Radiology Information System) components.

Image Uses

Once images of patient conditions are captured and stored, these images are available to healthcare providers for documentation, diagnosis, communication, tracking of patient conditions over time, analysis by software programs that quantify the image content, and teleimaging. Documentation, diagnosis, communication, and tracking are existing clinical processes that are enhanced with the use of electronic images. Image analysis is a methodology used to quantify features that otherwise are assessed subjectively. Teleimaging is a means of storing and forwarding an image in order to communicate a patient condition, request a consultation, or make a remote diagnosis.

Maintaining Image Security

Strategies for capturing, storing, and displaying patient images and patient information must include security features that protect patient confidentiality. Before implementing an imaging program, the nurse informaticist must assess existing network security measures (firewalls) and educate users about the procedures necessary for maintaining security. For instance, clinicians might want to use store and forward technology, in which an image is stored on one computer and transferred to another via e-mail. If the image is to be forwarded outside of the existing network, the organization's information security officer should be consulted to evaluate transmission procedures and to verify that the proposed transmission will not violate the security of the patient data.

Maintaining Image Integrity

Editing images may change the gradations of color, light, intensity, subtleties in brilliance, and other image characteristics. Editing, in this context, refers to the alteration of an original digital file between the point of capture and storage. Traditional photography or medical imaging produced a "hard copy" image that has been quite difficult, if not impossible, for the clinician to alter. In electronic imaging, because the image is purely a digital file constructed of electronic measurements and mathematical calculations, it is easily altered by anyone with direct access to the file. Because electronic images do not have a traditional, physical counterpart to use to benchmark color, density, and saturation for comparison purposes, the original digital file should be stored in its unaltered state.

Most imaging applications in health care allow for post-storage manipulation of images that does not change the information contained in the original digitized file. The options available to the viewer of the image usually include the ability to make changes in brightness and contrast, reverse the black/white contrast to show a "negative" image, annotate an area of concern, and perform other functions that can be either discarded after the viewer has finished or saved as associated information. Nurse imaging programs that allow for the editing of images without securing the integrity of the original digitized file raise questions about the ethics of making changes to patient data.

General Healthcare Electronic Imaging Concepts

Development of Standards

For the disciplines that have been integrating electronic imaging into their practice, standards have been developed to ensure interoperability of equipment and appropriate image use by the clinician. The first of these issues, the development of imaging equipment, is monitored by the American College of Radiology and the National Electrical Manufacturers Association (ACR-NEMA) who have written the DICOM standards for functionality and interoperability of PACS based on clinician functional requirements. This DICOM standard is used by vendors as they develop PACS (Horii, 1996).

The development of DICOM standards has led to medical equipment that places DICOM headers onto the images that are captured. These headers provide a universal communication language among the various components of a PACS. Vendors traditionally developed proprietary communication protocols for their PACS products, causing interoperability problems (Bidgood et al., 1997; Lou et al., 1995). This proprietary approach meant that the user was required to buy all PACS hardware and software from a single vendor without evaluating various components from different vendors when acquiring and configuring a PACS (Horii, 1996). DICOM is based on entity-relationship models of how data pieces are related to each other. The goal of DICOM 3.0 is to provide a structure for how the components within PACS communicate with each other and how PACS communicate with hospital information systems.

The second issue is the clinical use of images. Healthcare professional associations have developed standards to describe how images are to be handled in different clinical settings. For example, the American College of Radiology has a standard for the use of images in telemedicine that defines equipment requirements and user qualifications. This type of a healthcare professional organization's standards directly affects the clinician's use of and interaction with the patient image.

Radiologists have the longest history of electronic imaging use and the most advanced clinical applications and professional association standards development. Today, nurses are also beginning to apply electronic imaging to clinical practice and share their experiences in the literature (McAfooes, 1997; McGuiness & Axford, 1997). Because of this, nursing professional associations must work to develop and apply standards for use of electronic imaging by nurses.

Nursing informaticists have the responsibility to guide professional nursing associations in the development of these standards. The standards should establish minimum quality requirements for data image capture, storage and archiving, and display. They should also address what additional patient data must be presented with the electronic image to create a sufficiently complete packet of information for clinical evaluations and decision-making. Standards for competence, expertise, and the ethical handling of such information also must be established.

The rapid evolution of technological concepts and terminology in the field of electronic imaging make it difficult to write standards that will remain applicable as the field advances. Therefore, nursing informaticists should probably focus their writing more on the establishment of criteria for general use and less on technology standards that will quickly be rendered obsolete by technological advances.

Telemedicine Applications

Telemedicine imaging applications for radiologists are compliant with the American College of Radiology telemedicine standards. Applications for visible light imaging are becoming widespread across many disciplines. At this time, there are no universal professional association standards for maintaining the integrity of the images.

Some telemedicine vendors have responded to this need for high-quality images displayed at geographically dispersed sites. Their products have high bandwidth data lines, capture equipment with very high-density resolution, storage capabilities with minimal data compression, and high-pixel rating display stations. Current marketing efforts for these products are primarily directed toward radiology and dermatology practitioners, not to nurses. Still, advanced practice nurses could benefit from use of these high-end systems when performing remote consultation or remote diagnosis.

Many telehealth applications currently used by nurses are systems that transmit many types of information, such as real-time video, audio, pulse oximetry, or blood pressure, as an analog signal over standard telephone lines. Series of static images are transmitted per second, with the frequency measured as a refresh rate. This type of transmission allows the nurse to interact with the patient, visualize wounds, watch the patient take medication, and observe other patient functions.

Naturally, the vendors and nurses would want to save some of this information for future comparison. To do this, they would convert analog images into digital files. This type of telehealth image should be carefully evaluated for image integrity related to resolution, data compression, and display issues. Before using images for remote clinical decision-making or remote diagnoses, research is needed to validate the ability of the imaging system to accurately represent the clinical condition and support diagnosis. Both nurse practitioners and their clients must be protected from the overuse and even misapplication of unproven technology. Nurse informaticists can participate in encouraging nurse professional associations to begin research and standards development in this area.

Image Analysis

Image analysis is a computer technique that takes advantage of the quantifiable data present in a digital film but imperceptible to the human eye. This technique has broad application in gray scale images generated from such scans as X-rays and mammograms (Giger & MacMahon, 1996). Electrical engineers have begun to evaluate whether or not image analysis is applicable within visible light imaging. It has been demonstrated that images of wounds captured under identical conditions using color calibration and measurement standardization can establish an objective value to subjective clinical assessment factors, such as erythema. (Hansen et al., 1997).

McGuiness and Axford (1997) have performed initial research about the clinical usefulness of wound images. Their recommendations for future research mention issues related to color calibration and image analysis to quantify erythema of clinical conditions. A great deal of research and development is still required in this area of study. Once images are analyzed and objective data are available to the clinician, the effect on clinical decision-making and patient outcomes could be measured with research methodologies. Future use of image analysis requires that the data currently lost by data compression techniques be preserved for objective evaluation.

Overview of Electronic Imaging in Nursing Literature

A compelling link between nurses and imaging is found in the interpretation of Ball et al. (1997, p. 40) of Reinhold Haux's first aim of his "Ten Aims and Tasks for Informatics":

Aim 1: Diagnostics: the visible body. Remote access to high quality digital images support new modes of care delivery. These can minimize cost, ensure access to specialists, and create new requirements for coordinating and managing care. Other developments include the incorporation of images of various types into electronic patient records. These advances will enhance the information available to caregivers, including nurses, and impact the ways in which they deliver care.

This visionary statement establishes a benchmark for future nursing imaging strategies. This type of foresight can motivate nursing leaders to prioritize the development and adaptation of quality imaging applications for use by nurse clinicians.

The first time the topic of imaging appears in the nursing informatics literature is in 1993, when Carol Romano published an article entitled "Imaging: An Innovative Technology." This article is a pioneering work that educates the nursing informatics community about general principles of electronic imaging that can apply in various ways, such as the scanning of documents or medical applications.

An example of innovative use of electronic imaging by nurses is described by McGuiness and Axford (1997). The foundation of this work is based on an assumption that data are more accurate when they are collected closer to the source that generates them. Building on this assumption, they used digital images of wounds captured daily over four days to test the diagnostic and treatment recommendations of both novice and expert nurses. Their hypothesis was that because traditional text documentation did not represent the visual/spatial assessment that took place in the clinical environment, electronic imaging had potential for better representing clinical assessment conditions.

The McGuiness and Axford (1997) study used experienced and novice nurses who were shown postsurgical ostomy images. Results indicated that expert and novice nurses who were shown only the day four image were more likely to have a correct diagnosis than were those shown the images from days two through four. The nurses who had the advantage of having all of the images to review were more confident of their diagnosis, even though they were more consistent in their inaccuracy. The novice nurses had better ratings for diagnosis, but the expert nurses were more accurate in the recommended treatment. It was suggested that the presence of digital images of wounds over time decreased the importance of the acquired clinical skill of long-term memory of clinical conditions. Although this work was performed in an academic rather than a clinical environment, it has direct clinical implications. The study may become a cornerstone for future nursing research that addresses the usefulness of images in a clinical setting.

Incorporating Electronic Imaging into Nursing Practice

Planning for incorporation of electronic imaging into nursing practice involves preliminary analysis as well as system selection. The preliminary analysis should identify the types of clinical nursing environments and the types of communications (text or verbal) between the environments that can be enhanced by imaging. For example, would a nurse practitioner-run clinic at a remote site that currently receives only written radiology reports benefit from having the actual digitized radiology images displayed? Can nurses better document the clinical condition upon which their decisions are made by using patient images? These types of practices will become more common as electronic images become more prevalent within clinical environments. This analysis of nursing need must be completed before system selection can be done.

System selection criteria should require support for image capture by nurses outside of radiology. This includes but is not limited to the ability to configure capture stations in various clinical environments and remote sites. The imaging system should interface with standard commercial off-the-shelf equipment and support image data compression, pixel rating, and resolution as specified by various professional organizations.

Selection criteria should include the ability to support the tasks nurses perform to assess, diagnose, identify outcomes, plan, implement, and evaluate patient care (Saba & McCormick, 1996). Additional criteria should include acceptable time requirements for storage and display that will be functional within existing nurse documentation and information-gathering activities. Because electronic imaging applications and PACS systems have traditionally been assembled by radiology departments, nurses may need to work with the radiology departments or consultants who have the experience of previous system configurations to develop an electronic imaging system that supports the dynamic patient care environments where nurses practice.

Innovation in Imaging

Developing innovative technology can be an exhilarating time within an informaticist's career, but innovation also brings risks, both organizational and personal. There are two aspects of innovation to take under consideration: the use of a promising but unproven technology and the organizational culture that supports innovation. When presented with technology that appears to improve existing processes or provide processes that did not previously exist, it is enticing to apply it to clinical use immediately. However, when a new system is implemented, existing procedures should be maintained, even if this produces redundancies.

Benchmarking of the imaging system against others used in disciplines with similar clinical functions can be performed. Once the innovation has been measured for reliability and its effect on patient outcomes, then the duplicative, existing system may be suspended from use. Formative evaluation is more appropriate than summative research because of the lifecycle of current technology. Valid research processes for the purpose of measuring clinical outcomes with prompt reporting of findings in the literature is preferred. Research questions should be phrased to elicit the value of the innovation; they should not be restricted to a singular product evaluation. During any innovation process, the development and research team should keep careful documentation of their experiences, challenges, solutions, and decision process.

The organizational climate that supports innovation is just beginning to be understood in the technology and healthcare environments. The most important requirement is that employees feel safe to explore nontraditional ideas within a climate of acceptance. Rewarding innovation should be based on the process undertaken by the development team, not on the success or failure of the innovation. It is the process of innovation that is important for the growth of new technology applications, not the failure or success of one or two individual projects. Partnering among professionals from diverse disciplines—clinicians, informaticists, engineers, health sciences researchers, vendors, and computer scientists—can help transform an innovation from a spark of an idea into an application with positive, measurable clinical outcomes.

The nurse informaticist has responsibilities to others when innovative technologies are being introduced. Technologies like electronic imaging promise potentially large benefits to the future practice of medicine and nursing. They also promise to create powerful undercurrents of resistance as new demands for learning and organization are introduced. Such disruptions are traumatic even for those who would otherwise support the innovation. In this situation, the nurse informaticist would be well advised to move slowly, test thoroughly before introduction, respond rapidly when flaws or failures inevitably appear, support users beyond the call of duty, and maintain a good sense of humor, even when things are falling apart. If one does this and builds bridges for support across a range of specialties, it is likely that innovations like electronic imaging can be introduced successfully to those who work in the clinical setting and the clients who are served.

Conclusion

Electronic imaging has the potential to support existing nursing practice and offer exciting new possibilities for influencing nurses' clinical decision-making. An understanding of general electronic imaging concepts will help the nurse informaticist adapt this new technology to current and future needs. Nurse informaticists can assist with the continuing development of standards by participating in defining functional requirements for image handling to meet the needs of nurses. Professional association development of standards for the clinical use of images will require partnering with nurse informaticists to produce standards that are both technically accurate and a useful resource for the nurse provider. Nurses are currently reporting experiences with electronic imaging in both academic and clinical settings. The clinical application of electronic imaging, as well as how nursing research defines the clinical usefulness of images, will influence future use of electronic imaging by nurses.

Questions

1. What are the components of a Picture Archiving and Communications System (PACS)?
2. What are the factors that affect images through the acquisition/capture, storage, and display process?
3. How do professional organizations influence the use of electronic images for their clinicians?
4. Briefly outline an implementation plan for an electronic imaging system. Do not research specific equipment, just have fun imagining a "killer app" to support your nurse provider. Include
   A. Nurse processes/environments that can be enhanced with the use of electronic images to justify implementation need

B. Image technical characteristics to be considered in the system specifications
C. The three areas involved in image handling
D. Image security issues

References

Ball MJ, Douglas JV, Hoehn BJ. New challenges for nursing informatics. In: Gerdin U, Tallberg M, Wainwright P, eds. *Nursing Informatics: The Impact of Nursing Knowledge on Health Care Informatics*. Washington, DC: IOS Press, 1997;39–43.

Bidgood WD, Horii SC, Prior FW, Van Syckle DE. Understanding and using DICOM, the data interchange standard for biomedical imaging. *Journal of the American Medical Informatics Association* 1997;4(3):199–212.

Dwyer SJ. Imaging system architectures for picture archiving and communication systems. *Radiologic Clinics of North America* 1996;4(3):495–606.

Giger M, MacMahon H. Image processing and computer-aided diagnosis. *Radiologic Clinics of North America* 1996;34(3):565–596.

Hansen GL, Sparrow EM, Kokate JY, Leland KJ, Iaizzo PA. Wound status evaluation using color image processing. *IEEE Transactions on Medical Imaging* 1997;16(1):78–86.

Horii SC. Image acquisition: sites, technologies, and approaches. *Radiologic Clinics of North America* 1996;34(3):469–494.

Lou SL, Wang J, Moskowitz M, Bazzill T, Huang HK. Methods of automatically acquiring images from digital medical systems. *Computerized Medical Imaging and Graphics* 1995;19(4):369–387.

McAfooes JA. Advances in digital video for electronic media. In: Gerdin U, Tallberg M, Wainwright P, eds. *Nursing Informatics: The Impact of Nursing Knowledge on Health Care Informatics*. Washington, DC: IOS Press, 1997;477–480.

McGuiness B, Axford R. Exploring nursing knowledge by using digital photography. In: Gerdin U, Tallberg M, Wainwright P, eds. *Nursing Informatics: The Impact of Nursing Knowledge on Health Care Informatics*. Washington, DC: IOS Press, 1997;281–287.

Romano CA. Imaging: an innovative technology. *Computers in Nursing* 1993;11(5):222–225.

Saba VK, McCormick KA. *Essentials of Computers for Nurses*, 2nd ed. New York: McGraw-Hill, 1996;246.

Section 2.2
Approaches

12
Informatics and Organizational Change

NANCY M. LORENZI AND ROBERT T. RILEY

It is easy to change the things that nobody cares about. It is difficult to change the things that people do care about—or when they start to care about the things that are changing!

Change is a constant reality in both our work and private lives. Children today take for granted such things as powerful personal computers that we could not even envision at their ages. Our societies, our professions, and our daily work lives are all changing, and the pace of this change appears to be accelerating, not slowing.

Nursing as a profession is undergoing rapid changes, and nursing informatics is a driving force in that change process. It is impossible to introduce a nursing informatics system into an organization without the people in that organization feeling the impact of the change. Informatics is about change—the change of data into information with a possible evolution into knowledge. Data become information only after the data are processed (i.e., altered) in ways that make the data useful for decision-making, and those enhanced decision-making capabilities will inevitably affect the organization. There is a simple but critical circular relationship between the organization, its informatics systems, and the change process. The organization and its people influence, shape, and alter the nature and use of the informatics systems, which in turn influence, shape, and alter the nature, operation, and culture of the organization.

Remember the saying, "Sometimes you get the bear; sometimes the bear gets you"? The analogy in change processes is that if we do not manage our change processes, they will manage us. The lower our feelings of control during the change process, the lower our "resiliency" will be (Conner, 1994). In turn, we will have a lower ability to bounce back from the stresses of the change and to be prepared for the inevitable next change in today's environment.

Change and Informatics

When using a manual system on an inpatient unit, the nurse usually serves as an integrator and reviewer. The physician scribbles something down on a piece of paper that is given to a nurse, unit clerk, or paraprofessional to do something with. A nurse typically "cleans it up" and transmits the information or order to pharmacy, radiology, laboratory, dietary, and so forth. Occasionally the laboratory or pharmacy will call the physician back. However, the nurse normally serves as the conduit for the information flow. When nurses fill this role, they have a total view of what is happening with the patient as they filter and organize information from various sources. This is a classic workflow design. What is the impact when a system is implemented that calls for the physician to enter orders directly into the system?

One Hospital's Experience

Originally presented by Dr. Bernard Horak at a 1993 conference on informatics and change, the following scenario was subsequently adapted by Lorenzi and Riley (1994).

In one hospital, the nurses did not like the new information system. They believed it reduced their role in the overall care process and took them out of the reviewer, case manager, and integrator roles they were trained to fill. The nurses said that their two most important roles were the nurse as integrator and the nurse as reviewer, and the new system usurped both roles.

These nurses became very concerned about the changes. In the old system, the physicians were used to issuing vague or approximate orders. For example, the physicians would scribble "d.c." or "d/c" for discontinue. They would order "X-rays," and the nurses would figure out that posteroanterior and lateral views were wanted. If the physicians tried to enter their orders as they traditionally did, they would either get nothing back or receive something they did not want. The physicians did not know how to order because they had not actually placed orders before. When the physician scribbled an order, the nurse knew the physician, knew exactly what was wanted, and would make it happen. With the new system, this was not possible.

Because there was a significant decrease in the role of the nurse as an integrator and reviewer of care, physicians began to make mistakes that nurses had previously caught, such as ordering incorrect drugs or incorrect dosages. There was lower coordination between the nursing plans and the medical care plans. In their new role, nurses tended to show less initiative in making treatment suggestions. In summary, the second overview and analysis by a trained professional was lost. On the other hand, some positive things did occur. Relieved of the paperwork of ordering, nurses had two to three more hours per day to spend on hands-on patient care.

Using This Scenario

The remainder of this chapter presents both theoretical concepts and practical techniques for dealing with informatics change processes. We suggest that readers try to relate each of the concepts back to this scenario, especially in terms of the role of nursing and nursing informatics in the modern healthcare organization.

Types of Change

Changes within an organization can often be identified as one of four types, with the definite possibility of overlap between two or more:

- Operational—changes in the way that the ongoing operations of the business are conducted, such as the automation of a particular area
- Strategic—changes in the strategic business direction (e.g., moving from an inpatient to an outpatient focus)
- Cultural—changes in the basic organizational philosophies by which the business is conducted (e.g., implementing a Continuous Quality Improvement system)
- Political—changes in staffing occurring primarily for political reasons of various types, such as when new management brings in "trusted" former associates

These four types of change typically have their greatest impacts at different levels of the organization. For example, operational changes tend to have their greatest impacts at the lower levels of the organization, right on the firing line. Personnel at the upper levels may never notice changes that cause significant stress and turmoil to those attempting to implement the changes. On the other hand, the impact of political changes is typically felt most at the higher organizational levels. As the term *political* implies, these changes are typically not made for results-oriented reasons but for reasons such as partisan politics or internal power struggles. When these changes occur in a relatively bureaucratic organization—as they often do—the bottom often does not notice the changes at the top. Patients are seen and the floors are cleaned exactly the same as before. The key point is that performance was not the basis of the change; therefore, the performers are not much affected.

Resistance to Change

It has been said that the only person who welcomes change is a wet baby. It seems to be part of the human makeup to be most comfortable with the status quo unless it is actually inflicting discomfort. Even then, people will often resist a specific change. This is probably the "devil you know is better than the devil you don't know" phenomenon. It is a shock for inexperienced managers the first time they see subordinates resist even a change that they requested.

Resistance Against What?

There can be countless reasons for resistance to change in a given situation, and the term *resistance to change* is often used very broadly. One of the first aspects that must be analyzed in a given situation is the difference between

* Resistance to a particular change and
* Resistance to the perceived changer(s)

In the first case, the resistance is actually directed against the changes in the system. In the second case, the resistance occurs because of negative feelings toward specific units, specific managers, or the organization in general. In this second case, virtually any change would be resisted because of feelings toward those who are perceived in favor of it. Both must be dealt with, but it is critical that we identify the primary one. Otherwise, significant energy can be wasted on fighting the wrong battles.

When a new nursing informatics system is introduced, three factors are very important:

* What is the general organizational climate—positive or negative, cooperative or adversarial?
* What has been the quality of the process used to implement previous informatics systems?
* What has been the technical quality of the informatics systems previously implemented?

Even if we are new to an organization, we inevitably inherit some of the organizational climate and history. Negative "baggage" of this type can be a frustrating burden that adds significantly to the challenge of successfully implementing a new system. On the other hand, the ability to meet this type of challenge is a differentiating factor for truly skilled implementers.

Intensity of Resistance

Resistance can vary from the trivial to the ferocious. Also, the very perception of resistance can vary widely from one observer to another. One might perceive an end user who asks many questions as being very interested and aggressively seeking knowledge. Another might see the same person as a troublemaker who should just "shut up and listen!"

We can safely assume that every significant health informatics implementation is going to encounter some resistance; however, the intensity can vary widely. In an organization with decent morale and a history of managing changes reasonably well, significant numbers of the people may be initially neutral toward a particular proposed systems change. However, there will still be a negative component to be managed. At the very least, this negative component must be prevented from growing. In other situations, the proportions of positive, negative, and neutral may vary widely.

The Cast of Characters

For any given change, people can occupy a wide range of roles that will strongly influence their perceptions of the change and their reaction to it. As on the stage, some people may occasionally play more than one role. In other cases, the roles are unique. Unless we clearly identify both the players and their roles in any change situation, we risk making decisions and taking action based on generalizations that are not true for some of the key players. The following categories provide one way of looking at the various roles involved in an overall change process.

- The initiator or instigator perceives the problem situation or opportunity and conceptualizes the change to be made in response.
- The approver or funder is the power figure who blesses and financially supports the proposed change.
- The champion or cheerleader is the visible, enthusiastic advocate for the change. The champion constantly tries to rally support for the change and maintain that support during periods of adversity.
- The facilitator attempts to assist in smoothing the organizational change process. The facilitator is sometimes involved from the beginning and sometimes is only called in for disaster relief once the change process has gone awry.
- The developer or builder is responsible for the technical aspects of the change (e.g., developing the new informatics system). These aspects can range from the broad technical conceptualization to the narrowest of technical details.
- The installer is responsible for implementing the change, including the necessary training and support activities.
- The doer is the "changee"—the person who has to perform his or her work in the changed environment.
- The obstructionist is a guardian of the status quo and typically conducts guerrilla warfare against the change. If the obstructionist is also a doer, the reason may arise from a personal fear of the change. However, the obstructionism may also arise from forces such as political infighting (e.g., over who gets the credit) or from institutional conflicts such as union resistance to a labor-saving system.
- The customer is the beneficiary or victim of the change in terms of altered levels of service, cost, and so forth.

- The observer does not perceive that he or she will be immediately affected by this change but observes with interest. These observations often affect strongly how the observer will react if placed in the doer role in the future.
- The ignorer perceives that this change has no personal implications and is indifferent to it. In the broadest sense, this category also includes all those who are unaware of the change.

An overview term often applied to all these roles is *stakeholders*. With the exception of the ignorers, all the categories have some stake or interest in the quality of the change and the change implementation process. The roles are subject to change, especially during a change process that extends over some time. For example, an initial ignorer might hear rumblings of discontent within the system and change to an observer, at least until the feelings of angst subside.

For those implementing change, the following steps are critical:

- Identifying what roles they themselves are occupying in the process
- Identifying what roles the others involved in the process are playing, being careful to recognize multiple roles
- Identifying carefully which role the speaker is assuming whenever communicating with those playing multiple roles
- Monitoring throughout the process whether any roles are changing

Magnitudes of Change

Change—like beauty—is in the eye of the beholder. A proposed change that virtually terrorizes one person may be a welcome alleviation of boredom to the next person. Also, the types and magnitudes of reaction are often difficult for an "outsider" to predict. When working with change and change management, it often helps to have a simple way of classifying the types and sizes of change.

Microchanges and Megachanges

A practical model that we frequently use divides changes into microchanges and megachanges, with no great attempt at elaborate definitions. A simple rule of thumb can be used to differentiate between the two: Microchanges are differences in degree, and megachanges are differences in kind.

In an information system, for example, modifications, enhancements, improvements, and upgrades would typically be microchanges, whereas a new system or a very major revision of an existing one would be a megachange. This scheme works surprisingly well in communicating within organizations as long as we remember that one person's microchange can easily be another person's megachange. Later in this chapter, we present a more rigorous analysis of the magnitude of change, which can be used when necessary.

Classic Change Theories

The rate of change in virtually all organizations is escalating, and health-care organizations—after a slow start—are no exception. The phrase *change management* has become fairly common, appearing in management articles everywhere.

Change management is the process by which an organization moves to its future state—its vision. Whereas traditional planning processes delineate the steps on the journey, change management attempts to facilitate that journey. Therefore, creating change starts with creating a vision for change and then empowering individuals to act as change agents to attain that vision. The empowered change management agents need plans that are (1) a total systems approach, (2) realistic, and (3) future oriented. Change management encompasses the effective strategies and programs to enable the champions to achieve the new vision. Today's change management strategies and techniques derive from the theoretical work of several pioneers in the change area.

Early Group Theories

In 1974, Watzlawick, Weakland, and Fisch published their now classic book, *Change: Principles of Problem Formation and Problem Resolution*. Theories about change had long existed. However, Watzlawick et al. (1974) found that most of the theories of change were philosophical and derived from the areas of mathematics and physics. Watzlawick and his coauthors selected two theories from the field of mathematical logic upon which to base their beliefs about change. They selected the theory of groups and the theory of logical types. Their goal of reviewing the theories of change was to explain the accelerated phenomenon of change that they were witnessing. Let us briefly examine the two theories that they reviewed to develop their change theory.

Only mathematicians or physicists can fully appreciate the more sophisticated implications of the theory of groups. Its basic postulates concern the relationships between parts and wholes. According to the theory, a group has several properties, including members that share one common characteristic. These members can be numbers, objects, concepts, events, or whatever else one wants to draw together in such a group, as long as they have at least one common denominator. Another property of a group is the ability to combine the members of the group into a number of varying sequences and have the same combinations. The theory of groups gives a model for the types of change that transcend a given system.

The theory of logical types begins with the concept of collections of "things" that are united by a specific characteristic common to all of them. For example, humankind is the name for all individuals, but humankind is not a specific individual. Any attempt to change one in terms of the other does not work and leads to nonsense and confusion. For example, the economic behavior of the population of a large city cannot be understood in terms of the behavior of one person multiplied by four million. A population of four million people is not just quantitatively but also qualitatively different from an individual. Similarly, although the individual members of a species are usually endowed with very specific survival mechanisms, the entire species may race headlong toward extinction—and the human species is probably no exception.

The theory of groups gave Watzlawick's group the framework for thinking about the kind of change that can occur within a system that itself stays invariant. The theory of logical types is not concerned with what goes on inside a class, but gave the authors a framework for considering the relationship between member and class and the peculiar metamorphosis that is in the nature of shifts from one logical level to the next higher. From this, they concluded that there are two different types of change: one that occurs within a given system that itself remains unchanged and one that changes the system itself. For example, a person having a nightmare can do many things in his dream—hide, fight, scream, jump off a cliff, and so forth. But no change from any one of these behaviors to another would terminate the nightmare. Watzlawick et al. (1974) concluded that this is a first-order change. The one way out of a dream involves a change from dreaming to waking. Waking is no longer a part of the dream, but a change to an altogether different state. To summarize:

- First-order change is a variation in the way processes and procedures have been done within a given system, leaving the system itself relatively unchanged. Some examples are creating new reports, creating new ways to collect the same data, and refining existing processes and procedures.
- Second-order change occurs when the system itself is changed. This type of change usually occurs as the result of a strategic change or a major crisis, such as a threat against system survival. Second-order change involves a redefinition or reconceptualization of the business of the organization and the way it is to be conducted. In the medical area, changing from a full paper medical record to a full electronic medical record would represent a second-order change, just as automated teller machines redefined the way that many banking functions are conducted worldwide.

These two orders of change represent extremes. First order involves doing better what we now do, whereas second order radically changes the core ways we conduct business or even the basic business itself.

Golembiewski et al. (1976) added another level of change, defining middle-order change as lying somewhere between the extremes of first- and second-order change. Middle-order change "represents a compromise; the magnitude of change is greater than first order change, yet it neither affects the critical success factors nor is strategic in nature" (Golembiewski et al., 1976). An example of a middle-order change might be the introduction of an electronic mail system into an organization. There is an organization-wide impact, but there is no reconceptualization of the basic business. E-mail is more of a tool for operational and communications efficiency.

Some personality types welcome changes that they perceive will make their jobs easier, whereas other personality types use their day-to-day work rituals to build their comfort zones. Personnel in one unit in a medical center started to code all of their continuing medical education courses with ICD9 codes. Even though these codes were never used and took a great deal of time to complete, the organization did not want to change the process as time passed because "we have always done it this way." The old process lasted through two directors. When a new director attempted to change the process, there was definite resistance to this change.

The five most important words to an individual involved in any change process are "How will this affect me?" This is true regardless of the level or degree of change or the person's organizational position. The most traumatic changes are obviously in the second-order change category, but one person might perceive changes in the first or middle order as more traumatic than another person might perceive a second-order change. One of the challenges for the change manager is successfully managing these perceptions. How the change manager implements the process of change can have a decided effect on the resistance factors.

Although Watzlawick et al. (1974) comprehensively presented the theories of change and offered their model of levels of change, they did not offer practical day-to-day strategies. We are interested in effective strategies for managing change and have reviewed many social science theories to determine the psychology behind the change management concepts and strategies that are used widely today. We believe that today's successful change management strategies emanate from several theories in the areas of psychology and sociology. Small group theories and field theories provide the antecedents of today's successful change management practices.

Small-Group Theories

The primary group is one of the classic concepts of sociology, and many sociological theories focus on small-group analysis and the interaction process analysis. Small-group theories help us to understand not only how to make things more successful but also how to analyze when things go wrong. For example, Bales (1954) presented in the *Harvard Business Review* a practical application of small-group research. Applying small-group principles to running a meeting, Bales makes the following suggestions:

- If possible, restrict committees to seven members.
- Place all members so that they can readily communicate with every other member.
- Avoid committees as small as two or three if a perceived power problem between members is likely to be critical.
- Select committee members who are likely to participate in varying amounts. A group with all very active participants or all very passive participants is difficult to manage.

We have all seen small-group behavior at work. For example, a job candidate is interviewed by a number of people. Information is then collected from the interviewers and is shared with a search committee. The search committee selects its top candidate, and that person is hired. If the person hired does not work out, a member of the search committee may very well say, "I knew that Mary would not work out, but I didn't say anything because everyone seemed to like her."

Many of the changes that new technology brings are discussed, reviewed, and debated by groups of people who usually fall within the small-group framework. If negative sentiments about a product or service are stated by a member of the group who is an opinion leader, the less vocal people often will not challenge the dominant opinion. For example, a medium-sized organization was selecting a local area network system. Although the senior leader wanted one system, some of the other people not only had other suggestions but also had documentation of the superior qualities of another system. During the meeting to decide which system to purchase, the senior leader stated his views first and quite strongly. Several of the lower-level staff members started to confront the senior person; however, when there was no support from any of the other people present, they did not express their strong preferences for their system of choice. When the system finally arrived, the senior leader's initial enthusiasm had dwindled. He then confronted the technology people as to why they had not made him aware of the shortcomings of the system selected.

These examples illustrate a key change management requirement: to effectively manage change, it is imperative for change agents to understand how people behave in groups and especially in small groups.

Field Theory

Kurt Lewin and his students are credited with combining theories from psychology and sociology into the field theory in social psychology (Deutsch & Krauss, 1965). Lewin focused his attention on motivation and the motivational concepts that underlie an individual's behavior. Lewin believed that there is tension within a person whenever a psychological need or an intention exists, and the tension is released only when the need or intention is fulfilled. The tension may be positive or negative. These positive and negative tension concepts were translated into a more refined understanding of conflict situations and, in turn, what Lewin called "force fields."

Lewin indicated that there are three fundamental types of conflict:

- The individual stands midway between two positive goals of approximately equal strength. A classic metaphor is the donkey starving between two stacks of hay because of the inability to choose. In information technology, if there are two "good" systems to purchase or options to pursue, then we must be willing to choose.
- The individual stands between two approximately equal negative goals. This certainly has been a conflict within many organizations wishing to purchase or build a health informatics system. A combination of the economics, the available technologies, and the organizational issues may well mean that the organization's informatics needs cannot be satisfied with any of the available products—whether purchased or developed in-house. Thus the decision-makers must select an information system that they know will not completely meet their needs. Their choice will probably be the lesser of two evils.
- The individual is exposed to opposing positive and negative forces. This conflict is very common in healthcare organizations today, especially regarding health informatics. This conflict usually occurs between the system's users and the information technology people or the financial people.

People can easily be overwhelmed by change, especially within large organizations where they may perceive they have little or no voice in or control over the changes they perceive are descending upon them. The typical response is fight or flight, not cooperation. Managers often interpret such human resistance to change as "stubbornness" or "not being on the team"—a reaction that solves nothing in terms of reducing resistance to change or gaining acceptance of it. Many managers do not realize that they are regarded as imposing "life-threatening" changes and establishing "no-win" adversarial relationships between management and those below in the organization.

Small-group theory is highly applicable in nursing informatics because of the way that medical environments are organized. The care of the patient or the education of students entails many small groups. Members of these groups converse and share information and feelings, and strong opinion leaders can sway others to their way of thinking relatively easily.

Kurt Lewin's field theory allows a diagramming of the types of conflict situations commonly found in health care. In this way, the typical approach-avoidance forces can be visualized (Lorenzi & Riley, 1994). For example, if I accept this new system, what will it mean to me? What will it mean to my job? Will I even have a job? How will it change my role? Will this new system diminish my importance? These anxieties are very clear and very real to the people within the system. One person's microchanges are often another person's megachanges. As the system designers think they are making a minor change to enhance the total system, an individual end user may see the change as a megachange and resist it vehemently. When designing the total "people" strategy for any system, it is important to involve the people from the very beginning and to clearly understand how groups function within the organization.

All of these social science theories assist the change management leader in understanding some of the underlying behavior issues as they bring health informatics technology into today's complex health systems.

Practical Change Management Strategies

Change management is the process of assisting individuals and organizations in passing from an old way of doing things to a new way of doing things. Therefore, a change process should both begin and end with a visible acknowledgment or celebration of the impending or just completed change. According to James Belasco (1990):

Our culture is filled with empowering transitions. New Year's Eve parties symbolize the ending of one year and the hope to be found in the one just beginning. Funerals are times to remember the good points of the loved one and the hope for new beginnings elsewhere. Parties given to retiring or leaving employees are celebrations of the ending of the employee's past status and the hope for the new opportunities to be found in the new status.

Based on our research, there is no single change management strategy that is effective in every situation. It is essential that the change management leaders take the time to know the desired state (vision-goal) and the relevant characteristics of the particular organization. Then they must develop the appropriate strategies and plans to help facilitate the desired state.

Over the years, we have evolved a core model for the major process of change management. There are many options within this model, but we believe that it is helpful for change leaders to have an overview map in mind as they begin to implement new information technology systems. The five-stage model that has proven effective for reducing barriers to technology change begins with an assessment and information-gathering phase (Lorenzi et al., 1990).

Assessment

The assessment phase of this model is the foundation for determining the organizational and user knowledge and ownership of the health informatics system that is under consideration. Ideally, this phase of the model begins even before the planning for the technological implementation of the new system. The longer the delay, the harder it will be to successfully manage the change and gain ultimate user ownership.

There are two parts to the assessment phase. The first is to inform all potentially affected people, in writing, of the impending change. This written information need not be lengthy or elaborate, but it will alert everyone to the changes in process.

The second part involves collecting information, with both surveys and interviews, from those involved in the change. The survey instrument should be sent to randomly selected members of the affected group. One person in ten might be appropriate if the affected group is large. Five to ten open-ended questions should assess the individuals' current perceptions of the potential changes, their issues of greatest concern about these changes, and their suggestions to reduce those concerns. Recording and analyzing the responders' demographics will allow more in-depth analysis of the concerns raised by these potentially affected people.

In the face-to-face interviews with randomly selected people at all levels of the affected portions of the organization, it is important to listen to the stories the people are telling and to assess their positive and negative feelings about the proposed health informatics system. These interviews should help in ascertaining the current levels of positive and negative feelings; what each person envisions the future will be, both with and without the new system; what each interviewee could contribute to making that vision a reality; and in what ways he or she might contribute to the future success of the new system. These interviews provide critical insights for the actual implementation plan. Often those people interviewed become advocates—and sometimes even champions—of the new system, thus easing the change process considerably.

An alternative to the one-on-one interview is the focus-group session. These allow anywhere from five to seven people from across the organization to share their feelings and ideas about the current and new systems.

Feedback and Options

The information obtained must now be analyzed, integrated, and packaged for presentation, both to top management and to those directly responsible for the technical implementation. This is a key stage for understanding the strengths and weaknesses of the current plans, identifying the major organizational areas of both excitement and resistance (positive and negative forces), identifying the potential stumbling blocks, understanding the vision the staff holds for the future, and reviewing the options suggested by the staff for making the vision come true. If this stage occurs early enough in the process, data from the assessment stage can be given to the new systems developers for review. When designing a model, this phase is important in establishing—and communicating—that the organization does learn from the inputs of its staff and that it acts strategically in the decision and implementation processes.

Strategy Development

The development phase of the model allows those responsible for the change to use the information collected to develop effective change strategies from an organizational perspective. These strategies must focus on a visible, effective process to "bring on board" the affected people within the organization. This could include newsletters, focus groups, discussions, one-on-one training, and confidential "hand holding," which can be especially important for professionals such as physicians who may not wish to admit ignorance or apprehension about the new system.

Implementation

The implementation phase of our model refers to the implementation of the change management strategies determined to be needed for the organization, not to the technical implementation of the new system. The implementation of the change strategies described above must begin before the actual implementation of the new system. These behaviorally focused efforts consist of a series of steps, including informing and working with the people involved in a systematic and timely manner. This step-by-step progression toward the behavioral change desired and the future goals is important to each individual's acceptance of the new system. This is the mechanism for tying together the new technology implementation action plan with the behavioral strategies.

Reassessment

Six months after the new system is installed, a behavioral-effects data-gathering reassessment should be conducted. This stage resembles the initial assessment stage—written surveys and one-on-one or focus group interviews. Data gathered from this stage allow measurement of the acceptance of the new system, which provides the basis for fine tuning. This process also serves as input to the evaluation of the implementation process. It ensures all the participants that their inputs and concerns are still valued and sought, even though the particular implementation has already occurred.

Conclusion

It is not always easy to know exactly why a particular individual, subgroup, or group resists change. However, experience shows that an intelligent application of the basic five-step change model—coupled with a sound technological implementation plan—leads to more rapid and more productive introductions of technology into organizations. This change process can be expensive in terms of time and energy, but nowhere near the cost of implementing a technical system that never gains real user acceptance.

Perhaps most importantly, overall success requires an emotional commitment to success on the part of all involved. We need the new system to be "our" system—not "your" system, "my" system, or "their" system. The people must believe the project is being done for the right reasons—namely, to further the delivery of higher quality, more cost-effective health care. If a project is generally perceived to be aimed at just "saving a quick buck" or boosting someone's ego or status, it is doomed to fail.

An MCI television commercial depicted a book editor—faced with adapting to major informatics changes—commenting that "Art is constant; tools change." In the same vein, the ideals of nursing are constant; the tools change. The challenge facing nursing informatics is to successfully implement those new tools in organizations that often do not welcome them.

Questions

1. Using your own words, define change management.
2. What might be some ways to help people celebrate remembering the past and moving to the future?
3. In the "Cast of Characters," which roles are nurses at various levels in the organizational hierarchy most likely to play? Why? What roles are nurses least likely to play? Why?
4. Why is the "feedback and options" phase so important in the change management model presented?
5. For the change scenario presented in this chapter, create a detailed change management plan that you think would lead to better results than those that were described in the scenario.

References

Bales RF. In conference. *Harvard Business Review* 1954;32:44–50.

Belasco JA. *Teaching the Elephant to Dance: Empowering Change in Your Organization*. New York: Crown Publishers, 1990.

Conner DR. Bouncing back. *Sky*. 1994(September):30–34.

Deutsch M, Krauss RM. *Theories in Social Psychology*. New York: Basic Books, 1965.

Golembiewski RT, Billingsley K, Yeager S. Measuring change and persistence in human affairs: types of change generated by OD designs. *Journal of Applied Behavioral Science* 1976;12:133–157.

Lorenzi NM, Mantel MI, Riley RT. Preparing your organizations for technological change. *Healthcare Informatics* 1990;December:33–34.

Lorenzi NM, Riley RT. *Organizational Aspects of Health Informatics: Managing Technological Change*. New York: Springer-Verlag, 1994;228–229.

Watzlawick P, Weakland JH, Fisch R. *Change: Principles of Problems Formulation and Problem Resolution*. New York: WW Norton, 1974.

13
Nursing Informatics Consultancy: How to Select a Nursing Informatics Consultant

EMILY M. WELEBOB

Healthcare reform continues to drive rapid change in the delivery and management of healthcare services. Whether organizations are meeting internal and external demands by selecting and implementing a new computer information system, assessing administrative and clinical workflow processes, or preparing an information systems strategic plan, they may require the assistance of a consultant. In 1993, 80,000 consultants in all industries sold $17 billion in services; this was up 10 percent from the previous year (Norwood, 1998). The demand for consulting expertise continues to grow as healthcare organizations assess new technologies and implement new delivery methods to improve access, delivery, and management of services.

How do healthcare organizations keep up with these changes, as well as design and implement the appropriate solution(s)? One answer is to seek and retain a nursing informatics (NI) consultant to help the organization with healthcare delivery and management solutions.

The Role of the Nursing Informatics Consultant

Nursing skills and experience have far-reaching applicability to other roles besides the traditional nursing role of delivering direct patient care. One of these new nursing roles is the nursing informatics consultant. In an NI role survey (descriptive study; n = 48; 40 percent response rate) completed by the American Nursing Informatics Association (ANIA) in November 1996, the majority (77 percent) of NI professionals practice in the hospital setting (Rosen & Routon, 1998). Another 12.5 percent were practicing in an NI role with vendors (8.3 percent) or consulting firms (4.2 percent) (Rosen & Routon, 1998).

Consulting is the process by which a person or group of persons (a consulting firm) uses specialized knowledge to help a client achieve a stated outcome (Biech, 1999). A consultant is a specialist within a professional area who completes the work necessary to achieve the client's desired outcome(s) (Biech, 1999). A nursing informatics consultant is a specialist who connects NI (nursing practice, computer science, and information management) with consulting skills and abilities.

Healthcare trends have driven an increased demand for nurse informaticians. These trends include staff downsizing, heightened business competitiveness, rapid and constant change, and advanced nursing education.

Staff Downsizing

Due to decreased utilization of inpatient hospital care and the resulting proliferation of ambulatory services, healthcare organizations have reorganized, reducing the need for traditional bedside nursing care. This has led to an increasing number of opportunities for nurses to explore the role of nursing informatics and consulting.

Heightened Business Competitiveness

Healthcare organizations are evaluating their operations and workflow processes to reduce costs and streamline healthcare delivery. Organizations are looking for consultants with knowledge and skills to help them achieve their business goals and remain competitive. For example, the emergence of integrated delivery systems is pressing clinical information systems to evolve from departmental systems to enterprise-wide systems. Integration of disparate organizations is a multifaceted process. Nurses are often uniquely positioned to help, due to their understanding of the care delivery process and the appropriate tools to manage information.

Rapid and Constant Change

The pace of change in health care is increasing. Healthcare organizations need to respond quickly and implement appropriate solutions while managing the changes those solutions bring. They may lack the time or resources to conduct a job search, hire an individual with specific skills, and allow for that person to matriculate into the organization as an employee. The consultant with the appropriate knowledge and skills can be hired and brought up to speed at the start of the project.

Advanced Nursing Education

Computer and healthcare information management knowledge and skills are highly marketable qualifications. Nursing education answered this market demand several years ago with the introduction of nursing informatics concentrations and graduate degree programs. Today, the American Nurses Association offers an NI advanced certification.

When to Employ a Nursing Informatics Consultant

The rapidly changing state of health care has increased the opportunities for nursing informatics consultants. Let us examine a scenario illustrating a case for hiring an NI consultant to assist with an operating room information systems selection project. Organizations seek the assistance of a consultant for this type of project for several reasons, enumerated below.

Savings

A one-time expenditure for a consultant may be smaller than the salaries and benefits paid to internal employees. Rather than hire a permanent employee, it may be more cost-effective to hire a consultant with specialized skills that are needed temporarily. A consultant can be hired as an experienced, temporary resource to work on a specific problem and reach resolution with efficiency. In this example, the NI consultant would have experience and knowledge in the operating room information systems vendor market, systems selection methodology, and project management.

Independent View and Objectivity

The organization may seek an outsider's viewpoint because of political and hierarchical issues and lack of experience and expertise. A consultant can help diffuse some of the risk inherent in change situations or high-profile projects. Consultants bring experience and can look at a problem in an unbiased manner. The NI consultant participating in the operating room information systems selection is unbiased about specific operating room information system vendors. He or she can act to resolve differences and assist in making a vendor recommendation as a nonpartisan individual if the project team members have a bias toward a particular information system.

Expertise

The explosion of both information technology and emerging healthcare delivery models has created change in the fundamental principles and processes of healthcare delivery. This rapid growth rate and large magnitude of change makes it difficult for any organization to keep informed of all the initiatives occurring throughout the healthcare industry. The consultant can expose the project staff to different practices from the healthcare field and share "lessons learned" from organizations with similar circumstances. During the operating room information systems selection, the NI consultant can tap into outside resources and vendor contacts and bring experience to the project from past participation on a similar project at another client site.

Acquisition of Human Resources

A lack of human resources and experience may restrict an organization's ability to directly employ all the personnel necessary to complete a specific project. Internal personnel may not have the time to complete special projects or research activities. Hiring a consultant to manage a specific area for a limited amount of time can fill leadership voids while an employment search is being conducted. The NI consultant can be part of the operating room information system selection just long enough to bring market and systems knowledge, conduct the system selection process, and bring the project to successful completion. The NI consultant role may be terminated once the project is completed—as in the example, once the operating room information systems vendor is selected, the project is completed and the NI consultant has achieved the project goal(s).

Choosing a Nursing Informatics Consultant

Knowing organizational requirements and the reasons behind them is essential when choosing a consultant. Nursing informatics consultants can be found as individual consultants, within specialty healthcare consulting firms who employ experienced healthcare professionals, or within large multidisciplinary consulting firms. The scope of the project, the desired time line, risk mitigation, and financial and personnel resources will determine the selection criteria for a specific consultation engagement.

Once organizations have the selection criteria identified, how do they find the consultant or consulting firm that is right for them? Two methods for locating consultants are search agencies or Internet searches, but the quickest, most reliable, and preferred method is word of mouth. One of the best ways to be assured of competent NI consulting is to check with colleagues who had a successful consulting engagement. Find out if the organization has a prearranged relationship with a specific consulting firm. Another approach is to explore various national professional organizations. Some that may be of help include:

- Advance for Health Information Executives, www.advanceweb.com
- American Hospital Association, www.aha.org
- American Medical Informatics Association (AMIA), www.amia.org, and Nursing Informatics Working Group, www.amia-niwg.org
- American Nursing Informatics Association (ANIA), www.ania.org
- American Nurses Association, Council for Nursing Services and Informatics, www.nursingworld.org/councils
- College of Healthcare Information Management Executives (CHIME), www.chime-net.org
- Computer-based Patient Record Institute, www.cpri.org

- Healthcare Information and Management Systems Society, www.himss.org
- Institute of Management Consultants, www.imcusa.org/imc.html
- National League for Nursing Council on Nursing Informatics, www.nln.org

After obtaining information about a consulting firm—how long the company has been in business, number of employees, financial stability, and market reputation—the organization choosing the consultant(s) must also determine the right consultant(s) for the project by

- Requesting a proposal to ensure that the consultant understands the problem
- Interviewing potential consultant candidates to find the right fit
- Contacting clients from a reference list (the proposal should include a client reference list of similar projects completed)
- Clarifying availability of the consulting staff; evaluating the skills and credentials of the consultant or consulting staff proposed by the firm; requesting resumes.

The process by which an organization evaluates and selects a consultant or consulting firm parallels the example given above of selecting an operating room information system. In both scenarios, the selection process entails conducting a market overview, determining selection criteria, interviewing potential candidates, and contacting references. It is essential for the organization seeking consulting assistance to diligently complete a consulting firm selection process to find the right consultant or firm at the right time and for the right price.

Working in the Client–Consultant Partnership

The client–consultant partnership starts during the initial contact and continues to grow throughout the project. After the consultant is hired, the initial meeting requires client and consultant participation. The client may want to present an overview of the organization and personnel involved in the project, clarify expected project outcomes and time expectations, and make the consultant aware of any "sacred cows" in the organization. Consultant activity may include presenting a workplan that includes the project's milestones and communication plan. Both of these plans must be approved by the organization.

Staff responses of consultation engagements can range from relief to suspicion to anxiety. The NI consultant must be able to understand the anxiety the staff may be feeling and help the staff grow and learn. Activities should be established by the organization to provide factual information that will dismiss rumors and worries.

Once the entire project team is actively engaged and the project is in full swing, the NI consultant's progress should be monitored and reviewed on a regular basis. Progress can be monitored by the workplan that was created at the beginning of the project. The consultant can complete project status reports and distribute them by e-mail, following an agreed-upon reporting schedule appropriate to the project length. Project status reports can be delivered weekly or biweekly, or the consultant can conduct actual meetings, depending on how the organization wants to be kept informed. Not only should the project status include project accomplishments, it should also discuss and raise awareness about actual or potential project issues and the resolutions.

Progress sessions may also be required to update the organization's steering committee on project status ("we are here"), including project accomplishments and barriers. Face-to-face update presentations should be utilized when project issues require discussion and decisions. In many consulting engagements, the NI consultant will have a "pre-meeting" with project champions or key individuals to raise or diffuse issues before a presentation. In this pre-meeting, information is received in advance so that the client can prepare or review the material to be presented and possibly make changes as appropriate. Consultants have expertise by virtue of their exposure to a variety of situations, but the client knows best what will ultimately work in the organization.

Engaging the NI consultant as an intellectual partner is another aspect of working effectively with consultants. Once an NI consultant is hired, full control of the project should not be relinquished. The client must always "own" the project and be updated regularly. The most effective way to enhance the client–consultant partnership is to facilitate the consultant's ability to create change. The client must provide the NI consultant with direct access to data, information, and individuals at different levels within the organization.

With the closure of a project, the NI consultant must complete a "knowledge transfer" with one or several of the project team members. This is a project milestone in which the client must validate that they have all documents, contacts, and information in relation to the project. A successful client–consultant partnership is one in which there is equality, growth, trust, and directness between both parties in an effort to accomplish a common goal(s).

Conclusion

Consulting is a profession with high expectations for both the client and the NI consultant. Just as nurses are taught from day one to assess, plan, implement, and evaluate, NI consultants must use this four-tiered process to guide their engagements. The combination of consulting, nursing, and information systems can assist healthcare organizations in identifying a problem/cause (assessment), identifying the solution (plan), and implementing the solution (implement and evaluate). Nursing informatics consultants can serve as invaluable resources, bringing expertise and successful conclusions to projects that healthcare organizations need to implement in order to stay in business and continue to deliver high-quality patient care.

Questions

1. Name the healthcare trends that have increased the market demand for NI consultants.
2. Why would organizations seek the assistance of an NI consultant?
3. Name possible sources for searching for a consultant or consulting firm. What is the best method for finding the right consultant for the organization?
4. Describe a successful client–consultant partnership.

References

Biech E. *The Business of Consulting: The Basics and Beyond.* San Francisco: Jossey-Bass/Pfeiffer, 1999.

Norwood SL. Making consultation work. *Journal of Nursing Admininistration* 1998;28(3):44–47.

Rosen EL, Routon CM. American Nursing Informatics Association role survey. *Computers in Nursing* 1998;16(3):172–175.

Bibliography

Beare PG. The ABCs of external consultation. *Clinical Nurse Specialist* 1988;2(1):35–38.

Berragan L. Consultancy in nursing: Roles and opportunities. *Journal of Clinical Nursing* 1998;7(2):139–143.

Nagelkerk J, Ritola P, Vandort PJ. Nursing informatics: the trend of the future. *Journal of Continuing Education in Nursing* 1998;29(1):17–21.

Shelley S. Interactive consulting: maximizing your consultant dollar. *Nursing Economics* 1994;12(5):272–275.

Simpson RL. From nurse to nursing informatics consultant: a lesson in entrepreneurship. *Nursing Administration Quarterly* 1998;22(2):87–90.

14
Nursing Considerations for the Selection of Healthcare Information Systems

MARY ETTA MILLS

Healthcare delivery systems continue to evolve toward the management of patient care and related costs, across a continuum of service needs and over the lifespan of each individual. As a result, there is increased attention on the best way to define, represent, and communicate healthcare data within and between delivery settings. Nursing has key responsibility and accountability in planning, evaluating, and delivering patient care services within this new framework. Consequently, nurses must participate in the selection of healthcare information systems that will support clinical and managerial decision-making.

External Requirements for Information Management

Any information management system must facilitate the organization's ability to satisfy external regulatory requirements and uniform standards of practice. Sources of these standards include the Joint Commission for Accreditation of Healthcare Organizations (JCAHO), the Computer-Based Patient Record Institute, and the Federal Health Reform Act. Their efforts focus on the ability of healthcare organizations to coordinate and integrate the information needed to provide efficient and effective patient care at a reasonable cost.

Joint Commission for Accreditation of Healthcare Organizations

The 1999 *JCAHO Accreditation Manual for Hospitals* provides a separate chapter that addresses the "Management of Information" (JCAHO, 1999, pp. 193–213). Within this framework of standards, the goal of information management is to "obtain, manage, and use information to improve patient outcomes and individual and hospital performance in patient care, governance, management, and support processes" (p. 193). Although not requiring computer support, the standards recognize that efficiency may be improved by computerization and other technologies. As outlined, the standards address the identification, design, capture, analysis, communication, integration, and use of information. Within the standards, criteria impacting information system selection include expectations for

- Ensuring confidentiality, security, and integrity of data and information
- Establishing uniform data definitions (such as minimum data sets and standardized classifications)
- Transmitting data in a standard format
- Integrating and interpreting capabilities
- Combining data and information from various sources
- Relating patient-specific data and information to care processes and outcomes
- Sharing information between systems
- Linking patient care and nonpatient care data (i.e., clinical and fiscal) over time and among all care settings
- Handling patient-specific data (e.g., demographic, assessment, treatment plan, advance directives, informed consent, therapeutic orders, procedures performed, clinical observations, response to care, medications ordered and administered, discharge instructions)
- Managing verbal orders and authentication of record entries
- Documenting detailed operative, postoperative, ambulatory, outpatient, and emergency care
- Integrating all relevant information from a patient's record from various locations
- Aggregating data (e.g., for use in risk management, quality improvement, operational decision-making, and planning)
- Using knowledge-based information resources (e.g., clinical and management literature, patient education materials, and comparative databases)

Nursing often is the network by which patient care is not only delivered but also coordinated. Central to guiding the selection process, then, is an information system's ability to support the coordination and integration of information needed for clinical and managerial decision making.

Accreditation standards for healthcare networks further emphasize the need for system-level interface and integration of information. In this regard, networks are viewed as systems composed of multiple healthcare delivery organizations. Guiding principles involve continuity of care and coordination of services supported by one-time data entry and immediate data availability to all users. Given that nursing care, facilitated through such modalities as critical paths, will eventually extend across care settings, information system selection must incorporate the possibility of data sharing across care delivery sites.

In the future, such technology as an "integration hub" is expected to support multiple information systems links. This approach would eliminate the need to develop point-to-point system interfaces. The hub would thus serve as a clearinghouse to route information. Nevertheless, at this time there are few products available to achieve the ideal system. The most popular are "interface engines, repositories, and data warehouses to address the integration issue and lack of timely information across the organization" (Health Management Technology, 1999, p. 33).

Computer-Based Patient Record Institute

The Institute of Medicine's (IOM) Vision 2000 supported the development of a computer-based patient record (CPR) and led to the creation of the Computer-Based Patient Record Institute (Dick & Steen, 1991). The goals of this project include the development of coordinated vendor standards and a uniform single patient record. Once there is a standardized approach to collecting nursing information at the level of individual healthcare organizations/networks, information appropriate to providing informed nursing care will be included in this process.

Federal Health Reform

The American Health Security Act of 1993 suggested a national framework for health information. Among its features were provisions for standard forms, uniform health data sets, electronic networks, and national standards for data transmission and confidentiality. The information system proposed was mandated to support consumer information, measurement of health status, health security cards, links among healthcare records, analysis of patterns of health care, health system evaluation, and data confidentiality and security. Although the Security Act was not supported by Congress, it set in motion the development of an infrastructure focused on

- Improving networks for linking hospitals, clinics, doctors' offices, libraries, and universities to enable healthcare providers and researchers to share medical data and imagery
- Database technology to allow healthcare providers to access relevant medical information and literature
- Database technology for storing, accessing, and transmitting patients' medical records while protecting the accuracy and privacy of those records.

Since that time, the Health Insurance Portability and Accountability Act (HIPAA) of 1996 has introduced concepts of uniformity in some electronic data interchange transactions, standardized forms, provider and payor identifiers, and uniform patient identification. Of issue has been the protection of "privacy and confidentiality of electronically stored, maintained or transmitted health information" (Marietti, 1998, p. 52) and, more specifically, to the choice of an individual identifier.

These initiatives emphasize the importance of nursing's involvement in setting the strategic direction healthcare information systems take at the local level. Knowledge of what future regulations will likely require is crucial, because this will facilitate informed selection and development of information systems that will meet nursing needs within an organizational context.

Information Systems Selection—Technical Details

Initial evaluation of an information management system is a critical first step toward identifying a system that will best meet organizational needs. The criteria on which an overall evaluation is based will generally include system function and features, functional architecture, references, quality of documentation, system design, risk, vendor support, vendor background, hardware and system software, and cost. Nursing is key to this evaluation process. Data systems personnel and financial analysts can assess the technical, mechanical, and cost feasibility of various systems, but nursing has the broad clinical and administrative perspective by which to critique the systems programs and information.

System Selection Criteria

Evaluation of information systems should include consideration of some broad-based requirements, as well as the ability to deliver specific information management functions. The following are some general guidelines.

Identify the Most Crucial Information Needs

Without trying to specify every data interaction that is currently performed, it is important to determine key categories of information that must be included in the information management system. Examples of priority nursing management information might include budget, patient acuity, reimbursement modeling, patient outcomes, case mix, and staffing. Clinical information priorities might include

- Nursing diagnosis/problems/assessments
- Order communications and results reporting
- Care planning/mapping, medication documentation
- Patient care flowsheets
- Patient education
- Discharge planning
- Procedure directory.

This list will help guide the review of proposed systems with respect to data availability.

Establish Data Requirements

The second step is to consider the most useful way of visualizing data and converting them into information supportive of clinical and managerial decision-making. For example, various forms of data might be better presented in one of the following formats: charts, graphs, tables, variance reporting, highlighting or colors, and trend tracking or forecasting.

Identify Types of System Capability Desired

System capability refers to the broad ability of the information system to meet departmental needs and organizational goals. Considerations might include the ability of the system to

- Draw relationships among data from divergent sources
- Provide a unified patient record across care sites
- Enable prediction and simulation of "what if" scenarios
- Adjust the format of information.

These are support areas of data management that expand the possible uses of recorded data. For example, data may have multiple uses as "system drivers" in which clinical assessment data may automatically feed into the calculation of patient acuity and determination of staffing levels. Another example might involve "information drivers" in which relationships are drawn between critical path variance and cost of care.

Utilize Usability Principles

Unless nursing staff can easily use the information system to support their activities in patient care, the system will lead to frustration, additional requests for customization, and delayed or ineffective system use. A series of "usability principles" was suggested by Nielsen (1990). These review criteria include

- Ensuring relevant information
- Speaking the user's language
- Minimizing what the user must remember
- Ensuring consistency
- Providing feedback
- Providing clearly marked exits, effective shortcuts, and helpful error messages
- Helping prevent errors through internal systems.

Future Expandability

Organizations must consider the ability of the proposed information system to support future initiatives. For example, as organizations continue to change dynamically, how will the selected system integrate with other health information units? Will the system smoothly accommodate wireless technology? To what extent will the system support a data repository where data can be captured and integrated? Will the system be compatible in offering telehealth services to distant clients? These issues will only grow in importance. Planning for their eventuality will promote more effective implementation of future strategic plans.

Information Systems Selection— Administrative Process

The knowledge that nursing brings to the administrative selection process includes details relevant to the interaction of departments participating in care management; the degree of systems enhancement that will be necessary; the ease or difficulty of implementation based on system complexity; the expense of staff education; and the potential for fully integrating system components. Most importantly, nursing can ascertain the system's potential to improve patient care. In this role, nursing provides a critical balance in facilitating the selection of a technically capable system that also yields maximum utility in a patient care environment.

The decision to implement an information management system represents a major financial commitment on the part of any institution. The potential of an information system to meet the unique needs of a specific healthcare facility is an essential ingredient for its long-term success in that environment. Both formally and informally, nursing can be an invaluable component in structuring the evaluation process, making recommendations for mandatory and desirable components, assessing a system's potential relative to the needs of practicing professionals, and making a selection with both the present and the future in mind.

Representation

Most importantly, nursing must be represented on the Information System Selection Committee or the Advisory Committee to this process. It is the responsibility of the chief nursing officer to make this expectation known and to identify appropriate clinical and management staff who can represent critical nursing knowledge. The development of information system selection criteria and vendor evaluation is time consuming, and the individuals participating in the process must be able to contribute the necessary hours.

Preparation

Before entering into formal committee discussions, take the time to determine current system availability, capability, and design. It will be important to conduct the following:

- Systems inventory
- Assessment of multidisciplinary systems in relation to their benefit to nursing
- Consideration of the nursing information system in relation to the healthcare organization's strategic plan and to nursing's strategic plan

Having access to information specific to current resources and future needs will serve to provide informed nursing representation to the organizational selection process. Furthermore, a detailed understanding of need will ensure that critical nursing information elements are included in any system selected.

Understanding the Request for Proposal

A document developed by the selection committee, the request for proposal (RFP) establishes a specified set of requirements and invites vendors to demonstrate how they might address those requirements to meet organizational needs. The RFP outlines the information management requirements that must be included in any proposed system, as well as other requirements the vendor is expected to provide. These might include such features as financing, equipment demonstration, staff training, system troubleshooting, and future software updates. Specific evaluation criteria are normally included in the RFP so that vendors understand the basis for system selection.

The better the RFP is understood by selection committee members, the more effective the process of discriminating between proposed systems and reaching an optimum decision will be.

Decision-Making

Because computer-based information systems will continue to revolutionize communications in health care and markedly impact nursing practice, nursing must participate in the information system selection decision. If the system does not meet nursing needs, there should be a right of veto. The context of communications must be structured to clearly define and facilitate the documentation of the nursing process, to streamline the clarity, availability, and integration of essential information, and to conserve nursing time so that it can be spent with the patient.

The only way nursing can ensure that the system selected will facilitate these goals is to participate actively in the administrative selection process.

A priority role for nursing will serve the best interests of the healthcare facility and the nursing profession. When that role has been a reality, information system selection has been proven farsighted and positive, and implementation has proceeded in a productive way.

Summary

Nursing is critical to the selection, design, and implementation of an optimum clinical information system. External standards from the JCAHO, emphasis on a computer-based patient record by the IOM, and federal healthcare information initiatives provide important considerations for the identification of nursing computing requirements and eventual systems selection.

The identification of system selection requirements should be based on the identification of the information most needed to support clinical and managerial decisions. Key to the selection of an information system that will support nursing is the preparation and involvement of appropriate nursing staff on the system selection committee. Data display requirements, system capability to transform and communicate data, and usability principles should be considered in developing RFPs and in evaluating proposed information systems.

Questions

1. What are the major requirements for future information systems as guided by accreditation standards and regulation?
2. What are the four key considerations for information system selection supportive of clinical and managerial decisions?
3. When and how should nursing be involved in the information system selection process?

References

Dick RS, Steen EB. *The Computer-Based Patient Record, An Essential Technology for Health Care.* Washington, DC: National Academy Press, 1991.
Health Management Technology. What do healthcare organizations want from a consultant? *Health Management Technology* 1999;20(2):30–33.
Joint Commission for Accreditation of Healthcare Organizations (JCAHO). Management of information. In: *Accreditation Manual for Hospitals.* Chicago: JCAHO, 1999;193–213.
Marietti C. Doing the right thing. *Healthcare Informatics* 1998(October):51–62.
Nielsen J. Traditional dialogue design applied to modern user interfaces. *Communications of the Association for Computing Machinery* 1990;33(10):109–118.

Bibliography

Whitten J, Bentely L. Information system development. In: Whitten JL, Bentely LD, Dittman KC, eds. *Systems Analysis and Design Methods*, 4th ed. Boston: Irwin-McGraw-Hill, 1998;70–115.

Zielstorff R, Hudgings C, Grobe S. *Next Generation Nursing Information Systems.* Washington, DC: American Nurses Publishing, 1993.

15
Project Management: Informatics

BARBARA A. HAPP

... where no plan is laid, where the disposal of time is surrendered merely to the chance of incident, chaos will soon reign.

—Victor Hugo

When Karen Scully, RNC, came out of the meeting with the client, she pondered the challenges ahead. The project kick-off meeting seemed to go well, but several new issues had come up. The client's expectations of the project outcome did not match the contract, and Karen's planned resources and schedule needed adjusting. Karen thought about the history of this project. As part of the internal Clinical Systems Planning Department, she had been designated project manager on this large information systems implementation. The vendor contract had been negotiated and signed, and a six person project team had been assembled before her appointment.

Karen understood the task to be the installation of a healthcare information system that would automate the Emergency Department (ED) activities in the acute care center of Hillside Health System, a not-for-profit integrated health delivery system. Karen's client was the Director of the ED. The go live date was just three months ahead. She closed her office door to review the Gantt chart and to think about revising the plans.

Purpose

The purpose of this chapter is to outline the process for successful management of projects related to informatics. Information is provided to support readers who are planning, organizing, or directing healthcare information system projects. This chapter outlines a practical approach to managing projects and delivering them on time and on budget while satisfying or exceeding clients' expectations.

Scope

Through the discussion of a case study, the essentials of planning, organizing, and directing informatics projects are introduced. A project management and healthcare informatics practice framework will guide the discussions. Project management is defined, and the essentials of leadership, team building, and risk management are applied to project management. As the architect, the project manager (PM) is the focus.

The material presented here is intended to be an overview. Discussion of very detailed project management and work design and specifications for software, hardware, or networking are beyond the scope of this chapter.

Objectives

This chapter has three major objectives:

- To define project management and describe a pragmatic project management approach for planning, designing, implementing, and evaluating
- To contrast the characteristics of successful and unsuccessful projects
- To outline current tools, methods, and resources used by PMs

Project Management: Definition and Approach

As Karen reviewed the contract, team composition, and client expectations, she thought about the project management definition discussed at the internal pre-kick-off meeting. She had described it as managing from start to finish, including planning and controlling to avoid common mistakes, identifying needs, defining requirements, budgeting, scheduling, allocating resources, and handling project politics. Now, project management included management of client expectations.

What Is Project Management?

Lientz and Rae (1999) refer to project management as the procedures, rules, and policies as well as the style of management and politics. A project is a well-defined sequence of events with a beginning and an end, directed toward achieving a clear goal; projects are conducted within established parameters (time, cost, resources, and quality). Projects are different from everyday activities, because achieving a project goal is a specific, nonroutine event (Catapult, 1995). Examples of projects include building a house, writing a book, and implementing a software system. Within the information systems lifecycle, examples of projects include development of strategic and tactical information systems plans, conducting a feasibility study, gathering end-user requirements, and acquiring or implementing the software application packages.

As it was explained to Karen, an ED task force had identified the system requirements, and an outside consultant had conducted the feasibility study. The Board of Trustees approved the budget, and the ED task force evaluated and selected the vendor after the lengthy request for information (RFI) and request for proposal (RFP) processes were completed. Karen's job was to direct the planning, implementation, and evaluation of this project. She was ultimately responsible for successfully implementing the ED information system on time and on budget.

In healthcare informatics, project management is the implementation of a solution. The context of project management within informatics practice is illustrated in Figure 15.1. Project management, the step after understanding client needs and developing effective solutions, is the implementation of effective solutions to solve the client's problem. It includes scoping the project, planning and organizing the tasking in a work breakdown structure (WBS), developing change management and conflict resolution strategies, managing the contract, reporting progress and issues, evaluating the project, and leading the team.

The basics of management (plan, organize, direct, control) and continuous quality improvement are the essential underpinnings of the framework. Focusing on the client and establishing a partnership is part of the task of maintaining professional credibility by doing valued project work.

A more specific framework for project management to include planning, communicating, managing, and evaluating is illustrated in Figure 15.2. Client focus is the central idea of the framework. Project management (the act of implementing effective solutions) is the continuous process of communicating, managing, evaluating, and planning. Strong leadership abilities are integral to healthcare informatics practice and project management. (See Block [1981] for detailed elements of the closely related practice of consulting.)

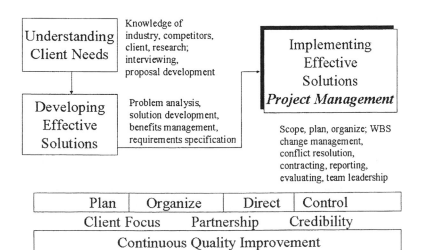

FIGURE 15.1. Healthcare informatics practice. Copyright 1999 Barbara Happ.

Project Management
Implementing Effective Solutions

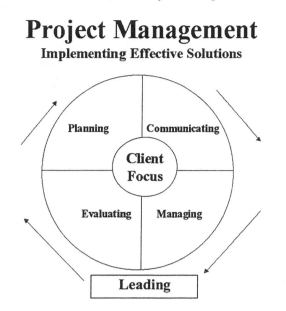

FIGURE 15.2. Project management. Copyright 1999 Barbara Happ.

Major Phases for Project Management

Karen continued to ponder the high-level project work plan on her desk (Fig. 15.3). A team member interrupted her thought process. The senior analyst needed information to update the project work plan and was in a hurry because she was going on vacation. Karen felt pressure to reiterate the plan tasks of the project, but she had many questions to ask the client before she could direct the analyst. Re-defining, validating, and planning were such a big part of this project, Karen thought. Now she had to restart by rereading the organization's strategic plan. Where did this ED project fit in? How important was the project to the success of the ED implementation? She learned quickly that a new ED system was a top priority and had support from the Board. JCAHO would be coming within one year of the project's planned completion.

The 10 major tasks for project management (see Fig. 15.3) for implementation of an information system generally fall into three major project phases:

- Defining and planning
- Implementing and executing control
- Project evaluation and learning

These are the ideal pragmatic steps in the management of projects. (Although this example is for the implementation of an information system, it can be adapted for project management of informatics projects in general.)

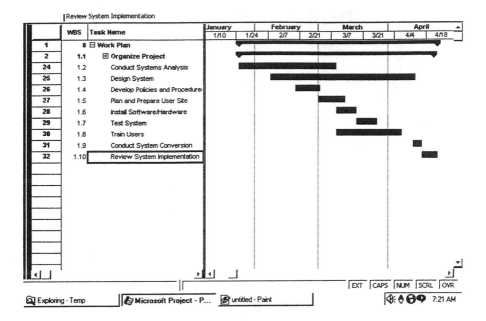

Review System Implementation

	WBS	Task Name	January		February		March		April	
			1/10	1/24	2/7	2/21	3/7	3/21	4/4	4/18
1	0	⊟ Work Plan								
2	1.1	⊞ Organize Project								
24	1.2	Conduct Systems Analysis								
25	1.3	Design System								
26	1.4	Develop Policies and Procedure:								
27	1.5	Plan and Prepare User Site								
28	1.6	Install Software/Hardware								
29	1.7	Test System								
30	1.8	Train Users								
31	1.9	Conduct System Conversion								
32	1.10	Review System Implementation								

EXT   CAPS   NUM   SCRL   OVR

Exploring - Temp   Microsoft Project - P...   untitled - Paint   7:21 AM

FIGURE 15.3. High-level project plan work breakdown structure. Copyright 1999 Barbara Happ.

Phase I: Defining and Planning

The maximum potential for influencing project outcomes occurs early in the conceptual and definition phases of the project. Autopsies of most failed projects indicate that the disasters were "well planned" to happen from the start. Therefore, even in an era of uncertainty and accelerated speed, don't rush to execution with only superficial preparations—invest quality time in early planning. (Laufer & Hoffman, 1998)

Organizing the project involves creating a workplan and assembling the project team and steering and advisory committees. Conducting the systems analysis or impact analysis includes reviewing the current systems and processes and reporting on the effect the new system will have on the department, facility, and enterprise operations. A significant amount of time should be spent on this phase to ensure that a solid, successful plan is envisioned.

An essential element of Phase I is the review of the organization's strategic planning documents (including mission and vision statements), the business plan, and the information technology strategic and tactical plans. The organizational strategic plan containing the enterprise vision acts as the map for the organization. To ensure the success of a project, the information technology/information management project plan must corroborate with the organization's strategic plans.

The strategic plan generally lays out the current situation and the information technology and information management approach. The plan communicates the enterprise philosophy and direction for information technology use. The strategy is generally shared to gain maximum payoff from information technology investments. All enterprise projects must be in concert with these plans. The project manager should review the plans carefully and upwardly communicate all gaps that might exist between the organization's strategy and new projects. Identified risks should be documented and communicated appropriately to executives.

From experience, Karen understood the ramifications of misalignments. She began to question if she was managing a project that was part of the organization's strategic plan.

Ritter and Glaser (1994) underscore the importance of aligning business goals and information technology investments (managing and prioritizing the right information technology projects). The success of information technology projects is correlated with the alignment of technology support and critical business processes. This is a crucial component of project management. Without this convergence, projects may risk losing upper management support. Mitchell (1998) also supports this principle and encourages managers to match information technology plans with corporate business plans.

During the defining and planning phase, the project goals and objectives are documented. Project objectives are generally related to delivering a product (implementation of the system) and meeting cost and schedule plans. These objectives must be validated by the client and reviewed and evaluated regularly. Without objectives, a PM may be trying to "do a task right" without focusing on the right task.

The project goals are generally based on the expected benefits set forth during the feasibility study. Feasibility studies answer questions like: "Can we do this project?" "Should we do this project?" and "What is the return on investment?" One project goal may be implementing a system that decreases time spent on documentation and increases documentation accuracy. Another might be staying within five percent of the baseline schedule while maintaining costs within or below the planned budget. Data collection for benefits measurement outlined in the feasibility study may be scheduled nine months to a year in the future.

During Phase I, project risks (slip in schedule, underestimation of costs, etc. and so forth) are identified, and a risk mitigation plan is developed. The quality management plan (QMP) is developed and documented. The QMP outlines the processes to be followed to ensure that the project stays within budget and on schedule—and, most importantly, ensures client satisfaction. It includes checklists and project management tools for continuously evaluating and reporting progress. The QMP tool set includes an interim and final client satisfaction form. A maintenance process to review and update all plans is also developed during Phase I.

The creation of the work plan involves review of the technical proposal and legal contract where tasks are detailed. Tasks and milestones are organized, resources are scheduled to reflect the level of work and planned budget, and a leader should be assigned for each major task. The work plan details each step in a WBS (1.0, 1.1, 1.1.1, and so forth), which an automated tool like MS Project captures and displays for monitoring and reporting. Fig. 15.3 illustrates the high-level tasks for project planning. Although the WBS acts as the guide to task implementation, details (how to) may be added as management decisions evolve and information becomes stable. The WBS works as the general master plan. (Details about project management tools are incorporated into the tools and methods section of this chapter.)

A project kick-off should be scheduled with the client early in this phase. At the kick-off meeting, the client and team meet to review the high-level project plan, lay out deliverables, and establish the project review process. The project manager should seek agreement on a communications plan to facilitate reporting and issue resolution. The technical proposal/contract should be reviewed and discussed.

After Karen reviewed the organization's strategic plan and the project plans, she felt more confident about the project's alignment. She understood where the client was coming from and the problems this information system was to solve. Except for one area, the plans were in sync. The area of concern was the client's anticipation of the new ED information system organization's benefits. The client was worried about ED automated reporting for JCAHO.

After she made a note to discuss this point at the next weekly client meeting, Karen focused on gathering the information for the senior analyst's request. Although she had a mature team in place, a few needed coaching about planning ahead. Indeed, Karen needed a better communication system for the team. She had a beeper and e-mail and her office was co-located with the team, but the team seemed to need more face-to-face interaction with Karen and the client. She would plan accordingly.

Phase II: Implementing and Executing Control

In a dynamic environment, project management is not about performing according to plan, with minimal changes. It is about meeting customer needs, while coping successfully with unavoidable changes. Therefore, the planning system should be capable of coping with changes. (Laufer & Hoffman, 1998)

After the project plan is in place and the systems analysis or impact statement is reported, the next phase is the actual information system technical implementation. This phase includes designing the system; developing policies and procedures; planning and preparing the user site; installing, testing, and training; and conducting the system conversion. Quality management processes are refined and implemented, and the project is operationalized. Regular in-process reviews (IPRs) are conducted to continuously report project progress and to outline issues for resolution. In-process reviews are scheduled to report the actual progress compared with the plan. Resources, deliverables, budget, and schedule are graphically illustrated and the client briefed during IPRs.

Managing the project on a day-to-day basis involves many meetings and discussions with appointed task leaders. The PM must be visible and available for the team and client. Weekly client meetings and team meetings are highly recommended. The PM is responsible for continuous monitoring of the resources, budget, QMP, WBS, and timely resolution of issues. The PM must be a keen negotiator and politician to anticipate and settle issues before they impact the budget or schedule of the project. (Further information is given in the discussion of successful and unsuccessful projects.) Project managers often appoint a "second" or deputy from the team to act in the PM's absence. This enables respite for the PM and provides flexibility when urgent issues arise and the PM is not available.

Finally, the PM must be the leader and cheerleader for the project team. As the strategy setter, consensus builder, systems integrator, and change agent (Gadeken, 1999), the PM should reward and recognize members and cultivate the common team commitment (Facteau, 1998). Team members should also be held accountable for group behaviors. This means that roles, responsibilities, processes, and procedures must be flexible; common sense should prevail.

Although Karen's day was filled with client and team meetings, she spent part of each day walking around and talking informally with team members. She also scheduled time to review all reports and speak in person with the client and others involved in the project. She scanned the environment and identified key people with whom to maintain contact. For instance, because she knew that the chief financial officer was very interested in the project budget, Karen made sure that she had lunch with her every other week to discuss the schedule and cost. Her job was to stay on top of the details without micromanaging the effort.

With task leaders' input, Karen managed the decision-making. She knew where to gather reliable information quickly, and she made a note to check the frequency of the scheduled IPRs. For Karen, the IPRs were a means of formally briefing management about the project. Cost and schedule charts were prepared and issues outlined. Karen's manager and the internal client used this monthly opportunity to ask questions and support the resolution of important issues.

As a leader, Karen wanted to support the development of future task leaders and PMs. She made a note to speak with the managers of two task leaders. (In the matrix organization, the team members were "on loan" to Karen's project.) She also thought about the need the team had for celebrating each success or milestone. Positive team morale was high on Karen's list of project objectives; measuring and nurturing this objective was important to the vitality of the project. Karen knew that replacing original team members would change the schedule and perhaps the budget. At the same time, she acknowledged that she had to have the right skill mix to get the job done.

(Actual technical specifics from implementation are beyond the scope of this chapter.)

Phase III: Project Evaluation and Learning

The postimplementation review and project closeout activities occur in this last phase. The success of the project is generally based on the attainment of the project objectives. This is measured, reported, and discussed with the team and the client. A lessons learned document (from this project for the next project) is often constructed and shared, and the postimplementation benefits data collection is scheduled at this time.

The use of 10 basic and pragmatic steps, broken into three phases for project management, should provide the means for clear communication and amity between PM and team members and the client. The steps enable continuous quality improvement and act as a guide for current and future successful project completion.

Project Characteristics: Contrasting Successful and Unsuccessful Projects

Good project management includes managing people, processes, and problems while coping with uncertainty and change. Motivating and organizing the team and setting up an environment supportive of innovation are essential. Processes must be defined, developed, and maintained, and problems must be rapidly identified. When processes fail, problems must be scoped and solved. Successful projects have measurable outcomes, a good balance in management control, flexibility, and a well-defined purpose and scope.

Conversely, projects become risky when the purpose changes and the project plans do not. "Scope creep" is another threat to success. The PM who allows the client to add work without negotiating a trade-off of tasks may endanger the balance of project resources and schedule. Successful PMs integrate creativity and solid, tested problem-solving methods to keep the project on track. Selecting the right project, focusing on the client, and evaluating the project importance (strategic alignment) are essential. Communicating effectively, crossing political boundaries, keeping close track on project progress and team morale, and sharing bad news also support the success of the project. Lastly, remaining flexible, knowing when to end the project, and integrating a sense of healthy competitiveness are additional proactive activities for successful project management.

Cyr (1997) and Lancaster (1997) address essentials for problem solving and creativity. Cyr's steps (1997) on problem solving can be used in project management to turn issues into solutions. The basics include

- Defining the problem clearly
- Researching deeply
- Calling in help when needed
- Practicing problem solving

- Sketching out the problem
- Churning, or taking some time to go over the problem
- Stepping away for a time
- Keeping space clear
- Knowing when to walk away.

Lancaster (1997) suggests that leadership and team creativity can contribute significantly to project success. Building a tolerance for bad ideas, thinking big, seeking out diverse friends, and disciplining creative ideas may also help inventiveness.

McComb and Smith (1991) offer a framework to assess project risks. The analytical framework for linking observed systems failures to behavioral factors is presented. The factors are illustrated along two dimensions: planning/executing and technical/human. Planning factors include estimating and compressing the project. This framework is an excellent guide for diagnosing problems early in the project implementation.

Karen was a member of the Women in Project Management special interest group (sig@pmi.org) within the Project Management Institute (www.pmi.org) and was also enrolled in a philosophy course. These activities supported the enhancement of her critical thinking and PM skills and abilities.

Several authors contrast successful and unsuccessful projects. In a survey of software projects by the Standish Group (http://www.standishgroup.com/), projects were classified as successful (on time, on budget), project challenged (over budget, over time estimates), or project impaired (cancelled during the development lifecycle). The Standish Group (1998) survey of 23,000 software projects indicated that only one-fifth were successful. Successful projects engaged users, had executive management support, and had a clear statement of software requirements. Unsuccessful projects were plagued by restarts, cost overruns, time overruns, and content deficiencies. To avoid such difficulties, the authors suggest using shorter time frames and delivering software and prototyping the design and development ("growing" the software) frequently. Massaro (1993) reinforces the need for engaging end users in phases of software implementation.

Project Management: Tools, Methods, and Resources

Without a proper understanding of project management methodology, all software will do is help you document your failures—with great precision. (Lewis, 1998)

There is an abundance of resources for project management support, as well as a number of tools and methods to assist in managing projects. A method is a standard technique, framework, process, or procedure to guide how work may be accomplished. Technical or manual tools support the methods used to manage projects. An example of a method is the use of a WBS for planning. A tool or instrument like MS Project may support project tasking and reporting.

When selecting the appropriate methods and tools for a project, the PM or decision-makers should consider the organization's goals and constraints, the stability of the vendor, the cost, and the vendor support. Users must be prepared with tool training, a plan for tool integration must be developed, and managers must define and implement change management strategies. When problems arise, the PM should assess if the tool is being used correctly or if it is being forced to fit the needs of the organization. To avoid problems, the PM should start with a few tools and avoid changing tools and methods in the middle of the project.

Although automated project management software sales account for $900 million each year (Romberg, 1998), they do not guarantee project success. The manager of virtual project teams has special needs when it comes to tools and methods. Although virtual project teams share the same project goals, the geographic dispersion dictates increased use of telephony, automation, and the Web. Web-enabled versions of project management tools avail team members to update project plans, while managers make adjustments and develop reports on the Web.

Other resources include the Project Management Institute's *Book of Knowledge* (BOK) (www.pmi.org). The BOK can be downloaded (176 pp) and contains many interesting chapters and appendices for PMs to reference. It includes Project Management Institute PM framework and scope, cost, and quality chapters, several appendices, and a useful PM glossary. The Lientz and Rea (1999) text on project management includes a CD-ROM reference disk of handy resources, tools, and checklists on areas such as project evaluation.

For over 30 years, the federal government has successfully used earned value as a method to track project costs and schedule performance by comparing planned work with accomplished work. Some suggest that earned value is a proven methodology for measuring cost and scheduled performance on large projects with interdependent tasks.

Karen's department used a 10 step project management framework. She was familiar with this formalized approach and thought it was flexible enough to use for the ED project. The framework language was easy to understand. She selected MS Project because it was available on the network and familiar to several of the team members.

Conclusion

Karen and her team developed an effective project management plan to deal with known risks. Karen was familiar with leading projects and had selected the most effective tools. She identified areas where she needed help and resources for support. Finally, she knew that support was available from her team and upper management. As a PM, her days passed quickly, and each one was an adventure.

In this chapter, we have explored the essentials of project management. We have examined its definition, tools, methods, and resources, and we have followed a pragmatic approach from planning to implementation. As Karen's experience demonstrates, project management challenges the informatics practitioner's knowledge, skills, and abilities. The ideal PM will embrace these challenges with vigor and resilience, celebrating small victories and learning from every opportunity to excel.

Acknowledgments. The author gratefully acknowledges the technical assistance of the Spring 1999 University of Maryland Project Management: Informatics (NURS 698) class.

Questions

1. Define project management. What are its three major components?
2. Describe some characteristics of successful and unsuccessful projects.
3. What are some key issues the PM should consider when selecting the appropriate methods and tools for a project?

References

Block P. *Flawless Consulting.* San Diego: Pfeiffer & Company, 1981.

Catapult, Inc. *Microsoft Project4.* Redmond, CA: Microsoft Press, 1995.

Cyr D. How to solve almost anything. *Attache* 1997(November);46–48.

Facteau L. Moving the organization to operate within team-based approaches. *Seminars for Nurse Managers* 1998;6(4):177–182.

Gadeken O. Third wave project leadership. *PM Network* 1999;13(2):43–46.

Lancaster H. Getting yourself in a frame of mind to be creative. *Wall Street Journal* 1997;(September 16):B1.

Laufer A, Hoffman DJ. Ninety-nine rules for managing faster, better, cheaper projects. Lecture 1998 (October 14). Adapted from A Laufer, Simultaneous Management AMACOM, The American Management Association, 1996.

Lewis JP. *Mastering Project Management.* New York: McGraw-Hill, 1998.

Lientz BP, Rae KP. *Guide to Successful Project Management.* New York: Harcourt Brace, 1999.

Massaro TA. Introducing physician order entry at a major academic medical center: 1. Impact on organizational culture and behavior. 2. Impact on medical education. *Academic Medicine* 1993;68(1):20–30.

McComb D, Smith J. System project failure: the heuristics of risk. *Journal of Information Systems Management* 1991(Winter);25–34.

Microsoft Project 98: Step by Step (Step by Step Series) Inc. *Catapult,* November 1997.

Mitchell RN. Making a match. *Advance* 1998;2(1):27–34.

Project Management Institute. Book of Knowledge, (www.pmi.org). (Last accessed May 20, 1999.)

Ritter JL, Glaser JP. Implementing the patient care information strategy. In: Drazen EE, Metzger JB, Ritter JL, Schneider MK, eds. *Patient Care Information Systems*. New York: Springer-Verlag, 1994;163–185.

Romberg D. Project management tools cannot guarantee success. *Computing Canada* 1998(November 9);29–30.

Standish Group, (http://www.standishgroup.com/), 1998. (Last accessed May 20, 1999.)

16
Nurses' Responsibilities in the Implementation of Information Systems

Suzanne Jenkins

"Current industry statistics reveal that well over one-third of integrated healthcare delivery systems (IHDS) are in planning stages of implementing a computer-based record (CPR)" (Amatayadkul, 1998). During the past decade, the influence of nursing on the selection of such healthcare information systems (HIS) has continued to increase. Today's systems planning and implementation processes are based not only on the capabilities of information technology but also on the forces in the environment that impact health care.

History

Most computer decisions in the 1970s were financially oriented. Healthcare organizations saw the need for automating their patient billing process and other key systems, such as general ledger and accounts payable. Advanced technology led to increased sophistication of hardware and software capabilities and, concurrently, the information needs of the healthcare organization increased. More extensive reporting requirements, as well as the need for management reporting on productivity, became the norm.

Computer decisions in the early 1980s focused primarily on ancillary systems. Many of them were not integrated with the rest of the HIS and were categorized as stand alone systems. As a result, redundant patient information had to be entered into each system. The laboratory, pharmacy, and radiology generally had their own systems, including an order entry function typically done by their departmental staff. If terminals were placed on the nursing unit, clerks or nursing staff could enter the orders.

The trend for the 1990s and into the new millennium is documenting patient care at the point where care is being provided (bedside, clinic, physician office, rehabilitation centers, home). Although terminals at each bedside can be an expensive venture for a healthcare organization, many vendors are claiming both reduced nursing costs and increased quality of patient care. Terminals provide online flowcharting, vital signs, medication charting, and nursing care plans. The vendors claim that nurses can spend more time delivering care and less time charting and searching for charts.

Nursing has now defined additional needs and requirements for information systems. For many institutions, the ultimate goal is to have a "paperless" system. The entire medical record can be stored and accessed on-line from a terminal device. This concept allows consolidated, accurate information to be available at the user's fingertips. Patient charts from previous visits need not be tracked down, and medication and allergy records can be easily accessed on-line. On-line order entry means no more order or charge slips; all information can be captured automatically. As healthcare organizations "convert from the traditional medical record to the computerized patient record (CPR), physicians and other caregivers will experience some changes in how they both access and enter patient information" (Amatayadkul, 1998).

Also influencing the computer systems of the 1990s was the need for quality management and utilization management modules. Expedient, timely information about the patient is critical. Healthcare reform and managed care contracts are having a major impact in the financial arena and on the patient's length of stay. This ultimately impacts the type and quality of care provided.

Meeting the Challenges

The implementation of any CPR from selection through installation is never 100 percent problem free. Solving problems and overcoming challenges are what make every implementation unique and exciting. Unforeseen issues can occur at any stage of the implementation cycle, beginning with the selection of a system and moving through the next phases—installation, training, parallel testing, "going live," and even into postimplementation evaluation. The key to resolution is the identification of existing resistance factors. Once they are identified, plans can be made to eliminate them through teamwork, transitional strategies, and educational offerings.

The acquisition of a CPR is an expensive venture for a healthcare organization to undertake, and it requires a significant commitment from administration to support and guide the installation. Common barriers to overcome range from general mistrust of automation to misgivings regarding a specific system. Potential users may fear that implementation of a system will result in an increased workload without tangible benefits. These fears and inhibitions are some of the most difficult barriers to overcome. Together, they elongate the normal learning curve, increasing the time it takes to become familiar with the new system and realize its benefits.

Often, the politics surrounding a major acquisition like a computer system can slow or stall it. The very idea of change is sometimes threatening and can delay the installation process. Changing from manual charting (handwritten) to an automated system can generate insecurity and distrust, and changing from one automated system to another automated system often elicits resistance. A common complaint is that "the old system didn't do it that way," regardless of comparative merit. It is sometimes easier to train people who have never used a system than to retrain people who are constantly making comparisons to previous systems. Interestingly, though, the people most resistant to a new system often become its best promoters once they are knowledgeable about it and comfortable with it.

Besides assisting in expediting accurate patient information throughout the healthcare organization, an automated system should reduce paper generation. Most of the necessary information can be viewed on a terminal, and only legal documents of the medical record must be printed. Even though technology and security advances protect the "paperless chart," some healthcare professionals need a hard copy to reassure them their data input is secure. During the implementation process, therefore, it is advisable to allow moderate amounts of paper printing to promote security that reliable information is being transmitted throughout the system. A postimplementation evaluation should expose unused printed reports. This indicates that either the information is not displayed in a useable format or, more commonly, the information can be adequately accessed on-line and may no longer need to be printed.

Throughout the process, teamwork and cooperation among decision-makers are essential to a smooth implementation. Otherwise, in-house politics can have the largest negative impact on system implementation. Power plays among people and/or departments can bring an implementation to a virtual standstill. If one person on a committee of decision-makers is following a different agenda than everyone else is, all will experience frustration.

The duration of the implementation process can vary from a few months to a few years. Throughout the process, education and communication can prevent many negative perceptions. Defining specific goals and objectives early on will help the team members stay on track. Periodic checks and balances against the stated objectives will deter the team from losing sight of the mission. Too many tangential distractions will elongate the process, become costly and frustrating, and defer the benefits of automation.

The request for proposal (RFP) is one of the preliminary steps a healthcare organization takes when selecting a computerized information system. The healthcare organization generates a checklist of needs for each department or, alternatively, employs a consultant to assist in succinctly defining and communicating those needs to many vendors. In either case, nurses define the requirements to support the philosophy and practice of their department. Nurses must be involved in this process as information input comes from ancillaries and other organizational departments, as shown in Table 16.1. It is helpful during the checklist definition process to create

TABLE 16.1. Sample specifications for requests for proposals by area.

Registration
- Automatically utilize outpatient and emergency room data for inpatient registration
- Automatically utilize patient information from a previous visit recorded in the system
- Allow in the admission/discharge/transfer (ADT) system for the following fields: patient name, patient street address, city, state, zip code, home phone, birthday, sex, marital status, social security number, financial class, occupation, employer, employer address, and guarantor information
- Have a bed-hold feature for a specific time period for patients on leave of absence
- Provide the ability to add and delete beds and medical service units
- Allow placement of outpatients (i.e., same-day surgery) in inpatients' beds, maintaining accurate statistics

Order Entry
- Provide on-line ordering and result reporting
- Provide on-line real-time patient-centered scheduling
- Access status of tests and procedures ordered
- Change or cancel patient orders with audit trail
- Display possible conflicts between any current orders and those previously entered
- Print results to appropriate and multiple locations (e.g., patient's current location, doctor's office, consulting physician's office)
- List all orders not yet completed; sort for nursing unit, caregiver, and room number

Nursing Management
- Provide library of nursing care plans to which care items can be added, deleted, or otherwise made more specific
- Provide a predefined format for individualized care plans developed at the unit level
- Allow users to enter free text into the nursing care plan
- Provide worksheets for day-to-day and shift-to-shift planning of individual patient care
- Schedule nursing staff at the unit level and centrally
- Accommodate multiple versions of patient classification systems—for example, obstetrics, critical care, and medical and surgical, and generate acuity values as a by-product of charting
- Generate reports in terms of specific nursing care hours per day and per shift
- Maintain records for each employee, including credentials, competence verification, continuing education units, and illness and absence profile
- Store, update, and print nursing policies and procedures

Medication Charting
- Be able to display medications that are due both presently and at any time in the future
- Be able to document medication administration on-line
- Be able to provide on-line notification of overdue medications
- Be able to calculate required dosage based on patient-specific data such as weight, age, and so forth

Quality Management
- Set up defined criteria to which a patient treatment can be compared
- Generate a list of exceptions when patient data fall outside the established range
- Override previously defined criteria for the purpose of performing projects or reviews
- Log incident reports, including patient information, type of incident, place, and so forth

TABLE **16.1.** *Continued.*

Utilization Management

- Identify on a daily basis those patients who have met the healthcare organization's criteria for concurrent admission review
- Allow on-line completion of utilization review worksheet, including discharge date, length of stay, number of reviews, physician referrals, denials, diagnosis, and disposition of patient
- Allow editing of utilization review data for accuracy and completeness
- Generate a monthly log of patient discharges and the number of patient-days denied as specified by outside review agencies
- Maintain utilization review statistics reflecting monthly activity, for example, total number of discharges denied, discharges with denials by insurance carrier, admissions and discharges, emergency and elective admissions
- Maintain a log of denials by third-party intermediaries

scenarios that reflect the true working environment and existing organizational structure.

Nursing's involvement in defining requirements reflects its critical role as key integrator in the provision of patient care. When patients are admitted to a healthcare organization, they are deluged with questions, many of which are asked and documented more than once. It is the nurse who must integrate and collate all the information into a logical format and develop a comprehensive plan of care for the individual patient. Information the nurse collates is captured by registration, medical records, physicians, laboratory, pharmacy, radiology, physical therapy, dietary, and many other departments. The same information is fundamental to the utilization and quality management functions.

Integrating Systems

An integrated system should capture information once, sort it, and generate output in a readable, cohesive format. Nurses most logically determine the point of information capture, because they know what type of information should be captured at registration and what information nursing should capture. They can determine the critical points of integration that will improve the quality of information and eliminate duplication.

For example, many registration systems ask for patient height and weight during the admission process. Regrettably, admissions personnel are not the most accurate source of this information, and if entered into the system incorrectly, erroneous information will be accessed throughout the entire healthcare organization. It is the nurse who can best provide that information accurately, a task that is critical for the pharmacy when calculating drug dosages appropriate for the patient.

All of the departments that make up a healthcare organization are important and vital to the care of the patient, but they are generally focused on just one area (their own) and may tend to be myopic in their view of the patient. The nurse, on the other hand, is the focal point as caregiver for the patient, compiling all pertinent patient information and disseminating appropriate data to a department or person. It is imperative that the nurse, as the integrator of an HIS, work with the ancillaries in determining their requirements for computer systems and ensuring that those requirements are met.

Ancillaries interact with the patient on an individual basis, but the nurse coordinates the activities to best benefit the patient. Social services consultations are generally initiated by nursing based on the patient's need for financial assistance, postdischarge placement, or general counseling. Dietary consultations are also usually initiated by nursing. Nurses inform the laboratory of any pertinent medications prescribed for the patient that might affect normal results; for example, coumadin affects Partial thromboplastin times. Registration and medical record information are often corrected and updated by nursing personnel.

Nursing also interacts with departments that indirectly affect the patient's care, such as central supply, housekeeping, and transportation. Physicians write orders that direct the care provided to the patient, but nurses play an interpretive role for the physician and ensure that care is coordinated and integrated. The nurse, who needs access to all this information to provide quality care, is the most logical person to function as the integrator of the system (see Fig. 16.1).

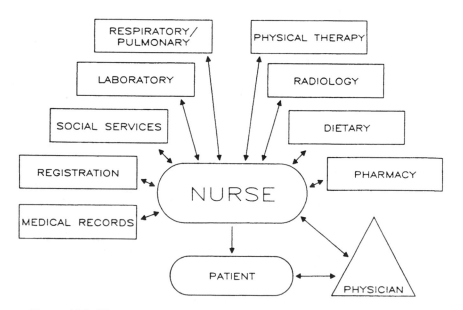

FIGURE 16.1. The nurse acts as the "hub" for patient information processing.

Implementing the System

The implementation of a healthcare organization computer system begins almost immediately after a vendor has been selected. Nurses can play an extremely valuable part in the implementation because nurses have more direct hands-on interaction with and knowledge of the different departments than perhaps any other member of the implementation team. Thus, the nurse can be a direct source of information to facilitate the implementation of a system—whether a standalone single application or multiple applications—in ways that might not be intuitively obvious to implementation planners. Nurses also provide helpful input into the restatement of policy and procedures and the workflow within healthcare organization departments during a system implementation. By contributing in these two ways, nurses can move a step closer to their primary objective: making optimal use of resources to provide quality care to their patients.

These contributions by nursing begin in the selection process, when requirements are first established. They continue throughout the standard cycle of implementation once a selection is made. Specific goals and objectives should be defined as soon as the implementation team is defined. Measurable outcomes should be identified, and distinction should be made between quality measures and quantifiable measures.

Preinstallatation

Before installation activities begin for the multidisciplinary work team, hardware for the system must be in place. Plan on four to eight weeks for delivery and installation. An organizational network must also be in place, and communication protocols should be current with the industry standard. A delay in installation of any of the infrastructure components will almost certainly delay the implementation process and goals, so make sure that adequate time is allotted before beginning installation activities.

Phase 1. Installation Kickoff

Developing a work plan that includes all departments and all tasks to be completed is one of the first and most important steps for a successful installation. An organization-wide kickoff meeting is coordinated to inform everyone of the goals and objectives of the project. Communicating expectations, defining desired outcomes, and letting everyone know about their respective roles and commitments will set the stage for the forthcoming events.

Determining communication channels (meetings, written status reports, automated tools for tracking progress of the project) and frequency (weekly, monthly, upon completion of milestone events that have been identified) is critical to project success. It is important to define periodic checkpoints to stop and take stock in progress that has been made and reaffirm next steps and delivery dates. Workflow assessment should be performed and process improvements identified so that CPRs improve productivity rather than enhance problems in the organization (Amatayadkul, 1998).

Phase 2. Training

Once the installation has begun, training commences. Typically, the vendor trains core healthcare organization staff who are responsible for the implementation in their organization. These core staff members are then designated to train "super users," who in turn train the end user. Because nursing is generally the largest group of employees in a healthcare organization to be trained and because accommodating multiple shifts is necessary, planning is of the utmost importance.

Training is most effective if taught in multiple short segments, two to four hours long. Depending on the complexity of the application, as well as on previous user experience, the sessions can be shortened or lengthened. Automated tools are available to record and replay standard training sessions for individuals or groups of users. This method provides standardization and consistency for training. Trainers must assess individual users to determine additional or follow-up training requirements. Upon completion of the formal training, exercises and assignments should be made to ensure that the users are familiar and comfortable with the new software. Changes in policies and procedures must be documented and reviewed.

Phase 3. Integrated Testing

Integrated testing involves a simulated dry run of what actually happens during the daily routine of a department. Test plans are developed to execute and record the desired outcomes. Interfaces to third-party systems must be thoroughly tested and documented. Testing printers and report output for content and accuracy are all time consuming but vital steps.

It is important to test the validity and reliability of the software and to ensure that new policies and procedures support the designed intent of the system. Information is sometimes duplicated during a parallel test. Patient orders may be entered into the system and may also be sent to the ancillary for verification purposes. Parallel testing may last from a few days to a few weeks to ensure thorough testing.

Phase 4. Going Live

The term *go live* is commonly used at the time the system goes into actual production. The parallel testing is complete, and data are being communicated on-line in real time. A help desk is usually set up as a focal point for logging issues, communicating resolutions, and escalating unresolved problems. The users should be well trained and fairly comfortable with the system. This is the phase when all the effort and hard work pays off.

Phase 5. Postimplementation Evaluation

There may be a temptation to shortchange the evaluation phase. This clearly is shortsighted. If all is going well, this final phase will help to fine tune the system just implemented. If problems exist, evaluation will help to avoid problems when additional applications are implemented in the future. In either case, evaluation can provide valuable insights to the healthcare organization and its many departments, especially nursing. Questions to be raised in evaluation include

- What reports are being printed, and why? Is there a use for them?
- What problem areas are procedural? Who are the problem users, and why? Is it because they do not understand the system? Do they need additional training? Do their problems result from not being involved in the implementation process?
- Is the system doing what the specifications say it is supposed to do? Is the workflow smoother? Is communication improved? Is there any increased efficiency in staff?

Nursing Involvement

By assisting throughout the entire process of implementing integrated healthcare organization information systems, nurses can apply the familiar nursing model of assessment, planning, implementation, and evaluation. Each is discussed here in detail.

Assessment

The scope of the project, the players, the time frame, and the needs of the healthcare organization are all analyzed and documented. Documenting the current workflow in each department will assist in determining the impact the computer system will have during and after the implementation. For example, it will show that because the system automatically notifies the nursing unit when a patient is admitted, a phone call from the admissions department can be eliminated. Similarly, clinical documentation can be accessed on-line, which will eliminate the need to find the hard copy of the chart when a physician phones to inquire about the last set of laboratory results and vital signs. The best-case scenario is that the physicians will directly access the results and vital signs by having remote and secure access to the system. These and many other time-consuming tasks are flowcharted during the analysis of the department workflow and identified as areas that will be eliminated with an automated system.

Planning

When the assessment phase is completed, roles and responsibilities are defined. The liaison nurse works closely with the vendor to identify checklists and checkpoints and to establish detailed work plans. Other events that may impact the planning and execution of the project are network installation, construction projects, Joint Commission for the Accreditation of Healthcare Organizations (JCAHO) reviews, and union strikes. Executive awareness and support for project implementation will help pave the way to success.

Another important step is establishing correct courses of action to follow when system problems arise. Nurses can help determine the chain of command, as well as who should be called when a problem has been identified. The vendor may be involved if the problem is software or hardware related. A solid plan is imperative to facilitate a smooth transition during any implementation.

Implementation

At this third stage, nurses can be invaluable. Coordination of scheduled activities within the healthcare organization and communication with the vendor is the focus of this phase. Critical path activities must occur on schedule to ensure a timely and cost-effective implementation. Healthcare organizations are responsible for more of the actual implementation activities than in years past when the vendor did many of the activities, thus making this phase key to the overall success of the implementation of a new system. A calm demeanor and problem-solving skills are advantageous during the actual implementation because last-minute issues often arise.

Evaluation

Postimplementation analysis ensures that all defined requirements have been met. Comparing the specifications of a system provided by the vendor to the actual system functionality will identify any delinquent areas. For example, if the specifications indicate that the system will generate a certain report and the system clearly does not produce the report, the nurse must decide how important the report is to the overall functioning of the department. The identified areas must be assessed as to the nature of the deficiency and prioritized. Plans must then be created and implemented to resolve any deficiencies. Often, a cost/benefit analysis is performed to identify improved areas of communication, reduced activities as they relate to cost, and an overall evaluation to determine improved productivity and quality care.

Roles Played

Nurses play a variety of roles during a systems implementation, roles that can be accomplished without a programming or technical background. It is far more important that the nurse have a solid understanding of healthcare organization policies and procedures and the ability to change those procedures to improve workflow of the departments. The two most important roles probably are communicator and coordinator. Other critical roles include mediator, decision-maker, and politician/marketeer. The following sections offer a glimpse of each of these roles.

Communicator

The role of the nurse as communicator starts before the implementation begins and does not end until the postimplementation phase is completed to the satisfaction of all participants. Many different tasks occur simultaneously during the implementation phase. If one link is lost in the shuffle, it can cause great distress and distrust of the system as well as delay of the implementation. The nurse can smooth the process and reduce confusion by identifying tasks and communicating with other involved healthcare organization staff members. Many people need to be kept informed of the status of the project, but at varying levels.

Coordinator

Nurses spend much of their time prioritizing needs and coordinating the care of the patient. This experience makes them ideal focal coordinators of an HIS implementation. Responsibilities of coordination include training, meetings with ancillaries, setting target dates, and defining a plan. Throughout the process, it is important to keep issues focused and to observe priorities. The nurse/coordinator may delegate as needed to ensure timely implementation.

Mediator

Many decisions must be made during the implementation process of a computer system. When multiple departments are involved, many issues cross departmental boundaries. An individual should be designated to mediate and facilitate compromise. Because nurses interact with and understand so many of the healthcare organization departments, they easily fit this role.

A side benefit of this arrangement is that it gives nurses a chance to see what happens on the other side of STAT lab results or the process involved in dispensing therapeutic medications or transcribing radiology reports. Conversely, the arrangement allows the ancillary department to better understand nursing responsibilities.

The first few times all department representatives meet to discuss system needs may call to mind hungry lions sharing a meal. A mediator will be essential. An effective mediator can help create a spirit of cooperation and a vision of how the rest of the healthcare organization operates, smoothing the implementation process. Ultimately, one person should be responsible for seeing that decisions are made and are made appropriately.

Decision-Maker

The role of decision-maker during the implementation of a system is crucial. The input of many people must be considered because the outcome affects the entire institution. A nurse with authority to make decisions must keep the project moving forward. Knowing healthcare organization policies and procedures aids the nurse during the decision-making process. Questions to be answered in decision-making center on access to information:

- Who are the authorized users?
- Who should print reports? Where? When?
- Will nurses enter orders or will ward clerks?
- What is the sign-off process of orders?
- Will orders be held in the system until a registered nurse reviews them? Or will orders be automatically released to the ancillary with verification taking place later?

These questions are just a few examples that require decisions. Ultimately, one person should be responsible for ensuring that decisions are made and communicated to all affected personnel.

Politician/Marketeer

Getting people involved is imperative, but it is also difficult considering the activity and workload in a healthcare organization. It is the responsibility of nursing to propagate positive information, solicit support, and promote the system. There are no hard-and-fast rules to follow to make this role successful, but a feeling of ownership of the system clearly helps in establishing a positive attitude toward the system.

The nurse's role as marketeer of the system can be an enjoyable one. Videotapes, buttons, and coffee socials are all methods of encouraging staff participation and support of the system. Skepticism may be prevalent initially, but curiosity usually overcomes the skeptics, and there will be ample opportunity to get everyone involved.

Keys to a Successful Implementation

All the roles the nurse plays during a system implementation have an impact on how well the system is received and utilized by the entire staff. For the implementation to be truly successful, six key factors must be in place:

1. Because a new system will change how nurses' workflow takes place, JCAHO now requires that nurse executives demonstrate input into an HIS system selection. If a healthcare organization's administration makes an independent decision without consulting nursing, system implementation can be greatly inhibited.

2. Solicit strong upper-management support. Nurses feel more confident and are more open to change if they know management is supporting their decision. A positive attitude at the top will generate a positive attitude throughout the institution.

3. Make sure that the time schedule is appropriate for success. Ask questions to determine whether adequate time has been allotted:

- What is the commitment of the healthcare organization?
- Is staffing adequate for training and coverage?
- Does the healthcare organization want to implement the system on one or multiple pilot units?
- Does the healthcare organization want to implement the system in one ancillary at a time or in multiple ancillaries?

The action plan should be closely coordinated with the vendor. It is important to define the responsibilities of the healthcare organization staff and the vendor up front.

4. Realize that mindset and attitudes can make or break a system. If the leaders of each unit are upbeat and enthusiastic, their positive attitudes will create a general feeling of security and support. No implementation is problem free, but most problems can be overcome by working as a team.

5. Designate a liaison person from the healthcare organization. Nursing representatives are often the best candidates for this role. The selected nurse preferably should be one who understands the healthcare organization's policies and procedures and who has the authority to make decisions. Subcommittees and working committees are valuable in some ways, but they tend to drag out the decision-making process and can delay the installation of a system. Nurses can accurately define the requirements of a system to meet the needs of the nursing department. They also add valuable experience of interaction with ancillaries, administrators, and physicians.

6. Highlight communication as an essential ingredient in the implementation process. Keeping the right people informed is a monumental task, but one that must be addressed. Weekly or monthly newsletters and/or meetings can be instrumental in a successful implementation. The risk of misinterpreting issues is decreased, and negative rumors are squelched. The project will also be more focused on critical issues that need immediate attention and resolution.

New Opportunities for Nurses

The increasing involvement of nurses in the implementation of healthcare organization information systems may be partially responsible for the current shortage of hospital nurses. Today, nurses are moving away from the bedside and into the boardroom. In some major metropolitan areas, per diem nurses are earning upwards of $50 per hour. Certainly there are at least as many nurses graduating from school today as there were 10 years ago, and there are more professional working women than ever before. Where are these nurses going, and why?

Many nurses are choosing to use their hard-earned degrees and experience to move into the business side of the healthcare industry. They are putting away their uniforms, donning business suits, and entering the healthcare market through a different door. This seems to be a natural path for many nurses, as they are familiar with the process, politics, and terminology that occur in a healthcare environment. This can be accomplished in many different ways and through many different roles.

Some are taking the experience they have gained from being part of an implementation team of an HIS, updating their resumes, and joining the corporate world. Others are part of the increasing enrollment in master's programs for computer sciences. It does not require technical brilliance to earn a degree in "Management Information Systems." This is just what it implies—managing information—and it is making nurses marketable in the healthcare industry.

New programs are emerging in the nursing informatics area as well. The computer industry is fast paced and forever changing—not an unfamiliar situation for nurses. Unlike nursing, it offers many opportunities for growth and promotion in a short period of time. Nurses associated with the computer industry can impact bedside nursing by facilitating the information processing related to patient care.

Nurses rarely give themselves credit for the multifaceted roles they play every day. They have marketable skills of which they are not even aware. They are analysts, consultants, politicians, and problem solvers. They are also logical thinkers and skilled communicators with experience in prioritization and organization. The following roles, which nurses fulfill in traditional patient care areas, can be effectively transferred to the computer healthcare industry.

Analyst

Nurses are trained to observe, to make decisions, and to act on decisions. Nurses have trained eyes for clinical and psychosocial situations. They have been taught to analyze the situation thoroughly before making critical decisions. They are adept at dealing with change—they do so every day. They have learned to be nonjudgmental and to ask critical questions to get to the heart of the matter.

In short, nurses are analytical. Their skills translate well into the role an analyst plays in the implementation process. An analyst must look logically at how the system works and how the healthcare organization will be impacted. Analyst positions are available in healthcare organization information systems departments as well as in the vendor community.

Programmer

Nurses who enjoy the technical side of nursing, where things are concrete and planned actions produce anticipated results, may be interested in learning to program. Many of the analytical skills developed through bedside nursing can be transferred, but some structured training is usually required to become a programmer. This is a highly sought-after combination in the healthcare computer marketplace today. It is much easier to teach a nurse how to program than it is to teach a programmer about the inner workings of a healthcare organization. Nurses quickly lose their stereotype in this industry, but they learn to keep an aspirin bottle handy for colleagues who come to them for a "professional" opinion on everyday maladies.

Consultant

The opportunities continue to grow for nurses in the consulting field. Healthcare consulting is a multimillion-dollar business because almost every healthcare organization purchasing an information system today uses a consultant to aid in the selection process. The nurse is the best resource for determining a healthcare organization's needs and deciding what vendor meets those needs.

Consulting contracts range from remote question and answer support to extensive analysis of the current workflow and requirements of a healthcare organization. Extended contracts may include long-range planning and marketing tactics for the healthcare organization to use in attracting patients. Nurses provide expert assistance in determining system requirements for a healthcare organization. The nurse's ability to take a large amount of data and organize it into a big picture is a positive asset in the consulting field. A certain level of detail is required, but the key is to take all the pieces and assimilate them into a larger concept.

Developer

Experience gained from being part of an installation team (either the healthcare organization side or the vendor side) provides credentials to develop new systems. The development of a system requires a healthy balance of technical expertise and practical user experience. The technical design by programmers is important to ensure efficiency of computer resources without degrading response time. Nurses can provide the workflow design and requirements of a system, as well as contribute to the human factor influence of how the screens should be designed. Neither side can work in a vacuum. Teamwork is essential to ensure the success of a newly developed system.

Sales and Sales Support

Nurses provide a tremendous amount of credibility and knowledge of healthcare organizations in the sales cycle of an HIS. Healthcare professionals feel more comfortable talking to peers who understand the issues facing healthcare organizations today. Medical jargon can be overwhelming to a non-healthcare person. Nurses provide the link of interpretation and communication between the non-healthcare person (sales representative) and the healthcare professional.

Other sales skills that nurses possess include the abilities to handle many different personalities and to use different approaches with people as the situation dictates. Product demonstrations require knowledge of that product as well as teaching skills that nurses have practiced and perfected over the years.

Marketeer

Nurses can apply their creative sides to marketing special products or total HISs. The strengths of interpreting medical terminology and knowing what healthcare organizations want to hear will assist any business in appealing to the marketplace. Having an inside track to the future of healthcare organizations makes nurses a valuable commodity. Suggestions to help nurses develop some background with computers include

- Attending healthcare computer trade shows
- Subscribing to journals (these will identify trade show dates and locations)
- Getting involved in a healthcare organization system implementation as an insider

- Attending classes at a local community college or university
- Joining a local network group

Summary

Nurses today have the opportunity to affect health care in many ways. They may choose to remain at the bedside, using hand-held terminals to deliver better care. They may elect to enter into the vendor arena, working to integrate information systems. They may also move into the corporate world and represent the interests of health care there. Wherever nurses go, one thing is certain: The computer will not be far away. To keep pace with changes in health care, nurses will become more and more involved with information management and the technology that supports it.

Questions

1. Identify three roles the nurse can play during a system implementation.
2. Identify four key factors to ensure a successful implementation.
3. Assimilate the nursing process (assess, plan, implement, and evaluate) with the implementation of a computer system.

References

Amatayadkul M. Preparing the organization for the computer-based patient record. *Journal of Healthcare Information Management* 1998;12(4).

Section 2.3
Applications

17
The Automation of Clinical Pathways

Kathleen M. Andolina

Clinical pathways have become an industry standard for containing costs, stabilizing quality, and preplanning routine patient care for many of the most commonly treated diagnostic-related groups (DRGs) in acute care settings. Table 17.1 identifies the most frequently benchmarked diagnoses in managed and nonmanaged care areas, lengths of stay, and mortality rates. The results would indicate that when managed care is well established, quality does not suffer. Although reasons are cited for reduced nursing and ancillary costs—including decreased lengths of stay, physician incentives under managed care, and the presence of managed care itself—stabilizing quality remains a mystery in these big picture snapshots (Center for Healthcare Industry Performance Studies, 1999, p. 54). Is it more than coincidence, then, that of the top DRGs listed, most have been subjected to clinical pathways initiatives in many large and small healthcare systems for the past decade?

Clinical Pathways Today

Clinical pathways are ubiquitous today. They are so much a part of the clinical management landscape that we barely remember how their appearance in the late 1980s helped institutionalize the collaborative framework we take for granted today. Nurse case managers, as both developers and promoters of clinical pathways, have continued to use them along with other providers and case manager groups.

Clinical pathways were originally developed with standard office software and spreadsheets, with which it was easy to publish, revise, and abstract data from the spreadsheet and grid designs. Data about length of stay, complications (variances), outcomes measures, and resource costs were fairly easy to abstract. At that time, case managers learned that it was more important to select several indicators for measurement. If an attempt was made to measure all variance data, it resulted in data overload. Today, clinical information systems (CIS) have expanded from desktop

TABLE 17.1. Acute care diagnosis-related groups (DRGs), average length of stay, and mortality in high and low managed care markets.

DRG	Description	Managed care penetration	Length of stay	mortality (%)
14	Cerebrovascular disorder (TIA)	High	6.30	9.53
		Low	8.20	11.09
79	Respiratory infections, inflammations with complications	High	8.36	13.64
		Low	9.61	15.42
88	COPD	High	5.33	1.91
		Low	6.05	2.19
89	Simple pneumonia and pleurisy with complications	High	5.87	5.60
		Low	7.03	6.46
106	Coronary bypass with cardiac catheter	High	10.23	4.51
		Low	11.06	4.06
107	Coronary bypass without cardiac catheter	High	7.61	2.83
		Low	8.03	2.60
112	Percutaneous cardiovascular procedures	High	3.67	1.17
		Low	3.90	1.10
127	Heart failure and shock	High	5.15	4.54
		Low	6.20	5.45
148	Major small and large bowel procedures with complications	High	11.77	7.19
		Low	13.14	8.82
174	GI hemorrhage with complications	High	4.57	3.30
		Low	5.46	3.86
210	Hip and femur procedures except major joint with complications	High	6.34	2.54
		Low	7.70	3.09

COPD, chronic obstructive pulmonary disease; GI, gastrointestinal tract; TIA, transient ischemic attack.

PCs and fax machines to powerful network platforms with multiple applications.

Today's information systems (IS) departments are likely involved with issues other than pathways. Key issues include integration decisions, which involve complicated analyses of whether to keep legacy systems and how to migrate to new ones. Innovative applications are so prevalent today that IS departments could be kept busy for the next several years linking communications, patient records, billing, cost accounting, patient scheduling, laboratory, pharmacy, telemedicine, case management, managed care, and practice sites to each other. Still, meager funding remains problematic for almost half of all the information technology units trying to achieve the business goals of healthcare organizations. A VHA survey of information technology units in not-for-profit members of the healthcare alliance found that 49 percent of 141 respondents called "lack of financial resources" the major challenge in trying to achieve goals (Benchmarking Guide, 1999, p. 78).

Despite these current concerns, options to automate pathways do exist. These include

- Maintaining the pathway on PCs for publication and statistical analysis
- Purchasing a pathways template-based application
- Mixing and matching applications that replicate the pathways processes (examples: clinical messaging products, electronic medical record, outcomes management products, pharmacy information systems)

With these options, the key question to answer becomes this: Does the clinical pathway provide the organizing framework, portal to other applications, or a selection within a menu or Windows-driven system? Whichever option is selected, the development of clinical pathways remains central to evolving clinical technology. Fortunately, clinical pathways can function in either high-tech or low-tech environments.

Features of Clinical Pathways

Clinical pathways are grids that define outcomes and interventions and plot these across time. The expected interventions and outcomes are written for a case type population (homogeneously defined group, procedure, or condition). Once written, the information becomes a comparison tool used to evaluate the actual individual patient progress. Clinical pathways emphasize the process of task and outcome timing. Where the individual patient departs or differs from the predicted plan of care, "variance" occurs.

Variance Analysis

Variance analysis is the act of evaluating care using critical thinking, both in real time and retrospectively. When variance is detected (via direct assessment and comparison with the pathway), caregivers analyze the reason for the variance, make care management decisions, and intervene when appropriate to do so. The variance data provide a rich source of information for both concurrent and retrospective continuous quality improvement and patient management. When the patient, provider, system, or community is the reason for the variance from the expected action or outcome, that category of variance is identified and addressed in one of two ways. If variance is analyzed in real time, it is subjected to clinical problem solving, either in the moment or at least within the length of stay. Retrospective variance analysis involves the process of predetermining what data will be selected for measurement, collection, aggregation, dissemination, and action as determined by the structures for continuous quality improvement (CQI) within the organization.

Timelines

The pathways include a linear timeline, identifying sequential or simultaneous activities necessary to move the patient and family toward the expected results. Timelines are described in anything from minutes (as in emergency department pathways), to around-the-clock shifts, weeks, or per encounter. The timeline feature and the fact that the pathway is a snapshot of one set of outcomes and decisions are what distinguish it from an algorithm. Algorithms may have time estimates attached, but the decision tree (yes/no) assessments are designed to result in numerous directional pathways. The clinical pathway is the best guess as to how an episode of care will transpire given a set of predefined activities, resources, and time.

Clinical pathways exist in numerous organizations under different names, including critical paths, maps, protocols, guidelines, evidence-based practice tools, case management plans, patient outcomes plans, anticipated recovery paths, and CareMap tools. This array of names indicates that the strategy is robust and has been adaptive. The development of the pathway and its full capabilities have been researched, chronicled, and promoted through the efforts of numerous large and small healthcare organizations, as well as the Center for Case Management, a clinical management consulting company located in Massachusetts. The Center for Case Management continues to oversee the progress of pathways worldwide and how they are integrated into CIS systems.

Terminology

Other essential features of pathways include a list of the problems, needs, limitations, or focus of care descriptions. Presently, there is no single standard for clinical languages. Although this gap will make it difficult to precisely benchmark pathways with each other, a single clinical language for health care is not likely to develop. Whole professional identities are structured into the languages used to communicate discipline-specific phenomena as well as to conduct research within respective fields. In fact, some of the earliest issues in developing pathways were based on arguments about terminology.

Defining a problem could become a linchpin issue around what tone a pathway was intending to express. Trying to prevent a patient from becoming dizzy became a complex exercise in naming. Was it to be "alteration in hemostasis" (nursing) versus "hypotension" (medical) versus "fall prevention" (functional)? More often than not, a merged terminology arose. While this did not settle the issue, merged language descriptions at least kept initiatives moving forward.

Such difficulties in reconciling terminology have given way to whole data language projects. The Systematized Nomenclature of Medicine (SNOMED) is a clinical vocabulary that has been developed and is now licensed by the College of American Pathologists. The Current Procedural Terminology (CPT) Coding, International Classification of Diseases (ICD9), North American Nursing Diagnosis Association (NANDA), and other key clinical language systems also are integrated, in part, into pathways. This assists with benchmarking and clinical repository efforts and supports multidisciplinary acceptance for the pathway.

Outcomes Descriptions

Finally, pathways provide descriptions of intermediate and discharge outcomes. The outcomes, plotted across time, correlate with the interventions stated in those time frames. Those new to pathways often made attempts to describe outcomes as tasks or process steps. It has been important to emphasize that outcomes (at least in the clinical care arena) are primarily developed from a patient-centered, functional point of view. Aside from research professionals, nursing has had a great deal of experience in describing outcomes.

Other disciplines also contribute functional language to outcomes statements. Physicians provide interim assessment criteria that must be achieved in order for patients to progress clinically. All providers interacting with a pathway have found it necessary to become comfortable describing, defining, measuring, and comparing outcomes. In addition, externally developed outcomes assessment tools either supplanted homegrown outcomes statements or at least complemented them in some way. Examples include the SF12, SF36, HSQ, HEDIS, OASIS, MDS, and a variety of patient satisfaction tools.

Outcomes-Based Practice

More of a style than a fully developed conceptual model or philosophy, outcomes-based practice provides a framework from which pathways operate. It is multidisciplinary and supports achievement of both cost and quality outcomes, with the patient and family as the unifying concern. It includes collaborative behaviors and a continuum view, relies on documentation tools and systems, yields data as evidence of the results of care, and focuses on intentional, proactive practice values. The expression of outcomes-based practice differs from organization to organization, but it usually starts with a commitment to as much value as cost and quality will provide. In addition, it requires identifying clinical case managers, system resources, some combination of caregivers with superb clinical skills, care management tools like clinical pathways, and a patient-centered focus.

What results from outcomes-based strategies is an organizational responsiveness to change, whether that change is administrative, regulatory, clinical, or financial. Organizations with fully collaborative practices and an outcomes focus will not make change decisions based on fear, panic, tradition, or politics (ideally) or by relying on rehashed data. Outcomes-savvy organizations will be responsive to data acquired through real-time, proactive systems of care and management. Clinical pathways, along with authorized and accountable providers using them, produce a practical strategy for achieving the best value for the cost.

Vulnerabilities of Pathway Initiatives

Pathways projects remain vulnerable to multiple pressures. Early initiatives often suffered from single-discipline ownership that had difficulty transitioning projects into wider and expansive applications. When it was necessary to expand inclusion, it often meant transitioning the leadership as well. The attitude of keeping it small, perfect, and tightly controlled could diminish both pathways expansion and innovation alike.

Upheaval in an organization is another reason for stalled initiatives. If organizations are in the midst of mergers, re-engineering, construction, downsizing, and fragmented continuums, they may suffer from overextended leadership and staff. In situations like these, it is likely that pathways will get lost in the shuffle. Underpowered information technology departments also mean delays in researching and planning for pathways automation and implementation. On a positive note, pathway programs are finding sponsorship in structures such as departments of case management or quality improvement and in centers of excellence.

Still, clinical pathways struggle for acceptability among providers themselves. Collaborative care remains a mystery to those who are individualistic operators at heart. Pathways may become politicized in battles for professional control or clinical agendas. Critics sometimes dismiss them as irrelevant, nice but unnecessary, or reductionistic, pointing to inadequate planning, poorly defined initiatives, or ineffective implementation strategies. Either way, pronouncements like these make it difficult to overcome inertia. Until technology has solidly engineered designs that help providers move in, out, and around in the pathway, providers may remain skeptical about its ability to save time and help them work efficiently. Finally, the potential for the pathway to survive long enough to make it into the next century's CIS frameworks depends on how integrated it will be with the overall CIS design.

Clinical Pathways Results

Despite those potholes, the results of clinical pathways have been well described. Clinical pathways support multidisciplinary communication and provide a central point where all disciplines can view the most recent "snapshot" of the patient's condition. In addition, clinical pathways, when developed by multidisciplinary teams, identify minimum practice standards, incorporate protocols, clarify accountabilities, and single out the most important tasks and outcomes to track. Since their inception, clinical pathways, by describing where the episode of care starts and stops, have provided a method that supports continuity of plan across complex systems. If accepted as part of the permanent medical record, clinical pathways are recognized as an official responsibility of the clinical staff, not merely a reference that sits on a shelf. In many instances, pathways have helped turn patient medical records into what they were originally designed as: a record of clinical process and results, a communication tool, and a database and a documentation device that protects patients, caregivers, and healthcare agencies (Nolin and Lang, 1994; Pozgar, 1990).

Clinical pathways support outcomes practice by forcing the definition of outcomes. The pathway is where the outcomes are tested to determine whether they are

- Simple and functional (everyone does what he or she is supposed to do)
- Engineered to respond to industry pressures (Health Plan Employer Data and Information Set (HEDIS), Joint Commission for the Accreditation of Healthcare Organizations (JCAHO)/ORYX, administrative, and regulatory law)
- Reimbursement focused ("medical necessity" based)
- Designed to support synergy, creativity, and knowledge dissemination (i.e., spiritual outcomes or "Center for Excellence" levels).

Table 17.2 summarizes the potential results from pathways systems.

Automation of the Clinical Pathway

An automated pathway system capable of supporting the results described in Table 17.2 would also need to support the development and maintenance of pathways as well. Progressive competence of the automated pathway product should be part of the planning and contracting process when a product is selected. Understanding the phases of implementing a pathway automation product is helpful to ultimate success. These phases include assessment and selection, implementation, evaluation, and redesign.

Assessment and Selection Phase

The assessment and selection phase is labor intensive and most critical to the ability to automate pathways. It is important to select a team of providers and IS staff to research products, features, and vendors. The team must understand the importance of input from a variety of end users, leaders, and anyone else expected to interact with the technology. Chief executive and financial officers will want to know specifics about what the product will improve, which specific costs it will address, and that the return on investment will be within three to five years. They will want to

TABLE 17.2. Results realized by clinical pathway initiatives.

Organizational Values

Patient centered–patient focused care	The best clinical pathways are constructed from the point of view that reflects a patient-centered approach. Despite pathways often being used to improve a particular process (e.g., discharge planning) or stabilize costs, the basic premise of the pathway is that it exists for the improvement of patient, family, and, sometimes, community outcomes. Keeping firm to that centeredness keeps the pathway from becoming a hollow process that merely reflects dutiful description of practices. Patient-centered care provides a platform that unifies the agendas of all disciplines, organizations, and patients.
Collaborative practices	Clinical pathways are collaborative endeavors. In the early days of pathways, all pathways were developed from scratch, with self-interest as the motivator. Now, pathways are used to benchmark collaborative inclusion as well.
Care coordination	Care coordination is expected across the continuum, whether the providers are in your network or not. The pathway can prompt specific activities (fax sent to primary care provider alerting about service contact, physician in the emergency room speaks to Attending before transfer). In addition, early action on scheduling will ensure coordinated access to ancillary services such as magnetic resonance imaging. Payors in particular will increasingly demand providers to notify and coordinate with primary care and other service providers. There will also be increased pressure to refer to services that will prevent or stabilize conditions. Pathways will need to address these aspects over time.
Inclusion of patient/family and teaching	Pathways describe the outcomes, making it clear what kind of teaching will be required. In addition, teaching content can be planned for maximum learning opportunity rather than as an ad hoc activity.
Provider satisfaction	Pathways provide the opportunity to make all providers more visible, acknowledge contributions to care, and, if designed properly, save time in documentation and care delivery.

Process Improvement Strategies

Case management programs and case managers	Case management programs often include pathways tools to manage the most common presentations of patients. Case managers are often in charge of developing the pathway and managing retrospective variance and step in only after the patient complexities interfere with progress as predicted on the pathway. Case managers provide input into the continual improvement of a pathway, increasing precision of the document over time.

TABLE **17.2.** *Continued.*

Resource management	Pathways describe and predict resources needed to get patient results. Pathways list equipment, tests, materials, staffing, supplies, and medications in varying degrees of detail. The resources and cost drivers become illuminated.
Timing of interventions	The timing of interventions, such as patient teaching, premedicating, or starting an antibiotic, can be critical to achieving reliable outcomes. Pathways when referred to provide the alerts needed by caregivers to consistently deliver on the expected activity.
Variance measurement and management Concurrent and retrospective continuous quality improvement (CQI)	Departures from the pathway are called *variances*. Although all variances are not measured, some, such as key tasks or outcomes, are. Reasons for variance can be categorized and identified from the variance database for each pathway. Data then drive the concurrent and retrospective CQI process and provide the paper trail needed to describe quality improvement to regulators and accreditors.
Discharge planning	For some organizations the mere act of moving a patient from one service site to another is a complex activity requiring enough detail to merit a whole pathway. Process improvement pathways may be useful in these instances to prompt needed interventions.
Documentation Single-entry data	Pathways represent a place to document some measurement data so that multiple providers can view it quickly. They reduce the need to search other chart sections and can replace routine progress notes in many instances.

Best Practices

Research	Clinical pathways can supply data for numerous types of research projects. The pathway itself is a form of "action research" in that it represents a hypothesis for care management.
Consistent, reliable practice patterns	Best practices are those activities and interventions that when replicated tend to produce effective outcomes over and over. Providers learn of best practices from a variety of resources: published practice guidelines, shared pathway program results, key leadership roles, expert knowledge within the ranks, and so forth. The pathway represents a realistic way to communicate best-practice patterns to all staff regardless of experience and becomes a vehicle for implementing practice change.

Growth and Program Success

Cost measurements	Data on care costs, drivers, stability, case mix, resources, value, and medical offset represent powerful information for program planning and forming business goals. Pathways support the acquisition of cost information and serve as a historical record of costs when saved and compared from year to year.

(Continued)

TABLE 17.2. *Continued.*

Outcomes measurement	Data from outcomes measurement ultimately point to the program's success or needs for improvement, a cornerstone to program evaluation.
Practice snapshot and calling card	Pathways provide a calling card for practices. When providers share important structural information about the populations they treat, it is not unusual to hear them speak telegraphically about what day an intervention is provided and what results they are getting. This can lead to discussions that help to change and develop practice patterns.
Centers for excellence	Pathways, when written for a number of related DRGs or product lines, provide a focus for "Centers of Excellence" activity. Pathways provide the ability to communicate practice patterns, resource use, and timeframes in efficient ways and to support the research activity that defines a "Center for Excellence" approach to care.

understand a vendor's track record, cost structures, service points, installations, and place in the industry.

There are some rules of thumb for proceeding:

- If possible, secure funding to send someone to the Healthcare Information and Management Systems Society (HIMSS) annual conference or case management/managed care organization conferences and plan to spend time talking with the vendors and viewing their products.
- Plan a site visit to a company developing such products, or view their installations.
- Be sure to understand the differences between niche and core vendors.
- Determine who the vendors are and how they differ on costs, service, experience, quality, delivery schedules, and contract agreements features.
- If the decision is made to go with a small automation product (template software or predefined pathways), then analyze these from an enterprise-wide perspective.
- Consider whether there is one place where it would make sense to have a small, low-tech solution rather than be included in the full enterprise installation.

Current pathway technology includes template designer discs, standalone products, modules that integrate with core vendor products, and applications that can be integrated with legacy systems. Table 17.3 identifies some current vendors with products that address both pathways modules and other related pathways applications have been available for several years. The products differ based on how they have been developed and for whom. When evaluating products in the development phase, be sure to look at the features described below.

- Preloaded templates. There are numerous templates for pathways. Most products provide distinct sections for outcomes, interventions, categories of care, variance screens, and so forth. Be sure to obtain hard copies of the templates for hand documentation or medical record storage.

TABLE 17.3. Partial list of current vendors with pathways and pathways-related products.

Vendor	Product	Installations
Oracle Reston, VA www.oracle.com	Clinical pathways	North Arundel Hospital, Glen Burnie, MD
Meditech Canton, MA www.meditech.com	Patient Care System (PCS)* links electronically to their *Enterprise Medical Record (EMR)* product	
MedicaLogic, Inc. Beaverton, OR www.medicalogic.com	Logician Software: references patient-specific protocols and offers alert messaging at each encounter	Diabetes and Glandular Disease Clinic, San Antonio, TX
McKesson-HBOC, Inc. San Francisco, CA Atlanta, GA www.mckhboc.com	Pathways Care Manager*	
AutoData Systems Minneapolis, MN www.autodata.com	Creates, scans and analyzes healthcare outcomes forms	
Axolotl Mountain View, CA www.axolotl.com	Elysium Access Clinical Messaging System	Baptist Health Systems, Jackson, MS
Hospital Computer Systems Farmingdale, NJ www.hcsinterectant.com	INTERACTANT Critical Pathways Module	
InforMed Medical Information Systems Inc. Van Nuys, CA www.infor-med.com	"Template"-free and concept- processing pelectronic medical rocessing	
HealthVISION Corp. Santa Rosa, CA www.healthvision.com	Clinical data repository, order entry, results review, clinical documentation	
CliniComp www.clinicomp.com	Clinical Pathways Administrator (CPA)	
PACE Health Management Systems West DesMoines, IA www.PHS.com	Clinical Pathways Manager (advanced patient care management systems)	Door County Memorial Hospital, Sturgeon Bay, WI

*Nursing Information & Data Set Evaluation Center recognized this product as meeting American Nurses Association standards and guidelines.

- Preloaded sample pathways. Providers often like to perform a comparative analysis with other pathways written by similar institutions. When included in the software, organizations can customize the pathways and save on development time.
- Access to clinical language dictionaries. Any terminology that is likely to be used by providers would be beneficial for the purposes of standardizing pathways, benchmarking, and research. SNOMED, NANDA, CPT codes, DRG, ICD-9, and the *Diagnostic and Statistical Manual of Mental Disorders*, Fourth Edition are some examples of clinical language products.
- User-defined fields. Customizing software to suit organizational needs can be costly when vendors are paid to do it. The more capacity an organization has to define, add, and delete fields, the more flexibility it will have in designing custom pathways.
- Preloaded dictionaries. Dictionaries of expressions and outcomes statements are useful when building the pathways grid. Usually, an organization can add its own unique statements to the dictionary as more and more pathways are developed.
- Ability to view patient progress. Healthcare providers must be able to evaluate the progression of patient care. Viewing progress on outcomes is important in such areas as pain control, functional states, ambulation distances, and self-management, and it allows providers to evaluate variance or success in interventions. In addition, having the ability to identify what care areas and providers are involved supports both the big picture view and collaborative care.
- Access to outcomes measurement tools. Does the product have access to outcomes measurement tools and data required by HEDIS, JCAHO/ORYX, regulators, administrative law, payors, and so forth? Will it require additional connectivity, or can it be pulled up? Can updates be acquired regularly? How can pathway outcomes link to an ORYX vendor? Having access to industry-wide outcomes tools even as references are helpful when developing the pathway to address external outcomes measurement concerns.
- Process for use. There are many ergonomic and design issues that make for user-friendly systems. Systems need to be designed according to the organization's intended plan for use of the pathways. For example, will the pathways software run on a stationary PC or a moveable laptop? Will it be close to the bedside or at workstations? Who will access it, and what are the security log-on procedures? When would providers be expected to access it? Will the computer be available during high demand times? What are the back-up procedures should the system crash? How available are support technicians? How many screens does one go through to back in and out of the system? Can you access two pathways at the same time? Is there remote access, an Internet connection, and access to e-mail and other applications?

- Ease of use. Until voice technology improves substantially and other advanced computer systems evolve, we are still a long way from transparent technology that is truly invisible to the provider. Until then, there are standard features like point and click technology, graphical user interfaces, pull-down menus, forced choice selections, shortcuts allowing quick access to and egress from the system, automatic save features, and alerts that message clinicians when a significant outcomes or assessment issue requires attention. Watch for "smartboard" technology—it may make writing popular again.

Implementation Phase

In the implementation phase, the product has been selected and the software modified for use. Process engineering has been conducted so that all providers expected to interact with the pathway are nearly ready to do so. In this phase, it will be necessary to provide training sessions on the product close to the "go live" date. Can the product accommodate implementation and ongoing training sessions? Can training be self-paced and readily available? How intuitive will it be for someone who has not been trained? How will other providers or case managers cover staff who are unavailable or away? Will training be provided by the IS staff, the vendor, or someone else? How involved will the vendor be in the installation and go live dates? What maintenance is required to keep the system moving?

Evaluation and Revision Phase

How did the system not perform as expected, and where are the glitches? Are the deficits in the system solved through other software products? Can they be self-programmed or purchased? Does the pathway vendor have an upgrade process, and will the equipment handle the upgrades? How often are the products upgraded, and what are the costs? What do the staff think? How well did the technology support the principles of outcomes-based practice, and how did it do on the pathways checklist (Table 17.4)?

Summary

Clinical pathways are a proven strategy for care management in complex environments. After 10 years of use, they are ubiquitous in health care and support outcomes-based practice. Automating pathways represents a formidable challenge for vendors, IS departments, providers, and executives. As clinicians gain expertise in using these map and case management strategies, they will be in a better position to speak authoritatively about where they fit and under what circumstances they are used. As automated vendors

TABLE 17.4. The Pathways Automation Survey: How does the system score?

Element	1	2	3	4	5
1. Automates, standardizes, and ensures quality of documentation					
2. Trends reports used to identify and reduce variance					
3. Promotes multidisciplinary, outcomes focus					
4. Realizes cost reductions through identifying resource users and cost drivers					
5. Enables real-time care review					
6. Ensures information is accessible, identifiable, and findable					
7. Supports timely data entry and access					
8. Provides information relevant to pathway users from different disciplines or roles					
9. Ensures information is reliable, accurate, and trustable (secure)					
10. Supports disciplined information (information that is concise and to the point)					
11. Communicates potential and actual problems					
12. Supports collaboration, communication, and coordination (can it print out notification letters to primary care providers in other systems or parts of the enterprise?)					
13. Supports communication with the patient and family					
14. Has the ability to see one day compared with the rest					
15. Has the ability to update clinical pathway, add problems and interventions, and customize care					
16. Performs variance analysis					
17. Supports documentation that is satisfactory to JCAHO and payor standards (i.e., for medical necessity)					
18. Supports clinical data repository goals					
19. Yields information used to update pathways (best-practice revisions)					
20. Trends data for CQI					
21. Nursing Information and Data Set Evaluation Center (NIDSEC) recognized *Scores*					

Highest total score is 105.

better understand how clinicians use these strategies in actual practice, they will be in a better position to create useful designs.

With today's technology, any configuration for automated systems is possible. However, the effort it will take to make it all work will be a collaborative, not a solitary one. Clinicians, executives, and vendors, who respond together to the challenge of building outcomes-based practice and the automated support for it, will see results that profit both industry and patient. The promise of patient-centered outcomes practice will only be realized through unprecedented collaborations, along with a deep understanding of the structure of care.

Questions

1. Describe at least four options for automating clinical pathways.
2. Describe the executive-level concerns that need to be addressed in the initial planning stages of automating clinical pathways.
3. How does a clinical pathway differ from an algorithm, and how might that make a difference in choosing an automated design?
4. How does variance analysis lend itself to outcomes reporting?
5. Argue for or against a single language format for describing clinical phenomena in pathway systems.

References

Benchmarking guide. *Hospitals & Health Networks* 1999 (January) www.hhnmag.com, (last accessed November, 1999).

Center for Case Management, *CareMap Creator*, South Natick, MA: Center for Case Management, www.cfcm.com 1998 (last accessed November, 1999).

Center for Healthcare Industry Performance Studies. In: **Benchmarking** Guide. *Hospitals & Health Networks* 1999 (January 1999); 54 www.hhnmag.com (last accessed November, 1999).

Nolin CE, Lang CG. *An Analysis of the Use and Effect of CareMap® Tools in Medical Malpractice Litigation*. Expert Library, Vol. 1. South Natick, MA: The Center for Case Management, 1994.

Pozgar GD. *Legal Aspects of Health Care Administration*, 4th ed. Rockville, MD: Aspen, 1990.

18
Point-of-Care Information Systems: State of the Art

SHIRLEY J. HUGHES

When we examine all the initiatives clamoring for attention in today's healthcare delivery organizations, we find that cost containment, best-practice protocols, disease management, outcomes measurement, and customer service programs are all identified as top priorities. Every one of these initiatives focuses on improved efficiency, improved effectiveness, or both. Whether we are talking about excellent customer service or outstanding patient care, we consider optimum efficiency and error-free execution of processes (effectiveness) essential components of what we do. Is it any wonder, then, that point-of-care information systems have moved beyond a "nice-to-have" option? Today, these systems are assumed to be an integral part of clinical practice. What seemed futuristic a few years ago has quickly become a requirement for clinical practice.

Requirements for patient care documentation and information access by healthcare professionals have continued to grow in intensity and complexity. In a healthcare environment where inpatients are more acutely ill, staffing is minimized, and care is more integrated across disciplines and care settings, the documentation requirements and the need to access meaningful information in a timely manner is much more urgent. The goal has not changed since the Institute of Medicine's report in 1991; records must be computer based and used actively in the clinical process (Detmer et al., 1997). However, today's healthcare environment demands that healthcare professionals have more and better automated information tools with which to provide efficient and effective patient care. These tools must be available and used as an integral part of the patient care setting, whether at the inpatient's bedside, the physician's office, or the patient's home.

Providing computer-based patient records and useful automated information systems tools to healthcare professionals involves significant technology, communications, and software challenges. The technology continues to evolve and expand. Long-distance healthcare services are becoming more commonplace. Information systems at the point of care are now used to send information to off-site consultants, who provide specialized and timely health care to remote and, in the past, underserved communities.

Intranet services are now used to reach out to patient populations at high risk for health complications (Charbonneau, 1999). In some cases, these new high-tech services are involving the patients in reporting their own health status via the Internet, posing questions to healthcare professionals via e-mail, and receiving on-line educational information to help them learn more about their disease and how to stay healthy. Involving the patients in documenting and using point-of-care information is becoming more and more feasible as our consumer communities grow more computer literate and technology becomes more affordable.

Point-of-care information systems are still lacking, however, when it comes to integration across care settings. The various point-of-care systems still tend to be focused toward specific care settings, such as critical care, anesthesia and surgery, general medical surgical inpatient units, the physician's office, and home health care. Most, however, are based on technologies that support integration with other systems, some have already been networked with other products to provide an enterprise-wide information system solution, and others are being expanded to address the specialized needs of multiple care settings.

Productivity and Quality

Collecting and recording data about the health status of the patient and communicating that data to other healthcare professionals is one of the key roles played by the professional nurse on the healthcare team. The recording function, however, has historically been a very time-consuming and paper-intensive task. Communication methods intended to convey accurate information to other healthcare professionals in a timely manner have not always been reliable. The nurse often spends significant time away from direct patient care simply trying to ensure that the patient's needs are communicated and the orders carried out. Point-of-care automation should serve to simplify these data collection and communication functions, make them much more efficient and effective, and increase availability of information across the continuum of care.

Point-of-care systems are seen as tools that enhance direct patient care. These systems should serve to

- Minimize the time spent in documenting patient information
- Eliminate redundancies and inaccuracies of charted information
- Improve the timeliness of data communication
- Optimize access to information
- Provide the information required by the clinician to make the best possible patient care decisions.

Capturing data at the source, either by the clinician or via a medical device (i.e., hemodynamic monitors, infusion pumps, and ventilators), is the first step in minimizing time spent charting and eliminating redundancies and inaccuracies. When a single data entry can be added to an electronic chart at the point of care and made instantly available to all involved in that patient's care, then time is saved and those data have been transformed into useful information. The data may even be presented in multiple formats and automatically trended or compared with other data elements. With this type of functionality incorporated into point-of-care information systems, nursing productivity is maximized, data are more accurate, and information is more usable and accessible by all involved in the care process.

Productivity is also improved when access to patient information is made easy. With a point-of-care information system, there are multiple "copies" of the patient's chart, one at every terminal. The nurse, no longer the "gate-keeper" of the chart, will spend no more precious time tracking down and filing paper documents, phoning test results, and dealing with interruptions to convey information already documented. The nurse also has immediate access at the point of care to information documented by others and needed for decision-making.

For proper administration of treatments and medications, the care provider must have complete and accurate information on physician's orders and guidelines for carrying out complicated procedures available at the point of care. Additional assistance, such as dosage calculations and potential drug or allergy interactions, may be needed for medication administration. An automated point-of-care system can provide this information to the clinician, along with prompts to ensure that the proper schedule and/or sequence of events is followed. These types of features provide busy clinicians with valuable quality checks and balances, which not only result in improved patient care and satisfaction but also have the potential to lower risks and the costs of liability insurance.

Timely access to on-line reference databases, incorporation of standards of care and best-practice protocols into the care planning process, and the use of standard terminologies and data storage techniques for quality studies and research are all important quality enhancement capabilities computers can offer the healthcare environment. As data are gathered in real time at the point of care and stored in a usable format in the computer-based patient record, not only is the patient's record more complete and accessible, but this wealth of data also can be used by researchers to help clinicians learn to do their jobs better. Future patients will benefit, as will the entire nursing profession.

User friendliness and ease of data entry are especially important concepts when applied to point-of-care systems. At the point of care, the clinician's primary focus must be on the patient, not on the computer system. An automated point-of-care system that requires more documentation or time than a manual system will not enhance the time spent with the patient; it will only increase the time spent in the patient's room. The most effective point-of-care information system is intuitive to the clinician, requires minimal time to use, and presents a minimal amount of intrusion into the patient environment. Neither the patient nor the clinicians should be inconvenienced. They should all perceive the system as beneficial to the care process.

Input Devices

The hardware solutions used for point-of-care information systems have varied depending on the environment and the users involved. At one time, a number of point-of-care systems vendors were attempting to develop or partner with hardware vendors to provide unique terminals for healthcare environments. This seemed a logical approach because portable interactive terminals or small footprint stationary terminals appeared to give the healthcare professional the best of all possible worlds. It seemed that terminals developed specifically for clinicians would be simpler to use than standard PCs and less intrusive in the patient environment. However, with the rapid evolution of PC technology, it became impossible for these vendors to keep up with the industry.

The advantages of using industry-standard PCs and related software far outweighed any other options. As it turned out, in many cases clinicians preferred full-function terminals. They found it cumbersome to switch from one terminal to another depending on the function they were using. They wanted to use the same terminal device for all functions.

Today, we see many full-sized PCs and workstations, as well as laptop PCs mounted on the walls, placed on countertops, or attached to carts in the patient rooms or clinic examination and treatment areas. Most portable and pocket-sized PC options are used by mobile healthcare workers for such specialized applications as home health, respiratory therapy, and case management. Besides the standard keyboard data entry, most systems offer some sort of pointing devices, and some offer touch screens. Bar code input is most often used for specific functions like capturing supply usage and for medication administration, validation, and documentation.

Voice recognition technology is not yet in wide use, primarily because it has some growing to do before it easily accommodates a large number and variety of clinicians with unique medical vocabularies and accents and incorporates the need for timely access to dictated documentation in a shared clinical data repository. Voice input is the method of choice for physicians, however, and there are those willing to put up with less than the ideal to reap the productivity benefits this method of input can provide.

The wireless communications technologies required for real-time interaction between the portable or mobile point-of-care terminal and the computer-based patient chart are available today and are being used very reliably in healthcare environments. For less intensive care, such as home health, downloading patient records into a portable terminal for the caregiver's reference and periodically updating the central computer database via modem is an alternative communication strategy that seems to be working well.

Point-of-Care Starts in the Community

As healthcare organizations continue expanding into integrated delivery networks, one of the biggest challenges is ensuring that patients and customers can gain easy access to the most appropriate services in a timely manner. The widespread use of local area networks, wide area networks, and the Internet has been a huge benefit in addressing these challenges. We see healthcare organizations offering informative Web pages and even on-line appointment scheduling to those patients comfortable with communicating in this manner.

Even more promising are the developments in the use of multimedia technology for telehealth applications. Although these applications are not exactly commonplace today, there are a number of exciting projects under way. Simply stated, these projects are applying multimedia technologies to facilitate communication of patient information from where the patient is physically located to where the care provider is located, often hundreds of miles away. The information communicated might include multiple components such as a live video of the patient, a radiologic image, and the patient's electronic record, all at the same time, as shown in Figure 18.1. The promise of this long-distance point-of-care technology is improved access to quality health care for the patients while lowering overall costs.

Call centers, normally staffed by nurses, are another form of community-centered point-of-care services. Too often, consumers find it difficult to navigate the healthcare environment on their own. They are not sure when to call the physician, which physician to call, where to go for care, and how to manage their chronic conditions. It is this type of confusing and costly situation that call centers are attempting to address.

A call center offers a centralized point of contact for provider referrals and appointment scheduling, a source of information to the patients to prepare them for their healthcare visits, and even a triage point for patient encounters to ensure that the patient is seen in the most appropriate care setting. HBOC is an example of one vendor offering an information system designed to support an active call center. This type of system provides database access for the nurse to review past encounter information, guidelines to use in assessing callers' symptoms, and an easy way of documenting the calls and encounters. The information needed to facilitate the treatment approval process with the patient's insurance provider is also made available. The benefits from these types of systems include not only enhanced customer service, but also decreased costs resulting from better "matching" of patient needs with services offered.

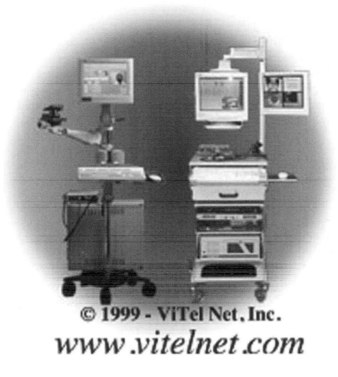

FIGURE **18.1.** Telemedicine technology integrates and supports multimedia. (Courtesy of Visual Telecommunications Network, Inc.)

Point-of-Care Systems in the Physician's Office

Point-of-care systems in physician offices and clinics are becoming more and more commonplace. Some comprehensive applications offering a completely computerized patient record are available. These easy-to-use applications provide nurses and doctors with templates and standard terminologies to facilitate documentation of history and physical examinations, observations, orders, and prescriptions. The availability of an on-line view of all of the patient's visits and phone contacts, instructions given, reminders for follow-ups, and immunizations is a major improvement in these care settings. The office triage nurse is much better prepared to make decisions and provide advice to patients with the point-of-care system providing immediate access to the patient's complete on-line record.

For example, the Epic Systems Corporation's EpicCare Electronic Medical Records System is used in a number of clinics and networked physician office environments. A PC is located in each examining room, each physician office, and at other central areas within the clinic. All are networked to a central database where the electronic patient record is stored. No matter which physician or nurse the patient sees, the same record is accessed and updated. Because the system's friendly graphical user interface was designed specifically for clinicians, it has been readily accepted by most. Clinicians have seen improved efficiencies and believe the quality of care delivered has also improved.

Point-of-Care Systems in Acute Care

It is unfortunate that so many information systems used in the medical and surgical inpatient setting have somehow lost their way to the bedside. A common approach to addressing the push for point-of-care systems has been to simply move the hospital information system (HIS) closer to the bedside (i.e., in the hallway or outside the patient room) so that the clinicians have more convenient points of access to the system. This has proven to be expedient because it provides the same functionality the clinicians are accustomed to at the central station, involves minimal development effort, and requires no additional user training. Unfortunately, it does not offer the advantages of point-of-care documentation (i.e., real time in less time).

Those who have moved their HIS all the way to the bedside have often found that the software solution developed for use at the nursing station is not necessarily the quick and easy tool needed for the point of care. Some of the features required at the point of care that may not be included in a system designed for the nursing station include security, confidentiality, quick data entry techniques, specific functions like validation of therapies, and expeditious retrieval of critical patient information. Usually, the clinicians access the system at central locations away from the bedside. This might be attributable to resistance to change, but more often than not, the system has not given the users an incentive to change. It has not made it easier for them to document as they go and/or the access methods for data review are not as helpful as they need to be for real-time use.

Clinical systems designed specifically for use in the acute care inpatient setting at the point of care are more focused on quickly capturing information normally jotted down by the nurse on the paper worksheet. Reminders of treatments and medications to be administered are provided to the nurse by the automated system. Validation of these therapies and/or warnings of potential error conditions are highlighted. Data access shortcuts are provided to facilitate quick access to critical information. Although these systems are designed specifically for the bedside, charting and data review may also be done at central locations. Typically, these systems are also tied into the HIS so that the need for data accessibility throughout the hospital is satisfied.

Some of the most effective acute care information systems are those designed specifically for use in critical care settings. These systems are designed to manage and display large amounts of data on critically ill patients. They include interfaces to medical devices to collect data automatically. The user interface is usually flowsheet oriented and provides numerous graphical and data trending capabilities. Because they have been designed for use within highly intensive care situations (i.e., anesthesia, post-anesthesia, and critical care), the user interface design has been fine tuned to eliminate unnecessary steps and optimize the usefulness of the data collected. Many of these systems use distributed architectures with multiple servers and redundant processors to ensure maximum system availability and quick response times for the users. They are normally interfaced to the hospital's HIS and laboratory systems to gather test results and provide access to orders.

Hewlett Packard's CareVue 9000 and the Picis, Inc., system are examples of these types of highly intensive care systems. The Eclipsys Sunrise Clinical Manager is an example of a product that has roots in critical care but has since expanded to include all of acute and ambulatory care (Fig. 18.2).

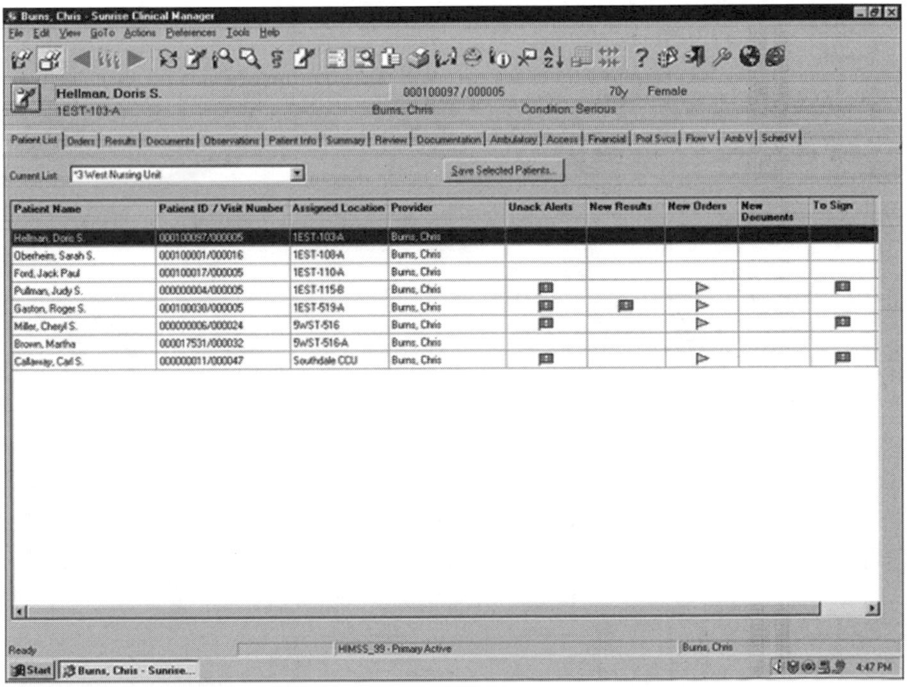

FIGURE 18.2. Use of graphics in critical care systems. (Courtesy of Eclipsys Corporation.)

Point-of-Care Systems in Home Health

Information challenges face home healthcare professionals who spend most, if not all, of their time working remotely (perhaps going into the office only once a week and in rural settings maybe not even that often). These challenges include administering care without ready access to the patient record (it is usually several miles away at the central office), spending hours catching up on the growing documentation requirements (often long after the patient care is delivered), and attempting to keep the billing records up-to-date and accurate. Again, the nurse is spending valuable time tending to information management problems instead of providing patient care. Point-of-care systems based on a central database and portable terminals can greatly enhance the efficiency of home healthcare providers, improve the timeliness and accuracy of the patient and billing information documented, and, with the patient record readily available, deliver appropriate care and make more informed decisions.

Patient Care Technologies, Inc. (PtCT) is an example of a point-of-care system developed for home health care. It uses a small portable terminal with applications specifically designed to support home health documentation requirements and patient chart review. The data are stored in the portable terminal and then transferred periodically by the users to the central database via phone modem (Fig. 18.3).

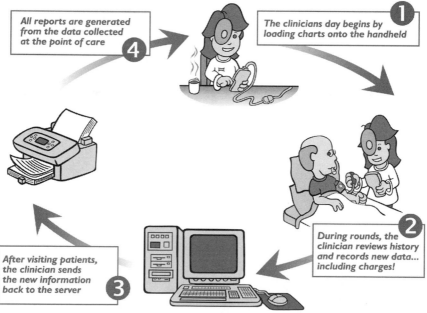

All reports are generated from the data collected at the point of care **4**

The clinicians day begins by loading charts onto the handheld **1**

During rounds, the clinician reviews history and records new data... including charges! **2**

After visiting patients, the clinician sends the new information back to the server **3**

©1999 Patient Care Technologies, Inc

FIGURE 18.3. Home health care. (Courtesy of Patient Care Technologies, Inc.)

Summary

Point-of-care information processing is certainly not a new requirement. It is a long-established one to which new technologies are now being applied. The major features included in the successful systems are those of fast and easy data entry, data accessibility across care settings, quality checks for accuracy of patient care, and, most importantly, nurse and patient friendliness. They are, simply stated, clinically focused. In addition, those systems most likely to stay "state of the art" in this ever-changing healthcare environment are based on industry-standard technology and communications protocols, provide flexibility and scalability, and support healthcare data standards. Healthcare organizations that use these systems have shown that point-of-care systems can provide significant quality and productivity improvements. Systems that enhance the safety of patients and increase the efficiency of nurses can also be cost effective in today's healthcare environment (Ball et al., 1995).

The databases of patient records resulting from point-of-care documentation provide a means for nursing informaticists to study processes and outcomes and learn more effective ways of caring for patients and promoting wellness. Over the next several years, as various point-of-care approaches and technologies in use today evolve, as new technologies are introduced, and as the computer-based patient record is established, nurses will find many opportunities to participate in and benefit from these systems. The challenge will be to effectively package the technology, clinical applications, and information management and storage capabilities into usable and reliable tools that are readily adopted by clinicians in patient care settings.

Questions

1. List the benefits of a point-of-care information system for nursing.
2. What benefits specifically are realized by capturing data at the source?
3. List three quality features typically provided by point-of-care systems.
4. What considerations do you feel are important when implementing a bedside information system?

References

Charbonneau MS, Fisher DC. Helping patients control their health through access to information. *Proceedings of the 1999 Annual HIMSS Conference and Exhibition.* Chicago: Health Information Management and Systems Society, 1999;3:87–94.

Ball MJ, Simborg DW, Albright JW, Douglas JV, eds. *Healthcare Information Management Systems: A Practical Guide.* New York: Springer-Verlag, 1995.

Detmer DE, Dick RS, Steen EB, eds. *The Computer-Based Patient Record: An Essential Technology for Health Care.* Revised edition. Washington, DC: National Academy Press, 1997.

19
Introducing Nursing Information Systems in the Clinical Setting

ANN WARNOCK-MATHERON AND KATHRYN J. HANNAH

The introduction of modern health information systems in clinical settings changes the environment and has a major impact on nurses, the single largest group of care providers in any healthcare organization (Hannah et al., 1999, p. 244). Individuals and organizational units may view such a change as threatening. This can contribute to decreased morale and reduced job satisfaction, which result in resistance to change. Other sources of resistance to change are detailed by Hannah et al. (1999, pp. 238–242) and are merely identified here:

- Oversell by vendors
- Unrealistic expectations
- Changes to traditional procedures
- Insufficient involvement of users
- System improvement as opposed to new approaches
- Fear of leaving the "Gutenberg culture"
- Fear of the unknown

As a consequence of the potential for resistance to change, nursing information specialists must be cognizant of the changes in procedures, functions, and roles that will result, and they must develop change management approaches that will promote nursing user acceptance of the health information system being introduced. Nurses need to be aware of and participate actively in the selection and implementation of the health information system (HIS) for their organizations, as well as the evaluation of the system implementation.

Few computer systems have been installed without the staff experiencing fears and frustrations. Anticipating potential reactions of nurses to the introduction of such a major change can facilitate successful implementation of HISs. If the reasons for these reactions are identified and understood, effective strategies can be developed to foster acceptance and support for the HIS from the nursing users. One strategy is to focus on the factors that make change rewarding rather than focusing on the resistance to change. Negative perceptions may result from a failure to respond in a complete or timely fashion to users' concerns about the system implementation or, interestingly, from unrealized or unrealistic expectations.

The balance between positive and negative reinforcement determines how nurse users of the HIS will react to change. When rewards, incentives, or benefits are perceived to outnumber drawbacks or disincentives, then acceptance will occur. Resistance, which occurs when the negatives appear greater than the positives, is expressed as a desire to maintain the status quo. The manner in which such issues as job security, professional status, and personal concerns about using the system are handled can tip the balance between incentive and disincentive.

In a classic work, based on the work of change theorists viewing change as rewarding rather than punishing, Kirkpatrick (1985) identified three key strategies to facilitate staff adaptation. These are

- Empathy. Empathy is described as a means of predicting nurses' perceptions of the proposed changes. A program to decrease negative perceptions and increase the positive ones will enhance the probability of a successful implementation.
- Communication. Communication is defined as the ability to "create understanding." By fostering understanding, the changes may be perceived to be more positive. Communication of a change should include all of those who need to know as well as all of those who want to know.
- Participation. Nursing acceptance of a new HIS can be facilitated by preparing nursing personnel for automation by soliciting their participation in the selection and implementation processes. True participation means that the users can influence the direction of the project, and the change manager must be prepared to respond to the concerns of the user. Participation also requires that the change manager ensure that those concerned with and affected by the change are actively involved, thereby promoting ownership and commitment.

Because organizational change and the use of information technology are interdependent, the introduction of a health information system requires that attention be paid to the health organization's culture as well as the human factors. Best practices (Adderly et al., 1997; Doyle & Kowba, 1997; FitzHenry & Snyder, 1996; Marasovic et al., 1997) for gaining nursing acceptance of the health information system include

- Involving nursing early in the preplanning (which includes nurses from all departments)
- Involving the nursing users actively in planning
- Designating a person in the nursing department at the senior management level to coordinate the implementation process within the nursing department
- Designating the nursing implementation coordinator as liaison between the nursing department and other departments

- Establishing a user's committee within the nursing department chaired by the nursing implementation coordinator; including the enthusiastic, the uncommitted, and the mildly negative on the committee
- Making resource people available as consultants to the nursing implementation coordinator and the departmental committee
- Developing a training program that includes explanation of rationale for the computerization, nurses' responsibilities related to the new system, expected effect of the system on nurses, and nursing care in the organization as well as actual use of the system
- Using professional colleagues and peers to train other nurses (i.e., a core group of trained nursing users train other nursing staff to use the system)
- Timing training to occur just before the new system goes live; allowing sufficient learning time; providing training time to all shifts.

Concerns related to resistance to change can be grouped into three areas, which—if properly addressed—can increase the probability of successful implementation of an HIS:

- Change management. Successful management of change results in increased probability of user acceptance of the system. Poorly managed change will generate resistance. When this occurs, attempts to circumvent changes will undermine the implementation of the system and the effective use of the system. Consequently, the organization will fail to attain the full benefits of the new HIS.
- Implementation process. A well-defined implementation process, including a project structure and formalized detailed implementation plan, is essential.
- Training of the users of the system. Preparing the nursing staff for introduction of the new HIS is crucial in establishing staff user acceptance and minimizing resistance. This can best be accomplished by designing a training program that will
  - Provide nurses with the basic principles underlying the HIS, including an understanding of computer systems
  - Inform staff of the rationale for system acquisition and selection of the specific system, including benefits expected
  - Define the roles and responsibilities of nursing personnel during and after implementation
  - Orient staff to the use of the system.

Management of the Implementation

For the implementation to progress, a means of allocating resources, making decisions, and reviewing progress must be established. Normally, these functions are the prerogative of a steering committee composed of the upper management of all the affected organizational units. Ideally, the chair of this steering committee is the project sponsor and a member of the health organization's executive management team with decision-making authority. User participation in the decision-making process enables the committee to direct the development according to the organization's needs and priorities. Additional functions of the steering committee include setting priorities, approving any significant change to system functionality or project scope, approving any major change in the project plan timetable, and resolving disputes.

The Project Team

The successful implementation of an HIS requires the participation of all affected individuals and organizational units. To integrate all these people into the project, a project team should be established. The project team will be composed of both information systems professionals and user representatives. The users will play an integral role in providing functional specifications and in supporting the implementation. Unless the project is carefully structured, the diversity of views represented will result in a counterproductive environment.

A project manager coordinates and leads the project team. Project managers require specific skills in order to deal effectively with the factors most likely to create problems for them in managing the project. Desirable project management skills include those necessary for communication, organization and administration, team building, leadership, and coping. Project managers must also possess technological understanding and functional knowledge of the system. In short, "to handle the variety of project demands effectively, the project manager must understand the basic goals of the project, have the support of top management, build and maintain a solid information network, and remain flexible about as many project aspects as possible" (Meredith & Mantel, 1989, p. 101).

Ideally, the project manager should be recruited from the user community within the health organization. Not all organizations, however, have individuals with the appropriate mix of skills on their staff, and some will not want to invest in developing such skills in individuals who will have little opportunity to use them within the organization once implementation is completed. In such cases, health organizations are increasingly retaining the services of consultants skilled and experienced in the implementation of HISs.

The Implementation Plan

Implementation of the HIS must compete for resources with other ongoing projects and normal work activities. Implementation processes tend to be complicated, and a plan serves as a map of the process to be followed. Three components that must be addressed when constructing a plan are identification of what is to be accomplished, the interdependencies of the tasks to be completed, and identification of the people who will carry out the tasks. The plan must identify time frames, personnel to be involved, specification of how problems are to be documented, and strategies for assisting users when problems are encountered. An implementation timetable listing all tasks, their expected start and end dates, human resource requirements, and interdependencies provides a useful tool both for planning user involvement and for tracking progress. Successful implementation requires notifying affected personnel about the implementation plan and providing clarification if necessary.

A clear division of roles and responsibilities for all individuals involved in the process is critical in order to

- Ensure availability of the right people at the right time
- Promote an effective and productive work environment
- Prevent costly duplication of effort
- Facilitate communication among team members
- Ensure accountability for project tasks to be completed.

When everyone knows what has to be done (implementation plan), who is responsible (definition of roles and responsibilities), and when tasks are to be done (implementation timetable), the likelihood of a successful implementation is greatly enhanced.

Training

In the development of the training program, consideration must be given to the needs of the organization, the clients to be served, and the needs and interests of the learner. The resolution of issues such as comprehensiveness of the training program and competencies required for successful completion of the program are inherent in the developmental process.

Nurses are inclined to view change with a certain amount of skepticism. It is necessary to identify common apprehensions of these nurse learners. It would be threatening to nurses if they believed that the patients' welfare might be endangered if nurses did not adequately understand the information technology. As a trigger for reviewing current nursing practice for congruence with evidence-based best-nursing practice, the implementation of a new HIS is highly acceptable. However, nurses likely would be resistant if they viewed the implementation of the HIS as the sole and unsubstantiated rationale for changing long-established nursing practices and procedures. If the "machine" is viewed as a barrier in the relationship between nurse and patient, resistance will develop. The expression and/or repression of their anxieties will impact training and the success of the implementation.

Nursing learners need to become competent in the use of the HIS equipment and the performance of its functions. Nursing staff must be provided with information about the use of the HIS and its benefits to nursing practice so that the learners become cognizant of issues related to the computerization of patient data. Myths and misconceptions about the system can be dispelled through the presentation of facts in the orientation sessions. At this time, computer terminology can be defined and issues related to computerization, such as ergonomics, confidentiality, and security of patient data, can be discussed.

Questions arise about whether a training program should attempt to influence nursing staff attitudes about the computer system in addition to presenting the information required to effectively use the system. A seminal work by Zielstorff (1976) has long provided recognized authority that if the affective components of an introduction to automated systems are ignored, an important adjunct to orientation is bypassed. Scarpa et al. (1992) conclude that strategies to promote attitude change during the introduction of computerized HISs are strongly recommended. The attitude of nursing personnel toward the system—and, ultimately, their morale—often depend on the quality of the training provided. Many health informatics professionals attribute the success or failure of an HIS implementation to the degree of user acceptance achieved.

It is reasonable to assume that the target population will be adult learners who may have predetermined opinions and/or anxieties about HIS training. They are mature professionals with a variety of life experiences and responsibilities. It is critical that the approaches within a training program be based on the principles of adult education in order for it to be effective.

Adult learners long have been described as

- Goal-oriented
- Persistent
- Highly motivated
- Geared to success
- Committed to family, work, and/or other responsibilities
- Limited in time allocated to educational activity
- Best able to meet educational goals using their individualized learning style
- Able to learn best when there is direct application of theoretical concepts and skills to the work situation.

Hepner (1993) outlined an approach for educating healthcare providers during implementation of an HIS based on guidelines for adult learners developed by Darkenwald and Merriam (1982). These included active versus passive participation and presentation of information in a logical sequence to enhance the learning process (Darkenwald & Merriam, 1982).

Several factors contribute to the complexity of the task of orienting staff. The nursing staff who need to be trained in the use of the new system may consist of administrative coordinators, nursing unit supervisors, head nurses, staff nurses, and unit clerks. Presenting information simultaneously to people of widely varied backgrounds and educational levels is a major challenge. One strategy for dealing with this diversity is to create learning groups that are as homogeneous as possible in terms of role, responsibility, and professional background. It is fair to anticipate that some in every group will oppose the introduction of a new health information system.

Defining objectives is essential, not only for specifying the material to be presented but also for evaluating the effectiveness of the course. Each objective should be clearly stated, limited in scope, and measurable, so that the learner can determine when competencies have been reached and so that the planners of the program can evaluate its effectiveness. Training objectives should include

- Providing nurse learners with basic information about computer systems, how they operate, what the benefits are to nursing, and the progress of the project to date
- Familiarizing the nursing staff with the functions of the nursing information system
- Familiarizing the nursing learner with the use of the hardware
- Promoting a positive attitude among the nurse learners toward computerization within the hospital environment
- Generating feedback from the nursing staff in identifying enhancements to system functions.

The training program should acknowledge the differences in knowledge and skills among the learners. By addressing these differences, providing factual information, and allowing the learner to express and interact in a stimulating environment, a training program does much more than teach nurses "how to compute." A training program provides the basis from which the learner may begin to grapple with the revolution of information technology in the healthcare setting—and, thus, it promotes a more sophisticated level of nursing practice. (See Shamian and Hannah, Chapter 21.)

Instructional Approaches

It has long been recognized that user training should be congruent with principles of adult learning, as described in the preceding section. "Training for any system end user should be as 'hands-on' and practical as possible to aid retention and comprehension" (Hepner, 1993, p. 235). A variety of methods can be utilized in presenting the hands-on training component of the program. These include live or videotaped demonstrations, followed by return practice by the learner that is guided by the facilitator. Presentation of material in a modular fashion allows the learner to control the rate of learning. Each module provides the learner with the information needed to successfully complete the function. This method of training allows for higher facilitator/learner ratios. To ease initial anxieties, all hands-on training exercises should be performed on fictitious patients. This allows nurse learners to stay more relaxed and provides the freedom to err without concern for patient safety. There is also no fear that the learner will corrupt real patient data during training.

Another training method is the use of self-paced multimedia tutorials (Hannah, 2000), which might be available from the vendor when a system is purchased. Reasons for considering a multimedia approach include organizational concerns about the traditional "trainer dependent approach" due to the volume of information that has to be presented. In addition, the facilitators often find that teaching the same class content repetitively is tedious. With multimedia tutorials, participants can work independently and at their own pace, at times convenient to them. Multimedia software programs can also help the facilitator manage student evaluations and tailor the course content to the participants' specific needs.

A multimedia approach provides several advantages from both a cost and a quality perspective. Tutorials have helped organizations realize cost savings by decreasing total training time and by reducing or eliminating the one-on-one training traditionally provided in departments such as emergency. From a quality perspective, there has been increased flexibility to schedule classes for participants, and the computer-based training (CBT) program could capture statistical data (Perez & Willis, 1989).

Preparation of Training Resources

As mentioned, to meet one of the primary objectives—that is, the nursing learner becoming competent in using the various functions of the system—hands-on experience is required. This can best be provided in a training room located away from patient care areas so that nurses are not distracted from learning by patient care requirements. Training rooms should have all the same equipment that learners will be required to use in patient care areas. Each learner should have an individual workstation and sufficient space for printed material and accessories. Arranging the workstations in a semicircle allows the facilitator to monitor several learners simultaneously.

Once the training facilities are ready, preparation of the training facilitators can proceed. Each facilitator should complete a basic training course and be provided with additional supervised time on the computer system. The facilitators should be knowledgeable in the content of information presented to the users so that the information and examples will be relevant to participants or users. Group sessions permit discussions on how to structure a session, the application of adult learning principles, and methods of dealing with a variety of situations that may arise. The training coordinator should evaluate each facilitator.

The material provided to learners should include a training manual detailing the steps required to perform necessary tasks and functions on the system. It is important that the learners become familiar with this manual during training so that they will be able to use it efficiently on the nursing unit. Self-evaluation and facilitator evaluation tools are valuable in generating input for the refinement of the training program. Additional training tools, such as audio and videocassettes or multimedia (computer-assisted) instructional modules, can be used to instruct learners on keyboard operation and troubleshooting sequences.

Scheduling of Training

The timing of training sessions requires careful consideration. The number of staff to be trained, the physical facilities available for training, the number of trainers, and the overall staffing situation within the healthcare facility are factors that affect the number of personnel that can be trained at any given time. Whatever the training rate, time should be blocked out immediately before implementation to allow review by the nurse learners who require or request it.

For each training objective, minimum competency levels must be determined. When the learner has successfully achieved the competencies that are the goal of the training program, access to the HIS is given. Should a nurse not achieve the minimum competencies, the training program should provide additional remedial activities.

In addition to the overall consideration given to developing institution-specific confidentiality and security policies and procedures, attention needs to be focused on reinstating access for the individual nurses absent during implementation of new functions and systems.

System Conversion

There are four basic approaches to system conversion:

- Direct or crash conversion. This occurs when the old system is stopped and is immediately replaced by the new system. Because the change is abrupt, this method of conversion places the greatest stress on individuals and the organization.
- Parallel conversion. This occurs when the new and old systems operate simultaneously for a period of time. The primary disadvantage of this approach is that the user workload is doubled. With this approach, provisions should be made to have additional staff available during the conversion period.
- Phased conversion. In phased conversion, parts of the new system are made available to users at discrete intervals. A major disadvantage is that

the new system can be used for only specific functions; other functions must be performed using the existing procedures.

- Pilot conversion. In this method, the system is initially made available to only a small part of the organization. At intervals, other units of the organization will receive access to the system. The disadvantages of this approach are the inability to move staff freely between organization units and potential communication problems when the functions that the pilot group performs must interact with those of groups not on the new system.

The four basic conversion approaches can be combined in various ways: for example, a crash conversion for a pilot group, a phased parallel conversion, or a phased conversion for a pilot group. Each of the conversion approaches has inherent problems. Giving careful consideration to the effect of the conversion method on the organization and producing a plan to address potential problems can minimize the difficulties.

Postimplementation Audit

Following implementation of an automated care planning system, Allen (1991) recommended that follow-up in-services be provided to address and resolve any additional problems. Meredith and Mantel (1989, p. 481) state that the word "audit" is usually associated "with a detailed examination of financial matters, but a project audit is highly flexible and may focus on whatever senior management desires." An internal postimplementation audit should evaluate, at minimum, the following:

- Training. The objective is to determine the effectiveness of the training program and whether users have encountered problems because of inadequate training.
- System functionality. The overall functionality of the system is rated on whether user requirements have been met. This will also determine what enhancements or upgrades to the system are required.
- Implementation process. The audit process views the success or failure of the implementation primarily as a learning exercise for future implementations. The lessons learned may be applied to the implementation of enhancements or extensions of the system. Questions that should be answered include
  - Were the budget and timetable estimates realistic?
  - What were the causes of missed deadlines and budget overruns?
  - What obstacles were encountered?
  - Does the system perform up to expectations?
- User satisfaction. If the users are dissatisfied, they will not use the system. Factors affecting satisfaction levels include the following:
  - What problems are users encountering?
  - How are or will these problems be resolved?

- What suggestions for improvements have users made?
- Do the users find the system easy to use? If not, what can be done to make it easier to use?

Problems identified in these areas, appropriately identified and documented, can be addressed after the review. It should also be remembered that the evaluation of these four areas is an ongoing process and that little items of frustration will have a long-term impact on the attitude of users to the system.

Conclusion

The implementation of HISs holds great promise for nursing practice. The nursing profession will benefit from the recent advances in information technology as nurses gain the ability to access information in a timely manner, thereby enhancing the decision-making process during the provision of patient care. To realize these benefits, nursing information specialists should

- Encourage involvement of nurses in systems testing and implementation
- Solicit feedback from nurses and respond to concerns
- Communicate with nursing staff during implementation
- Provide support during the implementation period.

This will enable nurses to cope with the changes in their work environment, to adapt to procedural changes, and to utilize the new tool, the computer system. By communicating, educating, training, and understanding the nature of user reaction to change, nursing information specialists are able to minimize the period required to reach a high level of nurse user acceptance.

Questions

1. Identify and describe the three elements essential to successful implementation of a nursing information system.
2. Discuss the impact of the implementation of a nursing information system on the organization.
3. Relate the principles of adult learning to the instructional approaches for training nurses to use the system.
4. Compare and contrast the four basic approaches to systems conversion.
5. What is a postimplementation audit, and what are its major foci?

References

Adderly D, Hyde C, Mauseth P. The computer age impacts nurses. *Computers in Nursing* 1997;15(1):43–46.

Allen S. Selection and implementation of an automated care planning system for a healthcare institution. *Computers in Nursing* 1991;9(2):61–68.

Darkenwald GG, Merriam SB. *Adult Education: Foundations of Practice.* New York: Harper & Row, 1982.

Doyle K, Kowba M. Managing the human side of change to automation. *Computers in Nursing* 1997;15(2):67–68.

FitzHenry G, Snyder J. Improving organizational processes for gains during implementation. *Computers in Nursing* 1996;14(3):171–190.

Hannah KJ, Ball MJ, Edwards MJA. *Introduction to Nursing Informatics*, 2nd ed. New York: Springer-Verlag, 1999.

Hannah RS. *Designing Multimedia for Health Care Professionals.* New York: Springer-Verlag, in press.

Hepner F. Teaching/learning strategies for a successful HIS implementation. Proceedings of the 1993 Annual HIMSS Conference. Chicago: Healthcare Information and Management Systems Society, 1993;231–241.

Kirkpatrick DL. *How to Manage Change Effectively.* San Francisco: Jossey-Bass, 1985.

Marasovic C, Kenney C, Elliott D, Sindhusake D. Attitudes of Australian nurses toward the implementation of a clinical information system. *Computers in Nursing* 1997;15(2):91–98.

Meredith JR, Mantel SJ. *Project Management: A Managerial Approach*, 2nd ed. New York: John Wiley & Sons, 1989.

Perez LD, Willis PH. CBT product improves training quality at reduced cost. *Computers in Healthcare* 1989;10(7):28–30.

Scarpa R, Smeltzer S, Jasion B. Attitudes of nurses toward computerization: a replication. *Computers in Nursing* 1992;10(2):72–80.

Zielstorff RD. Orientating personnel to automated systems. *Journal of Nursing Administration* 1976;6:12–16.

20
Healthcare Information Systems

BENNIE E. HARSANYI, KATHLEEN C. ALLAN, JOHN ANDERSON,
CAROLYN R. VALO, JEANNIE M. FITZPATRICK,
ELIZABETH A. SCHOFIELD, SUSAN BENJAMIN, AND
BARBARA W. SIMUNDZA

The 1990s were ushered in by the Institute of Medicine study regarding the quest for a computer-based patient record (Ball & Collen, 1992; Dick & Steen, 1991; Stead, 1999). This study has given rise to significant changes in healthcare information systems that will continue to accelerate in the new millennium. Ever-changing healthcare initiatives, evolving information technologies, and advances in healthcare informatics have resulted in the reengineering of patient-centered care and the transition from traditional healthcare delivery systems to integrated delivery networks (Collen, 1999; Drazen & Metzger, 1999). The healthcare information systems supporting these integrated delivery networks (IDNs) provide for the management and processing of patient-centered data, information, and knowledge across the healthcare continuum, patients' lifespans, windows of time, and diffuse organizational and geographical boundaries.

Concurrently, empowered consumers demanding access to quality and affordable health care and advances in Internet technology have spurred one of the most significant change agents in health care for the year 2000, tele-health (Atherley & Bilas, 1999). Increasing managed care pressures also ushered in the age of accountability, thus creating the demand for financial management analysis tools integrated with measurement tools for clinical performance (Miller, 1999). A key component to addressing healthcare delivery needs for the twenty-first century is the continued development of technological and information infrastructures for an integrated computer-based patient record, which will enhance patient-centered care within integrated delivery networks (Ball & Collen, 1992; Johnson, 1994; McDonald et al., 1992).

Patient-Centered Collaborative Care Delivery Framework

The patient-centered Collaborative Care Delivery Framework, in Figure 20.1, illustrates components of a collaborative healthcare perspective and the necessity for component integration. This integration requirement

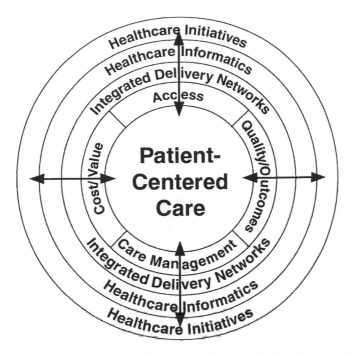

FIGURE 20.1. Patient-centered collaborative care delivery framework.

encompasses not only health systems and processes but also the integration of information technology providing the infrastructure for a computer-based patient record. Patient-centered care, at the core of the framework, cannot be achieved without considering the ever-changing healthcare initiatives, evolving information technologies, and emerging integrated healthcare networks. Healthcare informatics is an avenue for the definition, measurement, and evaluation of the healthcare delivery process (Hannah et al., 1994; Hays et al., 1994; Zielstorff et al., 1993). All of these aspects impact the access, care management, cost/value, and quality/outcomes of health care provided to the educated consumer.

A dynamic and cyclical process is reflected in the circular nature of this framework. The managed reengineering of healthcare delivery requires the ongoing exchange of information, as reflected by the arrows in each of the circles in Figure 20.1. Just as the integration of patient-centered data, information, and knowledge is necessary, framework component integration is necessary for today's healthcare information systems. The goal of this patient-centered collaborative care delivery framework is to facilitate cost-efficient quality care and outcomes valued by the consumer (Harsanyi, 1993; Harsanyi et al., 1994). The healthcare challenges for the twenty-first century will be to ensure a healthy population and to manage disease with the most cost-effective therapeutic options, affording minimal risk and predictable outcomes. Data-driven healthcare information systems will remain a strategic enterprise initiative, along with the pursuit of a computer-based patient record.

The healthcare consumer will become the new driving force behind healthcare initiatives, thus increasing the demand for integrated patient-centered data, information, and knowledge across the healthcare continuum. The next generation of the Internet will change healthcare informatics from supporting health care to transforming health care. Evaluation of the value of healthcare information systems will be based on patient outcomes and quality-years of extended life, not on financial return on investment (Collen, 1999). The goal of health care is to promote, restore, and maintain the health and wellness of the patient, family, and community.

To illustrate the use of healthcare information systems for access, care management, cost/value, and quality/outcomes, clinical scenarios are used to highlight relevant technological components of a computer-based patient record. This discussion is not meant to be all-inclusive.

Access

Healthcare initiatives, as a result of managed care, call for strategies such as wellness, disease, case, and demand management (Miller, 1999). Initiatives also call for universal consumer access to standardized essential services delivered in convenient, familiar, and nontraditional settings. Furthermore, initiatives call for care provider access to patient-centered data across the patient's lifespan, care continuum, and diverse delivery settings. For example, the emergence of integrated healthcare delivery networks is directly linked to this need for the availability of patient-centered data to all healthcare stakeholders, including the consumer. The computer-based patient record provides the avenue for this access.

For example, a nurse practitioner could easily sign on from home to an enterprise healthcare information system and gain access to key patient information to assist in managing a patient caseload. At this time, the practitioner could check a personal and professional schedule for the day and review clinical information regarding the first patient, Mrs. Patterson, a diabetic experiencing foot pain. At the primary care clinic, a patient care representative could quickly identify and reregister Mrs. Patterson while also surveying past encounters. Health coverage could also be identified and initiated.

While Mrs. Patterson is waiting, she can sign on to a terminal in the waiting room to access the most current information regarding diabetic nutrition. Concurrently, Mrs. Patterson's primary care physician would be using a clinical workstation and telemedicine technology to access existing clinical data, schedule the appropriate tests, examinations, consultations, and treatments, and create a referral to a podiatrist and a reminder for an annual mammogram. This would enhance Mrs. Patterson's satisfaction with the encounter.

One technological component in this scenario is the use of intranets and the Internet by consumers and providers to facilitate wellness and demand management. One goal is to Internet-enable client server applications as well as provide Web-based user interface tools and applications. On-line turnkey suites of Internet/intranet-ready applications that are seamlessly integrated into an easy to use personalized interface are now readily available. The cornerstone of these applications is the ability to access the latest health and wellness information from America's leading organizations, such as the American Academy of Family Physicians, the American Academy of Pediatrics, First DataBank, and the National Health Council. "Demand management, which focuses on reducing the need and demand for medical services, involves educating consumers and empowering them to change their care-seeking behavior" (Miller, 1999, p. 19). Applications affording self-assessments, education, functional/health status evaluations, and interactive computer-based instruction regarding self-administered interventions are now readily accessible to the consumer.

For example, when accessing self-management programs through the Internet, Mrs. Patterson can track blood sugar levels and medications and even plan appropriate menus and exercise routines (Fig. 20.2). Using an

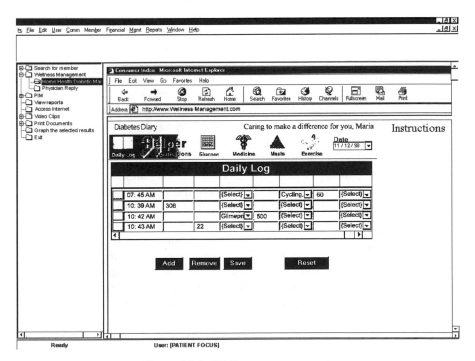

FIGURE 20.2. Wellness management.

integrated healthcare information system, Mrs. Patterson can also communicate with her physician regarding medical advice or Web-based informational resources. She can even connect to other diabetic patients for moral
support through on-line diabetic chat rooms or bulletin boards.

For care providers, telemedicine affords electronic communication and
information technologies to facilitate healthcare delivery when distance
separates the participants across the healthcare delivery network (Westberg
& Miller, 1998). Internet technology can also send daily updates on Mrs.
Patterson's health status to every member of her collaborative healthcare
team. Based on clinical information, her physician can be alerted when Mrs.
Patterson's blood sugar levels are elevated. Care guidelines can also be sent
to remind her about testing and screening examinations to detect early diabetic complications. The Internet can provide Mrs. Patterson with round-
the-clock access to medical support and information needed to maintain
her health regime. Future applications of the Internet for consumers and
care providers will include home monitoring, claims tracking, prescription
refills, on-line preregistration, nurse triage services, and a host of disease
management and wellness programs.

Disease management is enhanced by the second technological component of this clinical scenario, a patient/member demographic repository
shared by all stakeholders. A patient/member repository, using relational
database technology, includes key identification, demographic, and event
information. Care providers access this repository regarding information
about patients/members, guarantors, employees, physicians, and insurance
carriers. This repository facilitates the management of numerous business
functions, such as fiscal management, continuous quality improvement,
patient satisfaction, and care management.

For example, fiscal management provides reporting across member populations. The demographic repository streamlines the registration process
by providing comprehensive, complete, and accurate member information.
Consumer satisfaction is improved by care provider knowledge of the
member and the encounters with the healthcare organization. Care
provider management is also enhanced by a common, seamless access
(using point-of-care technologies) to the computer-based patient record.

As illustrated in Figure 20.3, a third technological component regarding
access and enhancing care management is electronic data interchange
service, including applications that provide an information conduit outside
the healthcare organization to other hospitals, payors, suppliers, external
case mangers, and employers. This conduit also provides bidirectional transmission and data translation into a format that all information systems can
use. Using open system standards, services like eligibility, financial settle-
ment, capitated membership, care support, care authorization, utilization
monitoring, and coordination of benefits and services can be integrated
easily.

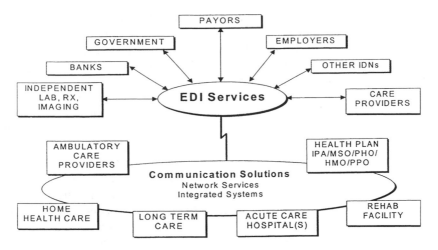

Figure 20.3. Electronic data interchange.

Care support services enable payors to communicate patient-specific information at the time care is provided. This can include details of benefit plan coverage, co-payment requirements, managed care rules, coordination of benefit rules, status of deductibles, and clinical guidelines. A by-product of this communication process is a database, enhanced by intelligent processing, that adds value and perspective beyond that which can be obtained using traditional individual operational systems. When integrated with a clinical repository encompassing comprehensive security measures, the care provider has an integrated view of financial and clinical information.

Care Management

As managed care changes the face of healthcare delivery, new care models that incorporate a patient-centered perspective have been introduced. Often described as care management, these models encompass patient-centered initiatives and processes that IDNs use to manage the health care of the populations they serve. The care models assume a patient management structure, integrating the appropriate access, resources, and expertise to address targeted patient populations.

To achieve care initiatives, the care provider needs rapid access to all patient-centered data, information, and knowledge at the point of care— hence the requirement for a clinical and demographic repository. Productivity tools, such as handheld devices, voice technology, integrated physiological monitoring, and telephony, are also required at the point of care. Automated patient assessment supports defining normal assessment values, displaying the most recent documented values, and charting by exception. Multiple types of data can be supported by logic-based access to electronic flowsheet and clinical decision support of data based on specific patient, clinician, and specialty. It is not the unique configuration of the data displays as much as it is the breadth, flexibility, and power of the review and analysis that creates the value for the care provider.

A key component of care management is the use of evidence-based standards and protocols for the healthcare management of individual patients as well as targeted populations. A technological component to delivering patient-centered services across the care continuum is the automation of integrated clinical standards and protocols, with orders, results, quality improvement initiatives, assessments, documentation, and clinical decision support. Automated clinical protocols support the definition and documentation of the enterprise's standards of care, associated variance management, and outcomes measurement. To automate changing care management models, technological requirements include the capability to define enterprise protocols, tailor protocols based on the patient's clinical profile, use a clinical pathway or map to identify and sequence the care and services, and evaluate outcomes across the continuum of care.

Automated clinical protocols provide the framework for organizing the treatment, identifying the outcomes, and structuring the evaluation of care. As illustrated in Figure 20.4, patient Louise Brady's automated clinical

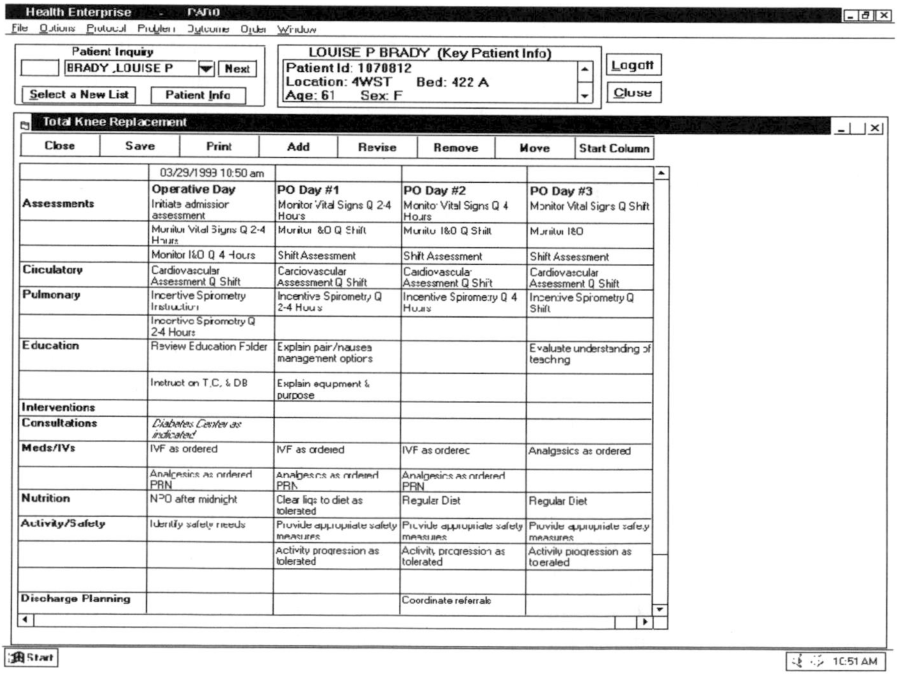

FIGURE 20.4. Automated clinical pathway.

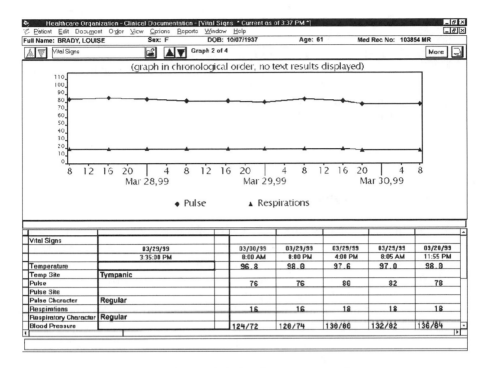

Figure 20.5. Vital signs/assessment graph.

pathway shows the exact timing of key events and patient activities that must occur for the patient to achieve the defined outcomes within the designated time frames. Technological requirements allow for merging of protocols to meet the complex surgical and diabetic care management of Mrs. Patterson.

Care management also requires that the care provider, using electronic flowsheets, can index large and diverse volumes of data as if creating folders in a file cabinet (Fig. 20.5). In addition, graphical displays of user-defined data, including flowsheets, worklists, reports, graphs, waveforms, and images, can be retrieved instantly from a clinical repository. For example, a case manager could tailor a list of patients for review and access integrated data comparing diverse variables. A case manager could also access an electronic flowsheet for an insulin-dependent diabetic and compare via graphical displays the administered insulin against the laboratory glucose values as well as the vital signs. Display formats can include lists, tables, abstracts, bar or line graphs, and columnar trending by data ranges, occurrences, type of observations, and display sequences. All data ranging from a longitudinal problem list to waveforms such as electrocardiogram (EKG) strips are retrievable via an electronic flowsheet and a common clinical repository.

From the consumer's perspective of care management, the computer-based patient record raises concerns regarding privacy. To ensure patient privacy, the Institute of Medicine report identified three sets of necessary activities: system security, data security, and data confidentiality (Dick & Steen, 1991; Kahn, 1998). Examples of technology that can address these issues are maintenance and presence of audit trails, encryption capabilities, access controls, firewalls, biometrics, and digital signatures (Buckovich et al., 1998).

Quality/Outcomes

The definitions of quality care and quality of life are changing due to escalating pressures from purchasers and consumers to measure the value of managed care. This change has resulted in continuous quality improvement initiatives, a consumer satisfaction focus, increasing care provider accountability, and outcome management. It also requires the availability of cost-effective therapeutic options with predictable outcomes for the consumer's quality of life across the lifespan. Concomitantly, comparisons with similar institutions and care providers regarding quality, lengths of stay, resource allocation, mortality, morbidity, and consumer satisfaction are resulting in the need for outcome benchmarking and analysis (American Nurses Association, 1991).

A clinical repository, consisting of a relational database, provides patient-centered data for a patient, Mrs. Bloom, across her lifespan, care continuum, windows of time, organizational boundaries, and episodes of care (Fig. 20.6).

The care provider needs this patient-specific atomic-level data, such as assessments and discharge plans, as well as agency-specific data and domain-specific data, such as policies and procedures and efficacy of various treatments for specific diagnoses for the management of quality and outcomes (Zielstorff et al., 1993).

Inherent in a clinical repository is the ability to capture the health interventions of the transdisciplinary team as well as consumer compliance. A clinical repository ensures consistent standardized data for outcome research regarding prevention, treatment, and education of the consumer. Providers are empowered with the information needed to determine the impact of the delivery system on the health of a population and have a solid foundation for cost-effective health management.

The data in the clinical repository require the constancy and standardization of data elements. Technology can provide a single source of information about the terms and concepts that comprise the healthcare vocabulary of an integrated healthcare delivery network. Technology, such as vocabulary engines, provides a single, integrated view of medical termi-

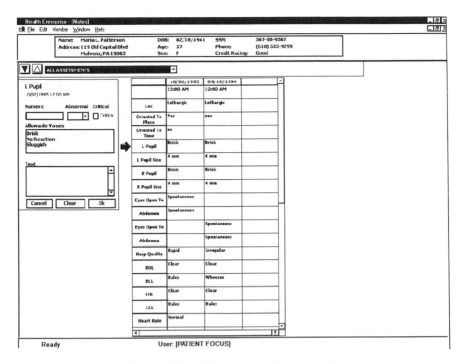

FIGURE 20.6. Clinical repository report.

nology across an IDN instead of a multitude of unrelated, unsynchronized master files.

Numerous theoretical frameworks, lexicons, nursing classification systems, and nomenclatures have been developed to describe the nursing process, to document nursing care, and to facilitate aggregating data for outcome measurement (Averill et al., 1998; Hannah et al., 1994; Zielstorff et al., 1993). Collen (1999, p. 4) predicts that

by 2008, national regulations will have imposed uniform medicolegal requirements in all states for licensed healthcare professional practice, established standards for medical terminology and data definition to permit nationwide integration of patient data, set minimum requirements for electronic claims reporting from computer-based patient records, and assigned universal identification numbers to all patients to permit linking individual patient records wherever the person receives care.

Data warehousing technology adds value to the management of quality and outcomes when clinical and financial data from disparate systems is integrated for analysis, enabling delivery systems to understand and manage costs, quality, and outcomes. The data warehouse maintains longitudinal data, allowing comparisons across time and patients and bringing a new dimension to research, treatment, and discovery of cost effective care (Nussabaum & Star, 1998). Furthermore, the ability to aggregate like patient population data for comparing clinical variances and outcomes improves care standards and treatment practices.

Documentation integration and compliance with quality improvement initiatives can be streamlined with on-line flowsheet charting, such as assessment documentation. Various documentation models and formats can be supported. Care providers can review pertinent patient-centered data, such as results, orders, medications, demographics, progress notes, vital signs, intake, and output values in a graphical flowsheet. By using allowable values for specific aspects, such as documentation of a pupil, the care provider can quickly document that section of a neurological assessment (Fig. 20.7).

Another major technological component of the computer-based patient record that impacts quality and outcomes is a clinical decision support application. Knowledge repositories include reference, algorithmic, diagnostic, treatment, cost, and outcomes. Rules engines act on all data and are capable of recognizing patterns of care that are integral to patient-centered care delivery and evaluation. Clinician-defined rules can provide alerts and reminders, give interactive feedback during order entry, and assist in the assignment and adjustment of protocols of care.

For example, Mrs. Patterson is also taking an antibiotic, gentamicin, and her serum creatinine level increases. In this scenario, a message would be sent to the care provider stating, "creatinine is increased, consider renal insufficiency due to gentamicin and diabetes diagnosis." Clinical decision support integration provides the ability to perform complex calculations, apply clinical algorithms, incorporate new knowledge from clinical research, and support wellness initiatives, thus enhancing quality improvement and cost-containment efforts for effective patient care management across the care continuum.

Cost/Value

In the twenty-first century, most insured Americans will be covered under managed care plans (MCPs). "Most MCPs will have merged to provide patient care services within vertically and horizontally integrated hospital and medical office facilities" (Collen, 1999, p. 3). Payor-driven cost containment, cost-burdened entitlement programs, government regulatory compliance, and funding cuts have all strengthened managed care as a prime architect in the evolving healthcare model. It has drawn momentum from the unrelenting rise in total healthcare spending, projected to reach $2.1 trillion in 2007 (Scott, 1998). Determining the cost/value of healthcare delivery in a managed care environment is an essential undertaking to ensure survival. The ability to aggregate financial and clinical data across the IDN while transforming those data into information and knowledge supports core initiatives of cost reduction and elevates the quality of care.

CLINICAL REPOSITORY FLOW SHEET
FROM 03/01/94 TO 1/14/99

PATTERSON, MARIA   MR#: 1030527   BDATE: 02/18/41   SEX: F

Active Problems 11/20/95 10 00	Medications 11/20/95 10.00	Allergies 11/20/95 10 00
Renal Artery Stenosis	Nephrocaps 1 tab/day	Penicillin
Chronic Renal Failure	NPH Insulin 70U q am	Sulfa
Coronary Artery Disease	Atenolol 25 mg po hs	
Congestive Heart Failure	Tenex 1 mg po bid	
Chronic Hypertension	Catapres 1 mg po bid	
Diabetes (IDDM) 7/88	Procardia 20 mg po bid	
Peripheral Neuropathy	Coumadin 1 mg po daily	

LABORATORY

	11/18/98 18 00	08/01/98 11 30	07/29/98 07:00	07/29/98 06:00	07/29/97 00:30	07/28/97 22.00	02/02/96 16 00	03/04/95 06 30	03/03/94 21 00
Chemistry									
Sodium	133"L	130"L	129"L	132"L	120"L		128"L	130"L	132"L
Potassium	4.7		5.6"H	5.0	6.6"H		5.8"H	5.2"L	5.0
Chloride	90"L	69"L	91"L	94"L	92"L		102	96"L	102
Bicarbon	19"L	21"L	25	22	25				
BUN	86"H		61"H				75"H	50"H	35"H
Creatinine	8.2"HH	7.8"HH	6.7"H	8.8"H			8.2"H	6.5"H	3.5"H
Glucose	154"H	130"H	108	154"H			91	145"H	140"H
CPK	84			45		30			
CPK-MB	3.3			3.0		3.6			
LOH	255"H			182		153			
LDH1	74			40		38			
LDH2	102"H			70		61			
LDH1/LDH	0.73	4.60		0.57		.061			
Glucose	154"H	130"H	108	154"H			91	145"H	140"H
Urea N		79"HH		74"HH					
Creatinine	8.2"HH	7.8"HH	6.7"H	8.8"HH			8.2"H	6.5"H	35"H
BUN/Creatinine		10		9			9	8	10
Calcium		8.8		9.0			9.0	8.5	8.9
Hematology									
WBC	14.9"H			17.5				10.0	10.5"H
RBC	4.18"L			2.84"L				3.10"L	3.3"L
Hcrt %	37.0			26.2"L				30.0"L	34.0"L
Hgb	12.0			8.7"L				10.0"L	11.0"L
MCV	88 5			92.2			93.0	88.0	88

DISCHARGE SUMMARY

Disposition   11/20/98 10:00

She is on a low potassium diet, no activity restrictions. She is to see Dr. Morehouse in about 10 days and the phone number was given. Visiting nurse will be seeing her to review the diet and medications.

Adam Martelli, M.D.

This was one of several admissions for this patient, a 57 yr. Old female with severe systolic hypertension and hyperkalemia. She was seen the night prior to admission because of uncontrolled blood pressure, chest discomfort. She has a past history of renal artery stenosis, several admissions for congestive heart failure, esophageal ulcers, aortic stenosis, coronary artery disease, and diabetes. She is dialysed 3x/week and she recently had an episode of bradycardia for which Dr. Morehouse saw her as an outpatient.

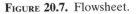

FIGURE 20.7. Flowsheet.

Adoption of data warehousing technology provides the infrastructure to centralize data and offers a collective view of clinical and financial operations throughout the healthcare continuum. A data warehouse is a strategic architecture designed to extract data from transaction systems, data repositories, and external sources and store them in detailed and summary forms. It employs common terminology for a consistent interpretation of enterprise performance and a standard data model to organize, group, and refine data. In the long term, building a data warehouse is a promising solution for the integration of financial and clinical data (Griffin, 1998).

Decision support applications can utilize the data warehouse as a data source and provide health managers with access to enterprise and facility performance information through powerful desktop analytical tools. For example, an executive information system empowers health managers with the ability to measure and monitor performance indicators and standards defined for the enterprise. A vice president of nursing, using decision support technology, can evaluate the effectiveness of a self-management education program for persons with diabetes. Graphical presentations can also denote patients self-administering insulin, admissions due to long term complications, admissions due to short-term complications, and the follow-up status and number of diabetic patients treated in the several treatment settings in the IDN. This early warning system can detect variances and suggest special studies to analyze the program's effectiveness.

Diabetes is a high-cost, chronic disease that results in increased inpatient hospitalizations and outpatient services. To validate initiating a care management program such as health maintenance screenings for vision care, the population at risk can be identified using decision support tools. This would include the ability to identify patients in a specific age range with a diagnosis of diabetes, a healthcare encounter within the last year, a creatinine level of less than 1.5 milligrams per deciliter (mg/dl), and those who have not had a retinal examination in the past two years. Armed with this information, a care management initiative can be implemented that addresses the IDN's at-risk population.

To further analyze a diabetic healthcare management initiative, the Vice President of Nursing can select one button on her clinical workstation and access colored graphs and alerts regarding staffing, productivity, and profitability. This enhances the management team's focus on immediate needs. Detailed operational data stored in an integrated relational database provide the administrator with access to structured, exception, and custom reports while also providing drill-down capabilities for performance analysis. The healthcare administrator can also evaluate the clinical effectiveness and utilization of services while analyzing value and costs for specific episodes of care. Performance can be measured using cost, efficiency, and treatment profiles.

Decision support applications facilitate comparisons of outcomes and resource utilization, resulting in the identification of discrepancies and their causes. For example, the vice president of nursing notices that patient volume in the diabetic care management program is decreasing the need for hospital admission, as illustrated in Figure 20.8. Using product line information, it is determined that preventive care programs and outpatient follow-up after the acute episode afford the greatest opportunities for improved health status and reduced utilization of emergency services. The diabetic services are repackaged as a comprehensive outreach program incorporating consumer education programs, preventive care, inpatient services, outpatient follow-up, and home care utilizing a network of providers

COMMUNITY HEALTH SERVICES ~ IDN
Efficacy of a Care Management Program for Diabetic Services

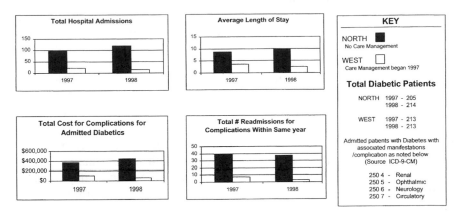

FIGURE 20.8. Analytical information for executive management.

and multiple services sites. This management initiative reverses the impact of an ineffective marketing strategy, promotes consumer choice and satisfaction, and reveals a new revenue opportunity. The integration of financial and clinical data is essential to maintain an appropriate cost/value balance and will challenge the IDN to respond with the appropriate technological infrastructure for the computer-based patient record.

Technology Perspective

The information technology industry is experiencing a period of massive reinvention driven by dramatic changes in human resource requirements, computing structures, and systems management. Concurrently, the movement into the twenty-first century has caused healthcare delivery networks to focus on their systems environments and the critical role technology plays in business operations. As a result of driving technological changes and Year 2000 projects, models of information processing, usage, and management will be forever altered (Mercer, 1999).

The seven key trends creating a significant impact on the information technology industry and affecting healthcare delivery networks are

- The growing staffing shortage within information technology
- Increased demand for information technology services
- Emergence of Windows NT
- Expansion of Internet use

- Growth of ubiquitous computing
- Growth of network computing
- Re-centralization of systems management.

Healthcare delivery networks are beginning to invest in manageability capabilities over functionality capabilities. To make technology operations more efficient and less costly, information systems organizations are increasingly consolidating data centers, server management, and the communications infrastructures, which includes electronic commerce (Mercer, 1999).

The trend toward centralized management is being driven by three key factors. First, Internet growth has inspired integrated healthcare networks to connect internal and external networks, maximizing information access and exchange. Second, mission-critical applications are being deployed on intranets, thus making continuous operation imperative. Finally, the rising cost of network-based PCs is becoming increasingly intolerable. Shifting software management to servers, which are centrally controlled, can potentially reduce overall management costs.

The growth of Internet use and ubiquitous computing provide opportunities to improve the quality of care via care collaboration, on-line patient education, management, and telemedicine. "Tomorrow's successful healthcare organization will be driven by a knowledge-based strategic framework that is customer focused" (Fitchett, 1998). Until the emphasis on managed care emerged, information was treated as a by-product of health care rather than a value asset. The creation of an information asset and the technology to support it is now the strategic goal of healthcare delivery networks (Mercer, 1999).

What, then, are the characteristics of the health information asset? The first is accessibility to information—that is, the technological form and connections that make information valuable and real to the care provider. The goal, establishing a common look and feel across application platforms, involves the creation of a standard user interface template that applications can employ. This creates a shell that makes the look and feel very similar between various applications, improves user navigation and use of the applications, and reduces training time and complexity. Technical approaches to support this common look and feel all share the goal of being Web-enabled, thin-client architectures.

The medium for the care provider's access to information becomes critical. A common and robust graphical user interface that is open, widely accepted, and easy to use is an indispensable component of any information asset. The more intuitive the user interface is, the more the care provider will use the asset. Information comes in diverse forms such as graphics, text, images, and sound; therefore, the user interface should be able to take advantage of these forms where appropriate to make information a strategic and tactical asset to all stakeholders. The second aspect of accessibility is the connection of the care provider at the point of care to the information through the effective employment of robust networks and platform infrastructures.

A second aspect for the creation of an information asset is the use of integration tools providing for the transformation of data into knowledge information. Knowledge information is a group of associated pieces of data that can be accessed and presented to the care provider that is consistent with their discipline and task and contributes to improved quality, productivity, and accuracy. To achieve this, data must be collected, stored, scrubbed, filtered, and translated at various points in the process. Raw information comes from many sources and must be assimilated into a useable asset. To translate and associate information from disparate sources, a common medical vocabulary is necessary. One approach to accomplishing this is to use an automated and intelligent vocabulary engine to translate and associate disparate medical terms into a common vocabulary.

Just as the medical vocabulary in health care can differ, so can the form of information. Automated engines are available to assist in the process of integrating diverse information forms such as voice and video at the point of care. For example, a physician simultaneously could view the results of a patient's tests while also viewing video clips of the patient using parallel bars in a gait study. Another integration tool is the application of intelligent rules to information, a process that provides an intelligent resource for the clinician. Automated rules engines that integrate industry-standard templates such as the Arden Syntax extend and enhance the capabilities of the information asset by providing a system of checks and balances in the care process. Information models for treating patients in clinical settings will differ from information models used to analyze generic, metric-based clinical and business information. It is important that standard tools provide for these models to be optimized for their specific purpose while remaining synergistic in the replication of information.

Finally, a knowledge base model for the business of health care is enhanced by the use of an information warehouse. The information warehouse is the natural collection and transformation point for information collected from many disparate sources across the healthcare delivery network, such as information created in episodic foundation systems. It becomes an enterprise information asset when it is combined with other sources to create a cross-episodic and trend-sensitive resource for clinicians and other users. This cross-episodic view can be referred to as "knowledge information," which forms a key characteristic of the information warehouse.

The information warehouse provides the means of identifying and following customers through the entire continuum of care within the enterprise or target market. It also provides a transformed medical repository of information that can be used over a lifetime to treat the patient and contribute to outcome-oriented health care. Because information comes in many forms, the information warehouse is engineered to accommodate the integration of multidimensional information. This may take the form of storing information in a relational database, storing pointers to other media storage such as optical disk, or simply having the ability to associate the information with other knowledge sources, such as external knowledge databases. It also provides an information model designed and optimized for the analytical aspect of information management. Just as the lifetime patient clinical information is critical to the quality care process, the analytical information model is critical to the overall wellness of the health business, whether it be an individual physician practice, a free-standing hospital, or a complete IDN. The analysis of health information must be capable of creating opportunities into sets of data, sometimes referred to as *data marts*, to be analyzed, refined, and summarized to address specific healthcare business needs.

For the creation of an information asset, however, what makes the information useful is the integration of application software and services that bring health business logic to the care provider's fingertips. Applications enable the automation of health processes and serve as the vehicle by which information is transformed into a practical ally for the IDN. For example, applications assist in the scheduling of patients and members across the healthcare delivery network while keeping all appropriate resources synchronized. They assist in keeping track of patient outcomes throughout the care process while automating the enterprise billing process. They also assist in performing statistical analyses of volumes of information and reporting the relative wellness of the healthcare delivery network. Furthermore, applications help integrate internal and external information so that decisions are based on the best information possible for healthcare delivery.

Tomorrow's information will be a distributed asset for the healthcare delivery network. Although there will certainly be centralized systems and processes, much of the information that is needed to manage the business of health care will be spread across platforms, entities, geography, and disciplines. The information asset must be maintained by employing tools, skill, and processes that minimize personnel requirements of monitoring availability, not only of servers, but networks and workstations as well. The integrity and reliability of the information asset must become a high priority of the enterprise management team. In the business of health care, the distribution of information can be risky and cumbersome without the proper infrastructure in place to ensure security and confidentiality of patient-centered information. The infrastructure must also provide a high level of access and performance in order for the asset to be used in the manner intended.

Finally, as in all information solutions, the asset will need to change over time. The infrastructure must be flexible enough to support the change without compromising the other necessary attributes of the information asset. Distributed systems contribute to productivity, but centralized information management tools and processes ensure that the asset remains

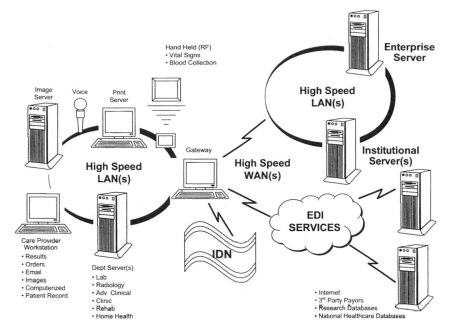

FIGURE 20.9. Integrated delivery network communication.

intact, synchronized, and consistent. This enables all stakeholders to confidently rely on the integrity of the information and enhance cost-effective quality care.

Summary

As is illustrated in Figure 20.9, the healthcare information system is expanding beyond the walls of the hospital into an IDN. The goal is to promote, restore, and maintain health and wellness of the patient, family, and community. The care provider must assume a leadership role in the design, implementation, and evaluation of healthcare information systems for clinical practice, education, administration, and research.

Questions

1. Discuss the barriers to achieving a computer-based patient record: legality, confidentiality, and security.
2. How does the patient-centered collaborative care delivery framework differ from the traditional hospital information system? How does the information system in your organization compare with the patient-centered collaborative system?

References

American Nurses Association. *Nursing's Agenda for Health Care Reform.* Washington, DC: American Nurses Publishing, 1991.

Atherley G, Bilas H. Telehealth: meeting the challenges in the year 2000. *Healthcare Information Management and Communications* 1999;9(1):16–18.

Averill CB, Marcek KD, Zielstorff R, Kneedler J, Delaney C, Milholland DK. ANA standards for nursing data sets in information systems. *Computers in Nursing,* 1998;16(3):157–161.

Ball MJ, Collen MF. *Aspects of the Computer-based Patient Record.* New York: Springer-Verlag, 1992.

Buckovich SA, Rippen HE, Rozen MJ. Driving toward guiding principles: a goal for privacy, confidentiality, and security of health information. *Journal of the American Medical Informatics Association* 1998;6(2):122–133.

Collen MF. A vision of health care and informatics in 2008. *Journal of the American Medical Informatics Association* 1999;6(1):1–5.

Dick RS, Steen EB, eds. *The Computer-based Patient Record: An Essential Technology for Health Care.* Washington, DC: National Academy Press, 1991.

Drazen E, Metzger J. *Strategies for Integrated Healthcare Emerging Practices in Information Management and Cross-Continuum Care,* 1st ed. San Francisco: Jossey-Bass, 1999.

Fitchett J. Managing your organization's key asset: knowledge. *Healthcare Forum Journal* 1998; 41(3):56–58, 60.

Griffin J. Looking into the future of data warehousing. *Advance for Health Information Professionals* 1998;8(23):17.

Hannah KJ, Ball MJ, Edwards MJA. *Introduction to Nursing Informatics.* New York: Springer-Verlag, 1994.

Harsanyi BE. Use of information systems to facilitate collaborative health care delivery. In: American Hospital Association, ed. *Proceedings of the 1993 Annual HIMSS Conference.* Chicago: Healthcare Information and Management Systems Society, 1993;229–240.

Harsanyi BE, Lehmkuhl D, Hott R, Myers S, McGeehan L. Nursing informatics: the key to managing and evaluating quality. In: Grobe SJ, Pluyter-Wenting ESP, eds. *Nursing Informatics: an International Overview for Nursing in a Technological Era.* New York: Elsevier, 1994;655–659.

Hays BJ, Norris J, Martin KS, Androwich I. Informatics issues for nursing's future. *Advances in Nursing Science* 1994;16:71–81.

Johnson G. Computer-based patient record systems: a planned evolution. *Healthcare Informatics* 1994;1(1):42–51.

Kahn MG. Three perspectives on integrated clinical databases. In: van Bemmel JH, McCray AT, eds. *Yearbook 1998 of Medical Informatics Health Informatics and the Internet.* Germany: Schattaauer, 1998:289–294.

McDonald CJ, Tierney WM, Overhage JM, Martin DK, Wilson GA. The Regenstrief medical record system: 20 years of experience in hospitals, clinics, and neighborhood health centers. *Computing* 1992;206–217.

Mercer O. *Key Trends in Information Technology.* Unpublished manuscript, 1999.

Miller A. Managed care and its demands on data. *Advance for Health Information Professionals* 1999(March 15);9(6):18–21.

Nussabaum GM, Star AP. The best little data warehouse. *Journal of Healthcare Information Management* 1998;12(4):479–493.

Scott JS. Healthcare spending to reach $2.1 trillion. *Healthcare Financial Management* 1998;52(12):23.

Stead WW. The challenge to health informatics for 1999–2000. *Journal of the American Medical Informatics Association* 1999;6(1):1–5.

Westberg EE, Miller RA. The basis for using the Internet to support the information needs of primary care. *Journal of the American Medical Informatics Association* 1999;6(1):6–18.

Zielstorff RD, Hudgings CI, Grobe SJ: *Next-Generation Nursing Information Systems Essential Characteristics for Professional Practice.* Washington, DC: American Nurses Publishing, 1993.

21
Management Information Systems for the Nurse Executive

JUDITH SHAMIAN AND KATHRYN J. HANNAH

Ensuring effective as well as efficient care became a central function of the chief nurse executive during the last two decades of the twentieth century. Concomitantly, the public is demanding more accountability, more involvement, and more information about healthcare services. They want evidence that care is delivered when it is necessary, where it is required, in the most competent and cost-effective manner, and with interventions that lead to the desired outcomes. Access to information is increasingly recognized as a corporate strategic resource that is key to making appropriate allocation decisions and is the source of required evaluative data for the public.

Financial applications were the first computer-based management information systems available in healthcare organizations and thus, were accessible to chief nursing officers. Although the benefits of financial systems are easily observable and measurable, the usefulness of other management information systems to nurse executives continues to increase. Nurse executives are recognizing the value of information and the necessity of making informed resource decisions based on data and information. The spiraling complexity of patient care problems, the shift from the hospital to the community as the base of care, and the pressures for quality care that is fiscally responsible all have prompted nurse executives to desire timely access to relevant, reliable, and usable information.

To meet these challenges, new management methods and automated tools are required. Manual data processing is no longer an effective means of supporting management decision-making. The advantages of automation extend beyond its number crunching capabilities and great speed and include enhanced accuracy and increased detail, flexibility, and standardization in reporting.

Nurse executives generally have a variety of automated tools for examining and monitoring components of expense and clinical data. They get salary and supply budget reports, workload measurement reports, length of stay information, resource utilization and quality management data, patient demographics, and other staff and financial documents. The difficulty with these indicators is that little is revealed about the level, quality, appropriateness, cost, or clinical outcomes of care delivered to a specific patient. Information about ambulatory care is either not available or is in a format inappropriate for comparison with inpatient information. The materials are presented and viewed in a linear and singular fashion, and there is a lack of standardization of indicators and terminology across institutions. This makes benchmarking and identifying best practices difficult or impossible. Additionally, the data often are outdated because of the time lag between the episodes of care and the processing of information. Overall, nurse executives are left to cope with management information systems that are rich in data and poor in information.

In this chapter, we examine how automation and computers can assist nursing administrators with decision-making that enables them to provide organizational leadership. We discuss the definition of management information systems and cover a variety of management information systems and other computer applications that may be valuable to the nurse executive. Following a review of these applications, we present some considerations to ensure that information is useful, relevant, and challenging to the nurse executive in the development and use of new applications.

Management Information Systems: A Definition

Management information systems have been developed largely in the business and industrial sectors by management scientists, but they are relevant to nursing and all other health professions. A management information system has long been recognized as an array of components designed to transform a collective set of data into knowledge, which is directly useful and applicable in the process of directing and controlling resources and their application to the achievement of specific management objectives (Hanson, 1982). Austin (1992, p. 327) defines a management information system as a "set of formalized procedures designed to provide current information for management planning and control." More simply, a management information system provides information to assist the manager and administrator in the decision-making process and broadly includes financial, physical, clinical, and human resources information. The level of involvement in the decision-making varies.

Often, the agement information system is limited to applications that merely process, store, and retrieve data. Other applications provide the user with presentations of aggregated, synthesized, and summarized information with which to consider and estimate the impacts, consequences, or outcomes of alternative decisions through modeling. Finally, another group of applications allows nurse managers to electronically network with personnel within their own work setting as well as with colleagues globally. These applications, which include office automation, local area networks, intranets, and the Internet, allow the chief nurse executive to communicate interactively, seek input, ask for information, or announce a decision once it has been reached.

From the nurse executive's perspective, the primary intent of a nursing management information system is to achieve the highest quality of patient care by providing information to support the effective and efficient allocation of resources (Hannah & Shamian, 1992). Although this description could apply to both manual and automated systems, the remainder of this chapter addresses the most common functions of automated management information systems.

Management Information Systems Applications

Increasingly, the nurse executive's role in resource allocation and management is being facilitated by the use of management information systems. With recent advances in computer software, nursing management applications support decision-making, strategic planning, policy formulation, and issues management, and they provide a mechanism for communicating decisions. Automated systems now play a critical part in fiscal, clinical, human resources, and office management. Specific systems include fiscal resource management, patient care services costs, quality and patient care process management, workload measurement, personnel management, staff scheduling, and interoffice and intraoffice networking.

Fiscal Management

Operating Budgets

Nurse executives may have access to information about both the expenses and revenues of their institutions. Computers can easily store and manipulate the range of data required for budgetary purposes. In most healthcare institutions, nursing personnel costs are a major portion of the institution's operating costs. Examples of other budgets within the purview of the nurse executive, either indirectly or in collaboration with other departments, are supply, capital equipment, renovation, and information technology budgets. Management information systems collect, summarize, and format data for use in administrative decision-making related to nursing and nursing-influenced budgets. Periodically produced reports allow for the monitoring of budgets, identification of budget variances (difference in actual versus planned expenses), and assistance with planning future budgets. The reports can be numerical or graphic displays and can include trending of specific budget information. One advantage of the use of automated financial systems is the speed at which data can be retrieved, compiled, summarized, and presented in a consistent, meaningful, and comprehensive form. Another benefit is the ability to design reports for individual needs and situations. This facilitates the ongoing monitoring of activities within the institution and preparation of reports for other corporate staff or departments, the board of trustees, or outside agencies.

Costing Systems

"The most basic function of cost accounting is the determination of the costs of running the organization" (Finkler, 1991). Cost accounting systems assist in the understanding of costs and cost behaviors of a defined unit. In health care, these systems primarily have generated retrospective cost information with the department as the unit of analysis. Although these historical data are still important, there is a shift in the use of these systems to project what costs should be and to establish cost standards. Also, there is movement toward costing out nursing care for specific patient care groups, as well as determining the cost of an entire episode of care for a designated patient group.

Given the increasing emphasis on cost control, nurse executives understand that in order to compete for limited resources, they must be able to cost out nursing services as well as nursing's contribution to defined patient care processes (Johnson, 1989). There are many cost accounting systems used to determine nursing's contribution. These include using per diem, diagnosis, or diagnostic-related groups or workload measurement and patient classification systems to determine cost. As in other components of management information systems, the actual costs associated with collecting the cost data and access to usable and valid data are issues in determining the costs of nursing and patient care processes. Integrated management information systems are critical to the ability of a nurse executive, and the entire organization, to obtain and use cost information for decision-making about the allocation of resources.

Human Resources Management

At the most basic level, computer applications can be used to accumulate data about the employment and educational history of each staff member. Information stored may include absenteeism rate, sick and vacation time status, highest degree obtained, certifications, contact hours, and performance appraisals. Personnel databases are useful for accreditation purposes, to locate a staff member with special skills, or to monitor adherence to institutional requirements for annual educational endeavors. Also, an automated system allows easy retrieval of personnel information to determine staffing assignments via a workload measurement system.

Workload Measurement

Nurses' salaries and benefits generally are a significant portion of the overall institutional budget. The challenge for the nurse executive is to be cost-effective while ensuring that nursing staff is available to meet patient needs. Patient census data were used in the past to forecast the appropriate level of staffing. As patient care needs have increased in complexity, however, this single measure has become inadequate. Other factors such as personnel mix, ancillary support, environmental factors, physician practices, and care delivery models (approach) must be considered in determining effective staffing requirements.

Workload measurement systems have been developed to address the multivariate indicators of patient complexity. The workload systems provide both direct and indirect estimates of nursing care within a particular medical case type by day and over time. The ability of the computer to rapidly store, manipulate, and retrieve large volumes of data is essential.

Examples of systems include GRASP, Medicus, PRN 80, and ERIC. The various systems differ in their theoretical basis and approach. For example, in the GRASP system, time standards for nursing activities carried out for and with patients are measured; nursing hours of care are defined as the sum of all activities. The Medicus system defines a patient type through the application of indicators, and nursing hours of care are developed for each patient type. There is no standard within nursing for workload measurement, and comparative differences have been found among the different systems (O'Brien-Pallas et al., 1992).

Staffing Systems

In healthcare institutions, immeasurable time has been spent creating staffing schedules. Even with the use of master rotation plans, manual scheduling does not seem to eliminate all the problems of alleviating perceived biases in assignments, balancing adequate staffing with cost, and integrating special requests. Thus, automated staff scheduling is a potentially useful component of a nursing management system. Possibilities range from using the computer to print what is essentially a manual rotation schedule to adjusting staff on a shift-by-shift basis by considering patient acuity, workload levels, and staff expertise. The more sophisticated scheduling systems require an up-front investment of intense planning and data gathering. Necessary information, such as identification of levels of staff expertise and criteria for determining patient acuity and nursing workload, must be established. Personnel policies, including elements of union contracts, must be defined. A computer application is then configured to integrate all the information and schedule nursing staff by units.

The ability of the computer to manipulate large numbers of variables consistently and quickly makes personnel time assignments an excellent use of this technology. Advantages of the use of automated scheduling include less time spent on scheduling, unbiased assignments, and advance notice of staff shortages. Of most interest to the nurse executive is the availability of information about the relationship between staff size and characteristics on quality of care.

Clinical Management

Quality Management

Total quality management, continuous quality improvement, and more recently, outcomes measurement or evaluation have superseded the previous quality assurance movement. Nurse executives use these processes to assess the overall quality of patient care within their institution and to receive and communicate opportunities that enhance patient care and organizational effectiveness. Additionally, such external agencies as the Joint Commission on Accreditation for Healthcare Organizations, Medicare, Medicaid, and the Canadian Council on Hospital Facilities Accreditation require the monitoring of specific quality indicators.

Institutions use a variety of approaches to gather information to evaluate the quality of patient care. For quality assessment, information needs might include patient care data, patients' evaluations and satisfaction with care provided, chart documentation, care plans or care paths, performance appraisals, and incident reports. Audit reviews are a major tool for any quality program, and audits of these potential information sources are reviewed either concurrently or retrospectively.

Nurse executives have found integrated hospital information systems very useful in the retrieving, summarizing, and comparing of large volumes of data necessary for quality improvement initiatives. Unfortunately, only a few healthcare institutions have systems that provide the capacity for on-line (computerized), integrated data retrieval, particularly concurrent data, for audit purposes. Costly, time-consuming manual systems or reports from isolated systems are still used for much of the data collection for quality initiatives. It is difficult to identify and analyze utilization patterns and outcomes in clinically meaningful groups of patients or phases of case, using either a manual approach or unrelated reports. Certainly, the scarcity of integrated hospital or health information systems is one of the obstacles to automated support for programs related to total quality improvement, continuous quality improvement, or outcomes measurement and evaluation.

Other obstacles include the lack of a widely accepted method for coding patient care activities and interventions and the focus on the process aspects of quality management rather than the outcome. The quality of the tools used to provide input is another problem with computer-based quality management programs. Most organizations lack relevant outcome indicators, and the validity of even the most widely used audit tools and criteria is largely unsubstantiated.

Patient Care Process Management

Nurse executives usually receive reports of performance measurements such as patient census data, volume determination, patient acuity data, and admission, discharge, and transfer data. Often, this information can be aggregated and summarized via an intranet or local area network connection from a personal computer to the healthcare institution's mainframe. Some institutions are automating their clinical process management tools, known as *care pathways*, *care maps*, or *critical pathways*. Care pathways, discussed in another chapter of this book, can be important tools for the nurse executive when planning resource allocations or determining the cost of nursing care related to a designated patient group.

Other Applications

Office Automation

Office automation is the application of computer and communications technology to office activities. The purposes of such automation are to improve effectiveness and efficiency and to control office operations.

Computerization and communication technologies are changing the work environments of all workers in health care, including administrative, clinical, and clerical staff. Office technology has the potential to affect most aspects of a nursing department's work, such as text processing, filing, meeting planning, and distributing meeting agendas and minutes.

Word processing via a single computer is a simple example of office automation. It involves the automated manipulation of text to produce office communications in a printed medium. Word processing offers many advantages. It reduces the time and expense invested in correcting or retyping text material and shortens the time needed to produce a finished document. Storage and retrieval of documents can be handled quickly and efficiently. It is possible to search for documents by keywords, titles, or date of preparation.

A local area network (LAN) allows the grouping of free-standing personal computers into a coordinated, multiuser computer system. Users of a LAN can communicate via computers between multiple sites, share information easily, and send a complete document electronically. An antidote to the usual "telephone tag," the LAN electronic mail (e-mail) makes it easy to schedule appointments, plan meetings, and ask and respond to questions. The capabilities for widespread distribution of agendas and minutes and database and software sharing are all possible via the LAN. Other advantages include ease in accessing information and increased accuracy, timeliness, and efficiency of information for decision-making. It is important for the nurse executive to understand that implementation of a LAN requires ongoing support in both the technical and educational domains. Also, the use of the LAN by the nurse executive will model, and thus encourage, the use of the system (Chapman et al., 1994).

Most recently, the development of intranets that take advantage of browser technology on the LAN are enabling nurse executives to exploit data and information available in their organizations.

Internet

The Internet is a network of networks that circles the globe. It is a "vast, sprawling network that reaches into computer sites worldwide. . . . [T]his interlinked web of networks defies attempts at quantification" (Gilster, 1994, p. 15). This international network provides an opportunity for the nurse executive to network widely and to gather information easily and quickly from colleagues across town, the country, and the world.

One of the most basic and frequently used functions of the Internet is e-mail. Through this function, nurse executives can ask questions, request or share information, or simply communicate and network with colleagues about common interests. Other Internet opportunities for the nurse executive include:

- Broadcasting messages and questions to colleagues who belong to on-line groups built around specific topic areas and receiving responses from around the world
- Accessing external databases for clinical and cost data from other institutions
- Obtaining sharable software
- Performing literature searches
- Conducting electronic meetings

A number of Internet sites that provide statistical, historical, clinical, and economic data, tools, and information brought a new perspective to the work of nurse leaders and executives. Nurse executives can access the Internet through an organizational LAN, a university connection, a commercial service, or a free service (Freenet), which some cities provide (Nicoll, 1994).

Nursing Management Information Systems: Issues and Challenges for the Nurse Executive

With the proliferation of computers, acquiring information has been influenced by the new speed with which information is obtained, ease of access, availability of new information or information in different forms, and the timeliness of information (Danziger & Kraemer, 1986). All of these contribute to the nurse executive's ability to use information to make timely, rational, evidence-based decisions. The primary advantage of automated management information systems is their ability to process more relevant data at a greater speed. This statement suggests that more is equated with better in the realm of management information. However, a distinction must be made between data and information.

Data are simply a string of characters, whereas information acts as a signal that predisposes a person to take action. The role of the computer, therefore, is to process data into a useful and relevant form, called information. Unfortunately, because of the lack of integration of the multiple information systems in healthcare institutions, much of the output of computers is data rather than information. Today's technology cannot synthesiz and integrate data to enable analysis, planning, and action based on information, not just intuitive reactions to data. A more desirable approach is an integrated system that defines the healthcare institution's output in relation to the number and types of patients who are receiving care. Once the output is defined in a more meaningful way—that is, patients versus departments—the cost or resources used to produce the outputs and the resulting healthcare outcomes can be explored in an integrated manner. Cost effectiveness must be the focus, not cost containment. Cost, quality, and outcome data all contribute to informed decision-making related to resource allocation.

Nursing must become the key figure, not the key target, in shaping the interface between cost and quality. Nurse executives must be "bilingual," understanding the outputs from both cost and quality information systems. They can be active participants in ensuring that organizations assimilate and incorporate a philosophy of balancing cost and quality. Integrated information systems can certainly advance or strengthen this balance. Clinically accurate decision-making that achieves a balance of cost and quality will depend on the integration of these fiscal, clinical, and personnel information components.

According to the 1999 HIMSS/IBM Leadership Survey, 71 percent of healthcare organizations planned to increase their information technology budgets in the next year. It seems timely for nurse executives to be active players in information systems decisions. To support this role for the nurse executive, selected issues and challenges with strategies are discussed in the following section.

Data Issues

The concern about reliability and validity of data is a significant and widespread issue involving all components of nursing management information systems, as shown in Table 21.1. It is a well-known axiom that the quality of output depends on the quality of input. The quality of input can be influ-

TABLE 21.1. Management information data issues, challenges, and strategies for the nurse executive.

Issues and challenges	Strategies
Reliability and validity	1. Conduct regular checks for accuracy and completeness of data sets 2. Monitor compliance of data input
Real-time versus retrospective	1. Document differences in decisions made when using real-time rather than retrospective data 2. Advocate for purchase/upgrade of systems that provide real-time data
Availability of necessary data to capture entire episode of care	1. Educate information services and fiscal personnel about the need to include outpatient data in all systems 2. When new systems are being purchased and/or developed, support systems that can integrate financial, human resources, and clinical data for both inpatient and outpatient care 3. Have nursing actively participate in the definition of cost, quality, and outcome components

enced by its accuracy, compliance, and completeness. A thorough initial assessment followed by ongoing assessment of the quality is critical. The nurse executive needs to ensure that data are sufficient and that accurate (vs. biased) data are being collected and used for decision-making. For example, regular monthly screening to document the consistent application of indicators and patient types is essential to valid and reliable workload measures.

Nursing costs have never been reliably projected because fluctuating patient acuity levels and the related needs for nursing care have not been incorporated. With the integration of fiscal, human resources, and clinical data, the costs for nursing care of individual patients will become available.

The availability of real-time rather than only retrospective data is closely related to the issues of validity and reliability. Historical data are important for understanding events over time (trending), but in the frenetic environment of healthcare today, nurse executives need management information systems that provide timely data for resource allocation and clinical decisions. Some management information systems, such as the financial components, can only provide data that are weeks or even months old. This lag leads to missed opportunities for timely decisions. The use of real-time data to determine staffing requirements or to adjust a care pathway based on a patient's clinical profile is vital to ensuring high-quality care that is efficient and effective, thus ensuring the quality/cost balance. Nurse executives are in a position to document the differences in the financial, human resources, and/or clinical decisions made when using real-time versus retrospective data.

Another issue relates to the availability of necessary data and the responsiveness of organizations to provide these data. One particular challenge in today's environment is the capacity of information systems to integrate data across the continuum of care. The core business of health care is shifting from the acute, inpatient setting to primary care and wellness (Shortell et al., 1993) and from single, isolated facilities or sectors to integrated delivery networks. Management information systems need to be better equipped to provide nurse executives with the quality and cost information about a patient's entire episode of care. The challenge will be the definition of the cost, quality, and outcome components, as well as availability of the data for processing.

Furthermore, there is a growing understanding that in order to build cost-effective care, administrators must make decisions that will lead to the best care possible in the context of available resources. This means that data on clinical and cost benefit analyses must be integrated and priorities determined. In this context, we are becoming aware of the possibilities with the use of health services research and secondary data sets. Large data sets are gathered from different sources in areas of clinical, human resources, and financial data so that best clinical outcomes can be examined. The growing interest in evidence-based management, policy, restructuring, and care delivery approaches have led to increased investment and interest in the use of secondary data sets. We are in the early stages of developing the science, methodology, and expertise among nurses that will maximize the possibilities of these data sets. The coming years will lead to growing funding in this area as the industry searches for answers to optimal effective care.

Collaboration and Relationship Issues

Strategic alliances are critical to the development of useful management information systems, as illustrated in Table 21.2. No longer can the nurse executive make decisions about resources in isolation. There is need for dialogue, collaboration, and working agreements among all senior administrators regarding identification and management of resources. These partnerships must extend to the priority setting and decision-making processes surrounding management information systems. Nurse executives can be champions for implementing user-friendly management information systems and leaders in articulating the potential benefits of merging financial, human resources, and clinical components of an institution's information systems. By doing so, they can ensure that resource allocation decisions are made on the basis of information, not just on unsubstantiated data, history, or feelings.

Nursing administrators may serve as role models for using data to make decisions. When making presentations to other senior managers or to nurse managers, the nurse executive should explicitly illustrate how data were used to arrive at a particular decision related to resource allocation. Similarly, the nurse executive might reinforce the significance of management

TABLE 21.2. Relationship and collaboration issues, challenges, and strategies for management information systems.

Issues and challenges	Strategies
Nurse administrator working with data and information in isolation	1. Form a strong partnership among nursing, other care providers, finance, human resources, and information services senior administrators to create integrated systems and information 2. Initiate dialogue and collaboration with all senior administrators regarding the identification and management of resources 3. Establish a solid nursing informatics expertise in information needs 4. Educate nonclinical administrators about clinical care 5. Take and make the opportunities to learn the language and detail of the data requirements of the finance, human resources, and information services departments 6. Ensure that nursing is an active participant in the selection, installation, and evaluation of any financial, human resources, and/or clinical systems 7. Articulate the benefits of merging financial, human resources, and clinical databases
Nurse executive as role model in use of data for decision-making	1. Explicitly use data to illustrate how resource decision was made 2. Require nurse managers to use data to substantiate resource and clinical decisions
Sharing data across institutions	1. Support a Nursing Management Minimum Data Set, including pursuing institutional backing for standardized data collection and processing 2. Access Internet to network and give and receive information from other nurse executives throughout the world

information systems and the available data by requiring nurse managers to use data to substantiate resource and clinical decisions.

It is useful also to have nurses with informatics expertise within the nursing department or to have access to this expertise through agreements with university faculty or consultants. Along with the nurse executive, these experts can educate others in the organization about clinical care, the value and meaning of data, and clinical systems requirements. Also, the nurse executive and nursing informatics experts must learn the data sources and requirements of other departments so that they can use all existing data and be knowledgeable contributors to decisions about creating integrated systems and information.

Because nursing is a major stakeholder in any healthcare organization, nurses need to be active participants in all components of the selection and installation of management information systems. A strong nursing presence is required in all phases. These include the needs and feasibility assessment, the requests for proposals, the systems design and software development, implementation, and evaluation and maintenance.

In addition to collaboration within organizations, interaction is needed across organizations. The ability to identify best practices and/or benchmark via shared databases would be of great benefit to nurse executives and ultimately to patient care. Huber et al. (1992) have proposed a Nursing Management Minimum Data Set.

A Nursing Management Minimum Data Set is a collection of core data elements that assist nurse managers and executives in decision-making about care effectiveness. The data set includes uniform elements so that comparisons can be made within as well as across healthcare institutions. Elements of interest include four dimensions:

- Structure, process, and resources
- Outcomes
- Personnel
- Relational database links

Nursing unit characteristics, Medicare case mix cost, staff resources, budget, patient and provider satisfaction, and average intensity of nursing care are examples of potential data elements. Integrated health information systems provide the opportunity for ease in processing, sharing, and comparing the Nursing Management Minimum Data Set, but issues related to its implementation are still significant. Critical to the success of such a venture is the determination of common terminology, definitions of data elements, and a uniform method for collecting and reporting data elements.

As the core business of health care shifts from the acute, inpatient setting to primary care and wellness (Shortell et al., 1993), management information systems need to be better equipped to provide nurse executives with the quality and cost information about a patient's entire episode of care. The challenge will be defining cost, quality, and outcome criteria as well as the availability of the data for analysis and the nurse executive's ability to interpret and use the information.

Conclusion

The ability to access vast amounts of information for clinical and financial management expanded significantly during the closing years of the twentieth century. The public is hungry for more information about best providers, best care, best hospitals, and other quality performance information. The coming years will bring an explosion of knowledgeable consumers who will challenge both the nursing and medical establishment and nursing and organizational management. This trend will provide added incentive for healthcare executives to develop and monitor clinical, financial, and other performance indicators.

Although we have discussed, conceptualized, and implemented various management information systems for nurse executives over the last two decades, we believe that the first decade of the twenty-first century will be the decade of knowledge. The challenge will be how to provide a meta-synthesis of the information and knowledge that will become available. By using systems and processes recommended in this chapter, nurses and nurse executives could measurably enhance their ability to use data in decision-making. For this to happen, the relationship between management information systems and nurse executives has to be a dynamic one. Continuous development and changes, both in the area of information systems and technology and in health care and nursing, provide fertile ground for ongoing development. Current and future innovations in information systems and technology will further empower nurse executives to achieve quality and cost balance in health care.

Questions

1. How are management information systems defined in this chapter? Would you change this definition in any way?
2. What are some of the advantages in using a computer system for staffing and scheduling?
3. What obstacles are there to using computers for quality management?
4. How are computers changing the work environment of healthcare workers?
5. What are some of the elements you would propose be included in a Nursing Management Minimum Data Set? Think about the information needs in your organization as a start.

References

Austin CJ. *Information Systems for Health Services Administration*, 4th ed. Ann Arbor, MI: Health Administration Press, 1992.

Chapman RH, Reiley P, McKinney J, Welch K, Toomey B, McCausland M. Implementing a local area network for nursing in a large teaching hospital. *Computers in Nursing* 1994;12:82–88.

Danziger JN, Kraemer KL. *People and Computers: The Impacts of Computing on End Users in Organizations*. New York: Columbia University Press, 1986.

Finkler S. *Finance and Accounting for Nonfinancial Managers*. Upper Saddle River, New Jersey: Prentice Hall, 1991.

Gilster P. *The Internet Navigator*, 2nd ed. New York: Wiley, 1994.

Hannah KJ, Shamian J. Integrating a nursing professional practice model and nursing informatics in a collective bargaining environment. *Nursing Clinics of North America* 1992;27:31–45.

Hanson R. Applying management information systems to staffing. *Journal of Nursing Administration* 1982;12(10):5–9.

Huber DG, Delaney C, Crossley J, Mehmert M, Ellerbe S. A nursing management minimum data set. *Journal of Nursing Administration* 1992;22(7/8):35–40.

Johnson M. Perspectives on costing nursing. *Nursing Administration Quarterly* 1989;14(1):65–71.

Morrissey J. Spending more on computers to help keep costs in line. *Modern Health-care* 1994(February 14);63–70.

Nicoll LH. An introduction of the internet, part 1: history, structure, and access. *Journal of Nursing Administration* 1994;24(3):9–11.

O'Brien-Pallas L, Cockerill R, Leatt P. Different systems, different costs? *Journal of Nursing Administration* 1992;22(12):17–22.

Shortell SM, Gillies RR, Anderson DA, Mitchell JB, Morgan KL. Creating organized delivery systems: the barriers and facilitators. *Hospital & Health Services Administration* 1993;38:447–466.

The Tenth Annual HIMSS Leadership Survey Sponsored by IBM. www.himss.org/Survey/ (last accessed November, 1999).

Section 3
Emerging Trends

Overview: Emerging Trends in Nursing Informatics

MARION J. BALL

As we examine emerging trends in nursing informatics as they pertain to information technology, we uncover an important distinction: Health care is migrating from an environment based on data to a continuum based on knowledge. Technology, however, cannot be viewed as a panacea for all of health care's information-based ills; rather, it is an enabler that will allow active, skilled users to make better decisions. To reap this benefit, we must stay informed of new directions and developments in technology.

Max Planck once observed that "in the correct formulation of the question lies the key to the answer." A key question to ask as new technologies are developed and implemented is, "Do nurses have the information they need?" In the past, we would have had to answer "no": Too often, work-flow was impeded by slow and inefficient manual processes that did not offer nurses quick retrieval of crucial patient information. In the coming decades, technology will help nurses alleviate more of that burden. It will enable the kind of informed decision-making that was not feasible before, allowing nurses to access information where, when, and how it is needed.

Trends

When we make a telephone call, we know that speaking to the party at the other end is the objective. Whether the call went through a satellite connection or a packet-switching system in another part of the country is irrelevant—what matters is the voice we hear on the line. The same should be true of information: Particulars like where it is physically located and which machine is processing the application should not be important, because the emphasis is on retrieving current, correct information at the time and place it is needed. As the trend from network computing to ubiquitous computing accelerates in the near future, this vision of information access will become a reality. No longer will nurses worry about how they will locate the needed information. Because computers and portable electronic organizers and clipboards will interface and share information, it will be instantly available at the point of care.

The consumer revolution is another emerging trend, one that will shape and be shaped by technology. With the advent of on-line resources, the consumer has awakened and the lion has roared. Just as the Gutenberg press freed the peasant to educate himself, the Internet and Web have opened doors for the consumer. Free on-line access to the National Library of Medicine, Medline systems and such resources as Health on the Net,

Intelihealth, and drkoop.com all provide valuable information for the consumer who wishes to be an active partner in his or her own health care.

Technologies

Whether they are used to educate nurses and patients or revolutionize the way daily practice is conducted, emerging technologies are exacting an influence on health care that will only deepen in the next century. What follows is a brief overview of technologies currently in use or in the first stages of implementation and acceptance.

Education

Technology has and will be used to enrich the education of nurses and increasingly vocal consumers. The Internet, which has already achieved widespread acceptance by healthcare consumers, is perhaps the most prevalent example. In 1998, over 60 million people searched the Internet for healthcare information, and about 91 percent said they found what they needed (Louis Harris survey, 1999). Nurses can also use the Internet to supplement their education, downloading on-line course material, linking to information-rich websites, and communicating with fellow practitioners through e-mail, newsgroups, and mailing lists.

Virtual reality is another technology that shows great promise in the education and training arena. VR has many practical applications in health care, from training nurses through vivid simulations to introducing anxious patients to the sights, sounds, and sensations of an upcoming hospital procedure. As technology improves, victual reality will have the ability to handle more complex data forms and create an environment with more realistic elements, such as peripheral vision and the sensations of temperature and pressure.

Daily Practice

As computers become ubiquitous, much will happen to change nurses' daily practice. Expert systems, modeling systems, decision support systems, and Web-enabled applications will provide access to vast quantities of stored data and visual information for the skilled user to retrieve and apply. Nursing has already begun to see the effects of these technologies and adjust to them. The use of graphical and cognitive user interfaces is becoming extensive and widespread. The multimedia computerized patient record (CPR) has been introduced in many healthcare settings: 68 percent of 993 respondents to the 1999 HIMSS Leadership Survey report that their organizations have either developed, begun implementation, or completed installation of a CPR. Telehealth is emerging as a new means of transmitting information to patients in their homes, at the bedside, at times most convenient to both them and their practitioners. Remote diagnostic capabilities through video store-and-forward technologies already are prevalent in radiology and dermatology.

Information technology can also enable patients to go one step beyond self-education, into skill development and healthcare decision-making. Interactive video programs and computer programs with touchscreens have helped patients manage such conditions as asthma, hypertension, and diabetes, increasing their skills and confidence, reducing the number of office and hospital visits, and freeing more time for practitioners. Newsgroups, which allow patients to interact with nurses available for consultation and others who share the condition, can also be a valuable source of knowledge and support.

Forecasting the Future

It is impossible to predict precisely which trends and technologies will have the most impact in the next millennium, but we can make educated assumptions. For example,

- Health care will continue to explore and use new technologies like smart cards, e-commerce, the Internet, and Web technologies.
- The consumer focus will sharpen, resulting in expanded use of consumer informatics initiatives like interactive digital TV, two-way pagers, WebTV, and personal digital assistants.
- Virtual reality will be increasingly used in both practice and training and education.
- The quantity of electronic resources will multiply exponentially, creating an urgent need for standards and monitoring tools to ensure its quality.
- Exciting developments in telehealth and telecommunications will save the practitioner valuable time and greatly improve the experience of the homebound patient.
- Technologies like cellular communication and wireless data networks will offer greater efficiency and connectivity.

Health care—and, indeed, the world—is in a state of flux. We have progressed from an industrial age to an information and knowledge age, one in which technology has introduced both benefits and challenges. The worst thing nurses could do to address those challenges is expect and wait for change: We are in the position to create it, and we must exercise that power. The field of nursing informatics has the capacity to do more than simply refine selected pieces of health care's business and clinical processes. Nursing informatics, its teachings, and its skilled professionals can advance and transform health care as a whole, leveraging technology to ensure better care for all.

References

Louis Harris survey, Internet increasingly used to find healthcare information. *Healthcare Financial Management*, 1999; April 22.

The Tenth Annual HIMSS Leadership Survey Sponsored by IBM, www.himss.org (November, 1999).

22
Nursing's Future: Ubiquitous Computing, Virtual Reality, and Augmented Reality

James P. Turley

Computers have revolutionized many areas and processes in health care. Today, laboratory systems would not be possible without computer-based automation: Large numbers of samples are tested, and the results are promptly and efficiently reported. Billing and finance are completely dependent upon computer-based information for insurance expensing, record checking, and, in many cases, for the scheduling of patients, equipment, and staff.

Computers have entered into a number of clinical arenas and are embedded in a number of bedside products. Intravenous pumps, ventilators, and monitors are managed by computers. Until recently, these machines ran independently of each other, but lately these products have begun to communicate, sharing information related to patient treatment and record keeping. Information services have been among the last areas in health care to receive assistance from computing technology. In the coming years, new generations of computers will become commonplace throughout the healthcare arena.

Nursing has not been on the leading edge of computer implementation in health care, but that may change in the near future. Ubiquitous computing, virtual reality, and augmented reality indicate new directions for computer use in nursing practice. This chapter reviews some of the possibilities for computerized nursing in the future, examines some of the problems, and explores some of the features.

It is clear that computers will become ubiquitous in the healthcare and nursing environments. Computerization in health care will progress in some unexpected ways. First is the idea of ubiquitous computing, as discussed by Mark Weiser of Xerox Corporation; second is the idea of virtual reality, for which examples exist in medical education, and projects are underway in industrial and defense areas; and third is the idea of augmented reality, which combines aspects of ubiquitous computing and virtual reality to provide what may be the critical elements for nursing. All of these are computer-intensive concepts, and all will impact the delivery of nursing and health care in the future.

305

Ubiquitous Computing

Weiser (1991, 1993) developed the concept of ubiquitous computing. The main tenets are conceptually simple but technologically difficult to implement. In ubiquitous computing, everyday devices can and will be augmented by computer technology. Once these devices have embedded computers, they will be brought into a mode where they can communicate with each other. The result will be a work area similar to what we already know and understand; however, the work area will be enriched because the devices will be able to communicate with each other and provide data in the format most appropriate for the user.

This process has begun and can be seen in areas of today's workplace. Many people carry electronic appointment organizers, microcomputers with the ability to store names, addresses, telephone numbers, messages, and a variety of other personal information. These personal organizers can be linked to desktop computers, a process that allows for the sharing of information between the two computers. For example, if a new office phone number is entered into the pocket organizer, when the pocket organizer is linked to the desktop computer, the desktop database will be updated by the pocket organizer because the pocket organizer has the most current information on the phone number. Similarly, the desktop machine can update the pocket organizer when it contains the most current information. These updates can occur automatically, or they can ask for input from the owner. Pocket organizers can be linked to remote fax machines and other computer-driven devices.

Currently, this linking is accomplished by running a cable between the two computers, loading special software into each and instructing each to pass information to the other. With coming advances, communication between the computers will become wireless and occur on a regular, less disruptive basis. The data will always be current, and no separate steps will need to be taken to ensure that there is consistency between the machines. Communication between devices will be independent of location, operating system, and manufacturer.

As this example illustrates, ubiquitous computing allows for the development of a number of independent computing devices that are brought together. These devices will communicate with each other to present information in a way useful to the user. Multiple devices will be developed in order to allow different approaches to the manipulation of information. One device may appear as a Post-It® note, while another device may display the same information as a record in a database. The result is that computers will be embedded into a series of everyday devices. Some of these devices can and will mimic devices we currently use; others will appear as new products. New devices can be developed to more completely reflect the way we are working and the way we want to work.

How will these devices function in nursing arenas? Computerized devices are not currently in common use in nursing areas; therefore, the future leads to speculation. A common device used on many nursing units is a clipboard, which is used frequently during the day to collect vital signs or to list reminders. The clipboard is an example of a device that can be computerized. The screen on the clipboard may contain a list of patients who need to have their morning vital signs taken, and the vital signs can be entered on the screen of the electronic clipboard using a pen device. The data entered on the clipboard would not only be stored on the screen but also immediately uploaded to the patient's electronic record.

At other times during the day, the clipboard could be used to record and calculate intake and output (I & O) information. Typically, this information is recorded throughout the day as it is gathered. At the end of a shift or the end of the day, the nurse sits down with a calculator to total the I & O and bring the balance forward, and the sheet is placed into the permanent record. With an electronic clipboard, the items could be entered and the clipboard itself would calculate the automatic running total. This total could also maintain a running I & O summary from the time the order for I & O was initiated to the current time. Likewise, if the I & O balance exceeded preset limits, the appropriate people could be notified immediately rather than waiting for the end of shift or end of day totals. The electronic clipboard could send messages to the pagers of the appropriate people.

The medication kardex is another element of nursing practice that could be computerized. Often separate from the patient record and located on the medication cart, the medication kardex is needed to examine the current state of medication administration. When nurses seek the medication kardex, it is never near the patient record. With an electronic kardex, the patient could be automatically identified using a smart card or a bar code on the wrist identification bracelet. Likewise, the medication nurse could be identified with a bar code on the institution's ID badge or with a smart card, and the medication itself could be similarly labeled. By simply scanning the device, the medication nurse could record the patient and the medication, as well as the time, date, and dosage of the medication.

The electronic kardex could update the patient record immediately, and searching for the kardex could become a thing of the past. With all of the medications marked and all of the patients coded, it could be possible for the electronic kardex to check each medication against the patient's profile, check for interactions among the medications, check the appropriateness of the dose, and record the time it was given and by whom. Eventually, the electronic kardex could notify physicians when automatic renewals are needed for medications (e.g. antibiotics). The electronic kardex could also notify the medication nurse 10 minutes before the time a critical medication was scheduled to be given.

Devices like electronic clipboards and electronic kardexes will communicate with beepers or personal information devices worn by staff. When a critical event occurs, the appropriate people could be notified immediately to prevent risk to the patient. Automated scheduling of these events could reduce the time and effort needed to renew medication orders and prevent missed or improper medication and other traumatic situations.

In other areas of the nursing environment, computers are currently embedded in existing systems. Bedside patient monitors, IV pumps, ventilators, and other devices are already computerized. These devices typically have limited ability to communicate with other devices; each is designed to be a standalone device reporting information with a series of beeps, whistles, flashing lights, or an LCD display of information. Although efficient, these devices are not intended for easy or intuitive communication. Future designs of these products will allow them to communicate with other devices. Eventually, they will communicate directly with the electronic patient record, storing appropriate data, and with the nursing caregivers providing status reports, warnings, and alerts. Appropriate and timely data will be displayed in appropriate ways and locations useful for the delivery of nursing acare.

Patient monitoring systems in the future will be designed to communicate with other devices, either through the patient record or directly with each other. A bedside patient monitor might note that a patient's blood pressure was dropping below a predetermined limit. The bedside monitor would then note that an intravenous (IV) pump was also connected. Looking though the patient record, the bedside system would note that a vasopressor was included in the IV solution and would direct the IV pump to increase the medication dosage. At the same time, the bedside monitor would send a message to the nurse caring for the patient about the status of the situation and what had been done about it. A note would be entered into the patient record that the bedside monitor had noted the drop in blood pressure, and the monitor would identify what rule or algorithm had directed it to change the IV flow rate, note that the IV flow rate had been altered, and record the time, date, and name of the nurse who had been notified. Such systems would include more complex decision-making than is currently available. However, prototype systems that include "artificial consciousness" are being developed. Artificial consciousness will give the computer-based decision systems a greater ability to self-regulate.

Similarly, the bedside monitors could communicate with ventilators; if pulmonary pressures started to rise, the bedside monitoring system could communicate with the ventilator to modify the settings. What is important in the discussion of all of these devices is the ability to communicate. Communication includes the need for standards in the communication process, the need for a level of embedded intelligence that can direct the communication, and the ability to document all that has occurred in the patient record as part of the communication process.

The technology that will allow this to occur is already being introduced into the nursing environment. Standards such as Health Level 7, MEDIX, and the Hospital Information Bus are creating the communication standards that all of these devices will use. The Computer-Based Patient Record Institute (CPRI) Concept Model Committee is developing a model for a computer-based record that will allow for the recording of patient information in real time. In addition, the CPRI Concept Model will direct the electronic record to attach to external databases and knowledge bases, which can be used inside the electronic record to assist with logical controls and communications like those described earlier.

Slowly, the healthcare arena will see the development of a patient-based local area network. The patient network will allow for the free flow of data and information around the patient. This will include information from the monitors and devices that are attached to the patient and are part of the interventions. Another nurse-based network will surround the nurse and support the planning, decision-making, and intervention strategies the nurse performs in order to deliver patient-centered care.

In the future, there will be a clear interconnection between the patient-based network and the nurse-based network. Similar networks will be developed for physicians, pharmacists, and any other healthcare providers who are responsible for the care of a given patient. The result will be a complex set of interconnecting networks, each connected to several embedded devices. These networks will make possible patient-centered care using "information on demand" as the critical focus for the delivery of care. The delivery of patient-centered care is knowledge and data intensive. New devices with strong communication orientations will finally act to support clinicians in their practice, improving patient outcomes.

Virtual Reality

Until recently, most examples of virtual reality (VR)—such as the holodeck on "Star Trek: The Next Generation"—have been defined, developed, and refined in science fiction. The major exceptions have been the use of VR in flight training simulators and games. However, recent developments in VR have generated possibilities for its use in health care.

Virtual reality can be defined as the generation of a complete environment. Larijani (1994) describes the six basic subsystems necessary for the development of a VR system. Each of these can vary in complexity, depending on the implementation. The six subsystems are

- Audio (earphones, acoutestrons, microphones, synthesizers)
- Visual (glasses, goggles, projectors, screens)
- Tactile (smells, pins, gloves, bodysuits)
- Hardware (host computers, peripherals)
- Electronics (power supply, signal conversion, accessories)
- Software (operating system, simulation software)

In a VR system, a person receives multiple sensory inputs that are either generated or mediated by computer. At a basic level, VR systems include binaural video screens that display pictures of a world designed using a computer graphics program. Stereo audio in the headphones may include synthesized voice, music, or other sounds that are purported to belong to the "designed world." Typically, these audiovisual worlds are displayed using a headset that includes the binaural video displays and the stereo headphones. In turn, the headset is linked to external sensors. Thus, when the person physically turns or looks up or down, the video display adapts and shifts in a similar direction. The sounds likewise shift as the head is turned; they seem to be forward or behind the person.

Newer technology will allow the display of more complex data forms in VR. Transducers embedded in gloves and body suits can give the sensations of temperature and pressure. Newer display technology can add peripheral vision. Virtual reality can be interpreted as the opposite of ubiquitous computing. In ubiquitous computing, computers are embedded in all of the devices that are part of the everyday experience. In VR, the person has become embedded in a computer-generated world. Even when elements of the visual world are from videotapes of a "real" situation, the person's interaction and experience of the generated world is moderated through the computer.

Holusha (1993) described the use of VR for the training of surgeons. Using VR techniques, a surgeon could practice an operation a number of times before approaching the first patient. Virtual reality could allow the surgeon to practice the same surgery using a number of different approaches. The system would even allow a recording of how the practice had been done so that the surgeon could observe the procedure that had just been performed. Certainly this decreases the risk to the patient and increases the ability to "play" with alternatives and explore variations on a procedure to produce the best surgical solution.

The National Library of Medicine (NLM) established standards for the development of organs and organ systems for use in VR (Merril et al., 1994). Derived from CT and MRI scans, this set of standards for electronic organs is referred to as the Visible Human Project. As these standards evolve, it will be possible for companies and organizations to assemble organs from different companies and establish a virtual patient.

With the development of more sophisticated feedback instruments, it will be possible for student nurses to "feel" the sensations as venous catheters and nasogastric (NG) tubes are inserted into virtual patients. The tactile information has always been the most difficult for instructors to impart to students. Virtual reality can allow all students to have the "same patient" so that they can discuss how things feel. When doing the same technique with different patients, individual variation could limit the amount of generalization when describing a procedure or situation. Conversely, the use of VR can allow the instructor to structurally change the experience for each student with a known amount of variation. This can assess each student's ability to discern changes in a situation that may be known only to the instructor.

Virtual reality may have some novel implications for nursing. Much of the data and information nurses use are very complex. Physician data tend to be abstract and independent of the patient. The results of laboratory tests (e.g., CBCs, blood gases) can be interpreted independently of the patient. Many physicians can do their diagnostic work using only the data gathered by other sources and do not need to see the patient directly. In contrast, nursing data are not as abstract. Nursing data are often embedded into the way the patient responds to a given situation or illness. Different patients do have different responses to the same stimulus. Patients one or two days after abdominal surgery can have widely varied responses to the abdominal pain. Some will cough and deep breathe regularly with little complaint, others will attempt short walks, and others will be reluctant to move at all. Unlike the data used by physicians wherein the relationships between the laboratory tests and the disease are patient independent, nursing data are often patient specific.

Nurses often work with cues that are less defined than, for example, the "postabdominal surgery patient." Nurses talk about patients as "looking good," "sounding poorly," and so forth. These data are completely embedded in the patient response to a situation. Nurses are often not able to decompose the elements of this gestalt (Turley et al., 1993). Even with the components, the complete response is often a more complex interaction among the components than an identification of the components alone.

Virtual reality techniques may allow for the capture of such patient-specific responses. These techniques may enable nurses to use more complex data for identifying the patterns of a patient response to situations than what are available currently. The use of paper records restricts the data types that can be used for the recording and identification of patient problems. Virtual reality techniques can be linked to electronic patient records, expanding the data types that are available for identifying and recording patient-specific responses.

As nurses continue to explore ways to understand, codify, and display embedded information, VR techniques will become increasingly important to the profession. Nurses' understanding of patient responses to situations can be modeled using VR. This will give researchers and practitioners new avenues to describe, investigate, and report on complex patient responses.

Virtual reality may also become an important tool in patient education. In complex situations such as patients preparing for surgery or MRI, no amount of verbal explanation or paper drawings can prepare patients for the experiences that they are likely to encounter. Virtual reality techniques can immerse the patients in the sound, feel, look, and sensation of the environments that they will be encountering. With that as a basis, nurses will be able to discuss a patient's response to the situation before the actual situation has occurred. Creating a "safe" experience for patients to experience a situation may allow for a better understanding of what is occurring and why, and it may increase patient compliance. Such approaches may be important to children who have a limited ability to conceptualize something they have not experienced. With VR, parents and children could both experience a procedure before it occurs, giving them a common basis to address the child's fears and concerns.

Virtual reality will not be the solution to all problems. It is simply the application of an existing technology to the fields of health and nursing. In and of itself, VR is neither a solution nor an obstacle. As with any other technology, VR will be more useful when it is seen merely as a technology. Any technology must be applied for a specific purpose. When the purpose is clear (e.g., the teaching of the tactile sense of intravenous insertion) then and only then can the appropriate technology be selected and evaluated regarding how well it meets that purpose.

Virtual reality as a technology can assist nursing with the processes of describing and understanding complex phenomena. Although useful for describing and presenting these phenomena, VR will not solve nursing's need to formalize its concepts and language. As a technology, it may prove useful in this process, but the work must be done by nurse investigators.

Augmented Reality

Augmented reality, a computing approach that has received little discussion, can be thought of as a combination of ubiquitous computing and virtual reality. With ubiquitous computing, the computers were embedded into a variety of products and tended to disappear as unique products. Ubiquitous computing works because of the focus on communication among the computing devices, which allows the data or information to be presented in a variety of formats. With VR, external reality tends to disappear as everything presented to the observer is mediated by the computer. Complex data and information can be presented in VR. By being immersed in VR, a person can sense, feel, and be immersed in a situation, not just look at the data. Augmented reality incorporates elements of both ubiquitous computing and VR.

In augmented reality (AR), the users have a headset or viewer that allows them to view both a computer-generated image as well as what is going on in front of them. External reality is not blocked out as it is with an enclosed VR headset. In AR, the user tends to wear a single earpiece, and there is a single-image video screen mounted to a visor. This is similar to rearview mirrors that bicyclists attach to their glasses or helmets. The cyclist learns to focus on the rearview mirror when necessary and ignore it while focusing forward the remainder of the time.

Systems using augmented reality have been developed for industry and military purposes. Boeing aircraft uses augmented reality to assist people who are involved with aircraft repair. The "manual," which has the complete set of instructions necessary for a repair, the associated diagrams, and flowcharts that contain the logic for troubleshooting are contained on a CD-ROM subsystem that the person wears. The CD-ROM is displayed on a view monitor over the right eye, and audio sounds can be played through an earphone into one ear. The repair person is free to focus either on the part of the airplane being repaired or on the monitor that displays the repair manual. The result is that the manual is available at the same time the work is being performed, and it is not necessary to interrupt the work. The real world is augmented with computer-generated assistance.

With AR, the user can decide on the fly how much time and attention should be given to the computer-generated view and how much attention should be given to the work being performed. As the worker becomes more proficient with the task being performed, it is likely that the worker will alter the allocation of time given to the electronic manual versus the time spent actively working on the engine repair. Several of the advantages of the VR system are available with AR:

- Complex data can be displayed.
- Audio and video data can be combined.
- Using sensors, the system can alter the display when the worker changes position or location.

The flexibility of AR, which allows the user to migrate between the computer-generated world and the "real" world, is one of its major strengths. Typically, the users of AR systems wear complete computer systems. Often the display is a small monitor that appears to float in front of the user. A CD-ROM is used to store large amounts of information, which is rapidly searchable. The size is no larger than that of a portable audio CD player. The CPU for the computer can likewise be shrunk to a package no larger than the CD-ROM.

Companies like NEC have created entry keypads worn like a wide bracelet on the wrist. With the combination of package shrinking and redefintion of the traditional keyboards, a wearable computer becomes a reality; in fact, in 1992, NEC hosted a fashion show of wearable computers. Although at first this seems humorous, the existence of a computer fashion show indicates the need to see the computer as part of the personal environment and not simply as an external device used in the office. Furthermore, exploring computing as a fashion issue will allow for innovative ways to design input devices. In the future, these wearable computers will be connected by wireless communication to other computers in the work environment. The AR worker will receive the most current information and data from other computers embedded elsewhere in the work environment.

This aspect of AR combines many of the strong communications features of ubiquitous computing.

Augmented reality may be the technology with the greatest application in nursing environments. As AR systems are integrated into the idea of personal networks and patient networks, AR technology can supply nurses with data and information while they are in the process of delivering patient care. Using AR, the nurse can have available the instructions for performing a complex task at the same time that the task is being performed. The instructions can be available in a hands-free form, which allows the nurse to focus on the patient while providing care. For example, if the nurse was involved in a complex assessment of newborns, the AR system could display pictures of what the nurse might be observing. Even if the nurse could not describe precisely what was being observed in the newborn, he or she could compare the newborn with photos of others and access more information from resources or compare the newborn's presentation with what it had been 24 hours or one shift ago.

Because nursing phenomena are complex and embedded in the patient situation, photos, videos, and sound may be necessary for developing comparisons and contrasts. On a paper record, normal values of laboratory tests can be printed as numbers per milligram percent, but nurses may need more complex data formats to display patient responses as normal. Augmented reality can do that. Admittedly, there may need to be some social and cultural modifications before patients easily accept nurses wearing AR systems.

Augmented reality will open a variety of new possibilities for nurses in clinical practice. Many of the applications for AR technology have not yet been considered. Augmented reality techniques will allow the nurse to have access to previous data, pictures, and sounds and to compare previous data with the current state of the patient. An electronic patient record would then provide for the recording of the current state, the previous state, and the changes that had occurred.

Summary

Ubiquitous computing, VR, and AR are technologies that have great potential to assist in the delivery of future nursing care. These technologies will greatly affect the teaching of nursing, the delivery of nursing care, and research into nursing practice, with simultaneous impact on the outcomes of nursing interventions. We must remember, however, that these are only technologies—and as such they are neither solutions nor obstacles. These technologies are important only to the degree that we understand nursing practice and what it is attempting to achieve. Within the goal of helping patients return to a life of health-seeking behaviors, these technologies can impact some specific areas, but they will not be solutions to all problems.

OUTPATIENT CARDIAC REHAB ASSESSMENT

_____ Age: _____ Date: _____

_____ Diagnosis: _____

ol ☐ College   Can Read/Write: ☐ Yes   ☐ No

n to see your doctor: _____

_____

_____

_____

_____

_____

r _____ ☐ Denies	☐ Cancer _____	☐ Denies
_____ ☐ Denies	☐ Diabetes _____	☐ Denies
_____ ☐ Denies	☐ PUD/GERD _____	☐ Denies
_____ ☐ Denies	☐ Hepatitis _____	☐ Denies
_____ ☐ Denies	☐ Other _____	
_____ ☐ Denies	_____	
_____ ☐ Denies	☐ Previous Surgeries _____	
_____ ☐ Denies	_____	
_____ ☐ Denies	_____	

For these technologies to have an impact on nursing, nursing must be willing to look outward and embrace technologies that can improve nursing practice. Nursing has a long cultural history of being technophobic (Turley & Connelly, 1993). In many cases, the reticence can be traced to the existing computer technology's failure to address the needs identified by nurses. Nurses cannot, however, stand by and wait for others to adapt technology to nursing practice. Nurses must seek out the technology that will improve the quality and efficiency of nursing practice. When the use of the technology can also improve patient outcomes, an ideal match will be found. The technology included in ubiquitous systems, virtual reality, and augmented reality may be that ideal match.

Questions

1. Create an example of the use of ubiquitous computing in any setting.
2. How does VR differ from ubiquitous computing?
3. What is the potential for AR in the field of nursing?

References

Holusha J. Carving out real-life uses for virtual reality. *New York Times* 1993(October 31);Section 3:11.

Larijani C. Homo faber or homo sapiens? *Virtual Reality Systems* 1994;1(1):7–10.

Merril J, Raju R, Roy R. VR applications in medical education. *Virtual Reality Systems* 1994;1(1):61–64.

Turley J, Connelly D. The relationship between nursing and medical culture: implications for the design and implementation of a clinician's workstation. In: Safran C, ed. *Proceedings of the 17th Annual Symposium on Computer Applications in Medical Care*. New York: McGraw Hill, 1993;233–238.

Turley J, Narayan S, Corcoran-Perry S. Practice disciplines, cognitive science and the other sciences the role of decision making. *Proceedings of QUARDET '93*. Carrete NP, Singh MG, eds. Barcelona, Spain: Cimne, 1993.

Weiser M. The computer for the twenty-first century. *Scientific American* 1991 (September);94–104.

Weiser M. Some computer science problems in ubiquitous computing. *Communications of the ACM* 1993(July):137–143.

23
Electronic Resources for Nursing

Susan K. Newbold

Since this chapter appeared in the second edition, the World Wide Web has become a major supplier of healthcare information for both nurses and consumers. Its impact cannot be underestimated. Today, nurses around the world are using their computers to access reference materials, to complete assignments for continuing education courses, to ask practice-related questions of colleagues through e-mail, to read messages posted to nursing-related bulletin boards or newsgroups, and to chat in "real time" with colleagues or fellow students. In short, computer networks have opened up a new world of communication and information for nurses.

In this chapter, we focus not only on what resources are available on-line but also on how nurses can access them. This is by necessity an overview because new resources are being developed and made accessible all the time. The fast-paced world of on-line communications changes so quickly that readers might find e-mail addresses or other references that have become incorrect since this volume was published. We will take the risk that some material may be outdated because we believe there is great benefit to be obtained from interacting with electronic resources. The author refers the reader to Appendix A, "Electronic Resources," for additional information related to this chapter.

The Basics of Being Connected

The term *on-line resource* is used to denote a resource that is accessible on a computer other than the one on which a user is working (a "remote host"). A user may connect to the remote host through a direct network connection (e.g., Ethernet for a campus connection to the Internet), a cable modem from home, or a dial-up connection (phone line and modem) to a machine that is connected via a gateway to other machines and networks. The term *on-line* does not necessarily imply "on the Internet," although often that is how the term is used. For example, an information source like a local nursing bulletin board system (BBS) could be quite useful even if it were

316

not networked with other computers. For our purposes, however, a user is not quite on-line to the outside world unless he or she can at least send and receive Internet e-mail.

Many local (non-nursing specific) BBSs provide Internet e-mail access and possibly even local "echoes" of Usenet newsgroups (see Appendix A), but few of them have full-scale Internet connectivity. The major commercial on-line networks such as America Online or MSN by Microsoft Corporation originally provided only e-mail access to the Internet, but all of them have either expanded their level of access or are planning to do so. New commercial vendors are continuously added to this list.

There are many ways to get on-line, and some of them are free. If a user has a personal computer connected to a campus or institutional network that has a connection to the Internet, he or she can probably take advantage of the full range of on-line resources, from e-mail to the graphical wonders of the World Wide Web. Few campuses or workplaces charge their users for access. If no direct network connection is available, users can achieve a similar level of connectivity and access by obtaining a personal SLIP/PPP account from a local Internet Service Provider (ISP). SLIP (Serial Line Internet Protocol) and PPP (Point-to-Point Protocol) are services that permit a modem and telephone line connection to emulate a direct network connection. Other types of access include

- A UNIX "shell" account on a host belonging to the user's institution (likely to be free), to a local "freenet" (free or minimal cost), or to a local or regional ISP (not free, prices and services vary)
- An account with one of the major commercial services, such as America Online or MSN (not free) or over 5,000 others available in the United States alone
- An account on a local bulletin board system (BBS) that has an Internet gateway (may be free, but costs and services vary).

The type of access will determine the resources available, the interfaces used to interact with the resources, and the costs incurred (if any).

Users need not have sophisticated or powerful hardware to access the majority of the resources currently available on-line. E-mail, real-time conferencing, bulletin boards, newsgroups, and retrieval of files and programs from Internet archives can all be managed adequately from a personal computer (PC) with a 486 processor, 8 MB of RAM, a monochrome monitor, and 100 MB or less of hard drive space. Other resources, especially the commercial on-line services and the more graphically oriented Internet resources, require significantly more computing power. These typically require a system with at least a pentium processor, at least 16 MB of RAM, a color (VGA or SVGA) monitor, and 100 MB or more hard drive space. Either a modem or a telephone line will be needed, as well as appropriate communications software (e.g., ProComm, CrossTalk, Kermit) to operate the modem, or a direct network connection (usually an Ethernet connection from a university or workplace) and the appropriate network software (usually the responsibility of the institution). Accessing the World Wide Web from home, using a personal SLIP/PPP account, requires the most computing power: a fast (i.e., 120 MHz) pentium computer with at least 16 MB of RAM, and a fast (minimum 28.8 bps) modem. Macintosh computers of comparable size may also be utilized.

Finding a provider can be difficult if there is no access through a user's school or workplace. It helps to know where to look. The commercial networks are easy to find; in fact, their user interface software often comes pre-installed on new PCs. Internet Service Providers and BBSs are harder to locate, especially in smaller cities. There are so many of them, springing up at such a rapid rate, that we would have to add a chapter just to list them all.

Uses and Benefits of On-Line Resources

On-line resources for nursing fall into three broad categories: communication with other people, reference materials, and continuing education. Access to these on-line resources offers the following benefits:

- Collaboration with other professionals
- Efficient retrieval of clinical, administrative, research, and educational information
- Support, both personal and technical, of users, their patients, and their institutions
- Ability to keep current
- Improvement of the state of nursing science

In the clinical setting, for example, a family nurse practitioner (FNP) practicing at a university-sponsored, nurse-managed center can use computer-mediated communication to ask a clinical question of colleagues or to search an on-line database for information. Perhaps the FNP would like to know how best to care for a client with terminal cancer. The FNP can look up current information with an on-line literature search, pose a question to a group of colleagues on an e-mail mailing list, post queries to the Usenet newsgroups alt.support.cancer and sci.med.nursing, retrieve a care plan on "hopelessness" from the CAREPL-L database of patient care plans, and browse the latest additions to the OncoLink website.

Similarly, nurse executives can use electronic communication to access external databases for clinical and cost data from other institutions (see Shamian and Hannah, Chapter 21) and share insights with colleagues on mailing lists devoted to healthcare management. The nurse manager can also benefit from support groups of other managers, where the nurse might pose a question on what computer systems are available for staffing and scheduling.

Nurse researchers may employ on-line resources for literature searching. At the University of Maryland, Baltimore, for example, both students and faculty have access to the Health Science Library Current Contents, Medline, CINAHL, and a host of other reference material from the library, from home as well as from their offices on campus. They can locate a book in any of the seven school libraries, reserve it on-line, and request that it be delivered to the nearest library. In addition, they can search publicly accessible catalogs in libraries around the world through the Internet. If they need additional material, researchers can pose questions on mailing lists or Usenet newsgroups related to their research topics. Calls for abstracts for conferences, grant funding opportunities, and other career-enhancing information regularly appear in on-line forums. Researchers with a variety of interests and at all levels of expertise can disseminate knowledge and encourage mentoring relationships and collaboration through online connections.

Nursing students and educators alike find the on-line world to be rich in resources. Recent topics on a mailing list for nursing educators included programs in community health education, computer-assisted instruction materials, textbook choices, recommendations relating to class size, and numerous job postings. The ability to access absolutely current information about who is doing what at schools around the world enhances decision-making and allows nurse educators to share techniques and materials that work. There are exciting new developments in distance education and in delivery of continuing education on-line. As a caution, the nurse who utilizes on-line information sources must be able to ascertain the reliability and validity of the content of the information.

Clinicians, administrators, researchers, educators, and students can all take advantage of the fact that professional nursing organizations have access to the Internet. The American Nurses Association, Sigma Theta Tau International, and the National League for Nursing all have e-mail addresses whereby messages can be sent and received. A growing number of other nursing and healthcare-related organizations, such as the *American Journal of Nursing* and the American Medical Informatics Association, are also accessible on-line.

Communication Resources

On-line electronic communication provides nurses with direct access to colleagues, professional organizations, and others (patients, family members, other caregivers) with common interests or concerns. Users can communicate with people individually or in groups, in public or in private, asynchronously or in "real time." In increasing order of complexity (and decreasing frequency of use), communication modes include

- E-mail
- E-mail mailing lists
- Usenet newsgroups
- Real-time interaction (UNIX "talk," individual and multiuser chat mode on BBSs or commercial services, as well as Internet Relay Chat and other Internet multiuser applications)
- Advanced real-time interactive video applications (e.g., video-conferencing with tools such as Cornell University's CU-SeeMe).

E-mail and Mailing Lists

By far the simplest and the most widely used application, e-mail is the gateway not only to one-on-one correspondence but also to discussion lists and other Internet applications. E-mail software is system dependent, and a technical description of how e-mail works is well beyond the scope of this chapter. The best way new users of e-mail can learn to use it (and any other on-line resource, for that matter) is to obtain a user's guide from the provider and seek the assistance of a friend or colleague who has some experience with it. A simple, one-to-one e-mail correspondence with another person is fairly straightforward, so we will not describe it in detail. The on-line world becomes more challenging and more rewarding when e-mail is used to connect many people at once through mailing lists.

Mailing lists are an advantageous way for a group of people with common interests to meet and converse. Dozens of lists cover specific medical and health-related topics (e.g., gerontologic health, traumatic brain injury, and endometriosis) and as of this writing, there are nearly 100 lists specifically for nurses and others interested in nursing issues.

Every mailing list operates basically the same way. First, after locating information about a list of interest, the user will follow the instructions given on how to subscribe to the list. Messages other people are posting to the list will begin to appear in the new subscriber's e-mail inbox. A user may then send an e-mail message to the list address, and a copy of the message will be sent to each person who has subscribed to the list. A subscriber can either reply directly to the sender and begin a private conversation or reply to the list address, in which case everyone on the list receives a copy of the reply. In the latter case, many people may reply to the message, and others may reply to those replies, creating a public discourse about the topic.

The conversational tone varies from list to list; some are very formal, with focused discussion resembling a professional meeting, and some are casual, chatty, and rambling. Just as the tone varies, so too do the expectations and level of discourse. Standard net etiquette ("netiquette"), however, would suggest keeping messages brief. This conserves network and personal resources, especially for those people who pay for their Internet access. It is also a good practice to sign each post, including an e-mail address. Some mailers strip such information from the headers of messages, which would prevent people from replying privately.

There are two types of mailing lists: manually maintained lists, in which a human being adds and deletes subscribers, and automated lists, in which members can subscribe and unsubscribe themselves, search list archives, and perform other useful functions by sending commands via e-mail to the software that manages the list. Most lists are automated, and the majority of nursing and health-oriented lists are managed by a software package called LISTSERV. Other common list managers are listproc, majordomo, and mailbase. The name LISTSERV, though, has become almost a generic name to refer to electronic mailing lists regardless of which software actually manages the list, much like "Xerox machine" refers to all photocopiers, regardless of brand.

All lists are run on a specific machine (a host) somewhere on the Internet. Whether manual or automated, lists actually have two addresses each: the list address and the administrative address. The list address will be in the form listname@host, and administrative addresses will be in the form LISTSERV@host (if they are LISTSERV lists) or majordomo@host (if the list uses the majordomo list manager). Requests to subscribe to or unsubscribe from the list must be sent to the administrative address. Each list has at least one human moderator, who is responsible for the smooth technical operation of the list and may or may not take an active role in on-line conversations.

As an example, let us examine one such nursing-related list, NURSERES. (See Appendix A for a description of others.) NURSERES is a list devoted to issues related to nursing research and nursing practice. Recent topics have included questions on locating instruments, research on spirituality in nursing, protocols for taking samples from catheters, and over-the-counter drug use among the elderly. It has over 1,000 subscribers from 19 countries.

The list is managed by LISTSERV software on a machine called kentvm.kent.edu. Thus the list address is nurseres@listserv.kent.edu, and the administrative address is listserv@listserv.kent.edu. If your name were Florence Nightingale and you wanted to subscribe to this list, you would send an e-mail message to listserv@listservkent.edu, with the single line:

sub NURSERES Florence Nightingale

Shortly thereafter, you would receive two messages from LISTSERV. The first tells you that your request has been processed, and the second is the welcome message that contains important information about how the list operates, including instructions on how to unsubscribe. Keep this message for future reference. Once your name is added to the subscription list, you will begin receiving messages in your e-mail inbox. Some lists (NURSENET, for example) are very prolific, and you will receive many messages each day. Limit the number of mailing lists to which you subscribe so that the mail does not become overwhelming.

Users can find a list on a topic of interest in several ways. Contacting a colleague in the field and asking them to which lists they subscribe is a good way to start. A newer way to look at what lists are available is to go to the URL (uniform resource locator) www.liszt.com and search the directory of over 90,000 mailing lists. To get an updated list of all nursing lists, go to this URL and key in words of interest, such as "nursing" or "informatics."

If no suitable list exists, a user may choose to create a list. This is possible with the software to manage the list plus a machine to house the list. This is how lists were started for nurses interested in substance abuse and subscribers to the Capital Area Roundtable on Informatics in Nursing (CARING) (see Appendix A).

Usenet Newsgroups and the Commercial Equivalents

Usenet (sometimes called Netnews) is a huge Internet-wide system of (conceptual) bulletin boards, called newsgroups, containing "posts" from readers all over the world. In other on-line contexts, like local BBSs or the commercial on-line services, the newsgroups might be called message bases, conferences, special interest groups (SIGs), or forums. Each newsgroup covers a particular topic, some of which are very broad (rec.music, for discussions about music) and some of which are very focused (alt.support.crohns-colitis, for support and information about Crohn's disease and ulcerative colitis). Unlike mailing lists, where a message is distributed via e-mail to a relatively small audience (usually less than a few thousand subscribers), a post to a Usenet newsgroup is distributed to every site that carries Usenet news and thus has a potential audience of over 10 million people. Also unlike mailing lists, where users have to subscribe and unsubscribe to get a feel for the list, Usenet newsgroups can be browsed quickly and easily using the newsreading software available on the host system.

There are a number of other important distinctions between lists and newsgroups, but conceptually they are quite similar. If a message is posted about job prospects for new nursing school graduates, people can either respond to it via e-mail or reply back to the newsgroup, creating a public conversation. As was said about e-mail, how users actually read and post to Usenet newsgroups is entirely dependent on the type of connection and the newsreading software available on the system. A service provider's support staff or a user's guide can give more information about newsreaders.

There are over 10,000 newsgroups on every conceivable topic within the Usenet system, and new groups are created nearly every day. Together, the newsgroups generate over 85,000 messages a day. To make it easier for readers to navigate the enormous volume of data, newsgroups are organized into a hierarchical structure. Each group is designated as part of a top-level category, followed by optional subcategories, which string together to form the name of the group. The major Usenet hierarchies are:

comp.   (computers, hardware, software, programming, and so forth)
misc.   (subjects that do not fit under any other hierarchy)
news.   (discussion and information about Usenet)
rec.   (recreation, sports, hobbies, games)
sci.   (science-related topics)
soc.   ("social" topics, relating to ethnic, religious, or cultural groups)
talk.   (discussions about political and social topics)

In addition, many sites carry the "alt." hierarchy, which—in addition to containing Usenet's most controversial subjects—also happens to include some of the newsgroups that may be of great interest to nurses. Other hierarchies exist as well, such as the bit.listserv groups, which are Usenet equivalents to certain mailing lists.

As an example of the hierarchical naming conventions of Usenet, the newsgroup for general discussions of nursing is called sci.med.nursing. Within the sci(ence) hierarchy, it is in the (med)ical topics subhierarchy and its specific topic is nursing. Other newsgroups geared specifically to nurses are bit.listserv.snurse-l (the Usenet equivalent of the SNURSE-L mailing list), for student nurses, and alt.npractitioners, for nurse practitioners. There are numerous other groups that may be of interested to nurses in specific practice areas, and some of them are included in Appendix A.

In addition to the Usenet newsgroups, some BBSs and the large network services like America Online have local conferences or SIGs on topics of relevance to nurses. Those conferences are only available to users who subscribe to those commercial systems.

Internet and the World Wide Web

Thus far, the term *Internet* has not been defined, possibly because the definition varies depending on how technical one chooses to be about it. For our purposes, it is enough to describe it as a vast worldwide collection of computers, networked together through the use of common protocols that define the way computers exchange data. The computers, of course, are of many types, most of them normally considered incompatible (like IBM mainframes and desktop Macintoshes), but they can "speak" to each other because the Internet protocols serve as a translator to a common language. Running on top of these low-level protocols are applications that take full advantage of the fact that millions of machines can now "speak the same language."

The use of the Gopher program, a simple, menu-driven application that allowed users to explore information stored on machines all over the world, has fallen out of favor with the emergence of the graphical user interface available for the Internet. The World Wide Web (WWW) has gained more and more acceptance in the on-line world since about 1993. The Web consists of collections of "hypertext" and "hypermedia" documents stored on machines all over the world. *Hypertext* is a term used to describe documents in which words or phrases within the document can be tagged as "links" to other parts of the document or to other documents entirely. Hypermedia describes documents that can include items other than just text, such as graphics, sound, movies, interactive search interfaces, and so on. Web browsers allow users to view these hypermedia documents and navigate among them, and they allow the links within documents to connect to documents in Web collections anywhere in the world.

Because the Web is a multimedia environment, most Web browsers use point-and-click graphical interfaces to display text and images. However, with a basic dial-up account and a slow modem (which would preclude use of the graphical browsers), users can still take advantage of the Web using a text-only browser. As of this writing, the two most popular graphical browsers are Netscape and Internet Explorer, and the most popular text-based browser is called Lynx.

When a user starts up a Web browser and tells it to begin at a certain location on the Web, the document that appears onscreen is called a *Web page*, and the top-level document for a site or an individual is referred to as a *home page*. The document often contains images, like university logos or photographs. Within the text of the document, some of the words or phrases will be underlined or displayed in a different color. These items are links to other pages on the Web; clicking the mouse on a link will cause the next page (which might be on a different computer) to be displayed onscreen. Some of the links do more than display Web pages; they play audio files or short movies (if the computer has the appropriate hardware and software installed), retrieve software and files from public file archives, allow the user to send e-mail to the creator of the page, and so on.

Very simply, this is what happens behind the scenes: Each link is associated with a URL, or uniform resource locator, which identifies the type of resource (Web page, archived file, and so forth), the host name (the name of the computer on the Internet where the file is stored), and the path to the resource on that host. For the most part, users do not have to think about URLs because the browser takes care of all the connections. However, when a user knows the URL for a nursing resource on the Web, the browser can be directed right to that resource. URLs for a number of nursing resources are given in Appendix A.

The Web is vast and growing at an extraordinary rate. For additional information on how to navigate it effectively, see Sparks and Rizzolo (1998) (who compare five popular general search tools and two metasearch tools) and the reference list for books available on Nursing and the Internet.

Real-Time Interaction

Real-time communication allows users to "speak" to each other directly and without the delay or time lapse incurred in e-mail communication. If e-mail is analogous to an exchange of letters, real-time communication may be seen as analogous to communication via telephone, with the caveat that users can only speak as fast as they can type.

Depending on the user's system and access to the Internet, various forms of real-time communication may be available. The UNIX "talk" command, for instance, allows real-time interaction between two people logged in to machines running the UNIX operating system, even if those machines are on opposite sides of the world. (Nearly all ISPs run UNIX.) A talk feature is available on networks such as America Online and is supported on most multiuser BBSs, but users can only speak to other members of the same service.

There are also ways to interact with groups of people. Some BBSs and all the large commercial providers offer multiuser chat programs that permit users of that system to talk with one another in groups. An example is the chat area provided by the Nursing Network Forum (see Appendix A). Every Tuesday evening there are real-time conferences with guest "speakers," and at other times members gather in the chat area for more social interaction. The most popular chat area on the Internet is the Internet Relay Chat (IRC). On IRC, people form "channels" in which they may talk about common interests, create links, or exchange ideas.

Advanced Applications

Real-time interactions that involve sound and video (the Internet equivalent of a video phone) require high-speed network connections that are presently available at campuses and large institutions and businesses. The higher speed lines now being installed in the home include the fiberoptic cable modem system. These types of applications allow users to see and/or hear someone who is sitting at a computer anywhere in the world. The rapid developments in the telecommunications industry make these types of applications accessible to the average user now.

Reference Resources

Databases

The Sigma Theta Tau International (STTI) Virginia Henderson International Nursing Library is designed to be a comprehensive collection of databases of nursing knowledge resources. There are eight databases as of this writing:

- Demographic Information. This is a database of nurse researchers that can be initiated and updated by the researcher
- Nurse Researcher's Projects

- Research Dissertations
- Research Conference Proceedings. This database contains abstracts of papers and posters presented at nursing meetings and conferences
- Research Grants Awarded by Sigma Theta Tau International. This database includes demographics, research information, and abstracts about projects funded by Sigma Theta Tau International
- Information Resources
- Table of Contents Databases. The Table of Contents from *IMAGE: Journal of Nursing Scholarship* and Sigma Theta Tau monographs comprise these databases

Another STTI initiative is the STTI *On-Line Journal of Knowledge Synthesis for Nursing*. This is the second on-line journal in existence. The editor is Jane H. Barnsteiner, PhD, RN, FAAN.

Except for the *On-Line Journal of Knowledge Synthesis*, access to the database is now free to members. Contact Sigma Theta Tau International Honor Society of Nursing for information at 1-888-634-7575 or 1-317-634-8171 (www.nursingsociety.org).

Archives and Databases from Mailing Lists

The archives of past postings to many nursing-related mailing lists can be searched for relevant information and thus can be thought of as on-line databanks. The list CAREPL-L is intended to be a searchable archive; the only messages distributed on the list are care plans. The creators and owners of the mailing list NURSERES have created a member database that serves as an excellent tool for linking nurses with similar interests. The information collected includes contact information, interests, and availability to assist with and/or collaborate on projects. Nurses seeking mentors or collaborators may retrieve the database by sending the command GET NURSERES DATABASE within the body of a message to listserv@listserv.kent.edu.

Software

Thousands of sites around the world maintain archives of software programs that are available for no charge or as "shareware," a try-before-you-buy honor system. Although there are currently few software applications geared specifically to nursing, there are some, and the wealth of applications available for personal use makes exploring these archives a rewarding endeavor. All types of programs are available, including educational software, planning, budgeting, and record-keeping software, and utilities to make the computer experience easier and more efficient. As new applications for nursing are developed, some will undoubtedly be made available in these file archives.

Continuing Education

There are many educational applications for electronic communication. The University of Maryland, Baltimore School of Nursing is offering continuing education credits for courses downloaded via the Internet. A student downloads the course (written instructions, reading material, a quiz, and course evaluation forms), studies the material, and takes the quiz. The student then mails in the completed quiz, along with a fee and forms, and receives credit upon successful completion of the quiz. The course materials can be found throughout the Web by performing an on-line search.

Distance education is being explored by a multitude of universities for nursing-related coursework. Efforts are underway at the Regents College to develop an entire master's program in nursing informatics, for full university credit, that will be delivered via computer, with the first offering during the Summer 1999 semester (D. Sopczyk, personal communication, 1999, dsopczyk@regents.edu).

One of the growing areas related to the Web and health care is the area of consumer informatics (see Chapter 24). A tremendous amount of sites for consumers have been developed. The key is to learn and to teach our clients how to judge the quality of a health-related site. Health on the Net (see Appendix A) has principles to guide the use of health information sites. The Health Information Technology Institute (hitiweb.mitretek.org/ docs/criteria.html) has worked with a body of nurses to develop quality criteria. The criteria are explained in detail and include credibility, content, disclosure, links, design, interactivity, and caveats.

Future developments on the Web include Internet 2, also known as the Abilene Project (www.internet2.edu), and the Next Generation Internet (NGI) at www.intewww.internet2.edu/html/internet2-ngi.html.

Conclusion

A wealth of material for, by, and about nurses is available on-line. One of the most exciting aspects of on-line connections is the support they offer for nurses working, teaching, and learning in isolated areas. All nurses and nursing students, whether they are in clinical practice, administration, research, education, or information systems, can take advantage of the world of on-line resources to enhance their education and career and to make meaningful connections with others who share the concern for excellence in nursing practice.

Questions

1. What are some on-line applications that may be of interest to you in your practice area?

2. List four benefits of using on-line resources.
3. Describe a scenario in which nurses in remote areas can use technology for education.
4. What are your criteria for determining a quality health information site on the Web?

Reference

Sparks SM, Rizzolo MA. World Wide Web search tools. *Image: Journal of Nursing Scholarship* 1998;30(2):167–171.

24
Consumer Health Informatics

Deborah Lewis and Charles Friedman

Advances in technology have made the delivery of healthcare information for consumers more complex and more exciting than ever before. Consumers now have many different ways to access healthcare information. The emergence of many more consumer health information resources gives individuals the opportunity to understand their health choices, prevent complications of disease, and develop their personal healthcare management skills. Nurses are challenged to understand how to best utilize these innovative approaches to support consumers' healthcare decision-making and enhanced healthcare outcomes.

In this chapter, we define consumer health informatics, describe information technologies used to deliver it, and provide examples of current consumer health informatics applications. We then focus on the challenges of integrating these new technologies, discuss strategies for doing so, and highlight nursing's role.

A Model for Consumer Health Informatics

Systems theory (von Bertalanffy, 1968) provides the framework for a definition of consumer health informatics. In this model, consumers are seen as co-evolving within the context of the larger social system. The system is defined as mutually interdependent components that interact in an integrated fashion to enable the system to function in pursuit of positive health outcomes. At the center of a shared health decision-making process is the consumer, who collaborates with others to convert information inputs to outputs by solving problems and making informed healthcare decisions.

Inputs from family, friends, and healthcare providers are integral to the process, as are the individual consumer's knowledge, values, beliefs, readiness to change health behavior, and current health status. Information technology, as a mode of message transfer, assembles and processes these inputs and facilitates the transfer of feedback across the system. Ideal system outputs include informed consumers who make choices based on personal

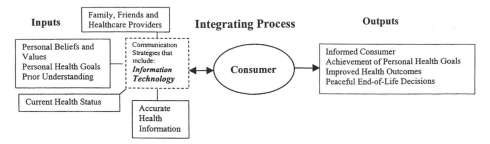

FIGURE 24.1. Model for consumer health informatics.

goals that lead to improved health outcomes or to peaceful end-of-life decisions.

In sum, consumer health informatics is the integration of consumer health information and information technology in an environment of shared healthcare decision-making that supports effective self-health action. As illustrated in the model shown in Figure 24.1, consumer health informatics can improve satisfaction with the process of care delivery and outcomes reflected in the health status of consumers.

Information Technologies

Information technology supports the consumers' ability to obtain health-related information through a variety of access strategies in a wide range of settings. Consumers can access resources using personal computers in their homes or using computers or information kiosks in libraries, hospitals, and clinic waiting rooms. Usually existing telephone lines or local and wide area data networks provide connectivity. Free-standing or networked computer workstations can provide information that is structured to adapt to the individual consumer's responses.

With computer graphics, virtual environments allow the individual to see and interact with a simulated three-dimensional world. E-mail and two-way video teleconferencing enable consumers to communicate with each other or their healthcare providers. Consumer informatics applications are being developed for newer electronic media, including interactive digital TV, two-way pagers, WebTV, and personal digital assistants. Emerging technologies, including cellular communication and wireless data networks, offer promise as modes of connectivity.

The willingness of consumers to consider information technology approaches is apparent in the proliferation of health-related websites. The Internet has made it possible to disseminate a broad range of current healthcare knowledge to consumers more rapidly than ever before. An estimated 41.5 million people are logging on to the Internet; nearly half of them spend time looking for health information (Council on Competitiveness, 1996; CyberAtlas, 1999a,b; Eng et al., 1998; General Accounting Office, 1996; Miller & Reents, 1999). HealthFinder, the federal government's consumer health information site, and OncoLink, an on-line cancer information resource, have logged over one million visitors in a single month. They are listed, along with other consumer health websites, in Table 24.1.

TABLE **24.1.** Learning interventions.

Primary author and year	Age group (years)	Disease and intervention	Outcomes
Horan (1990)	Adolescents, 12–19	Diabetes Computer-based instruction	Improved pre-lunch and dinner blood glucose results
Huss (1991)	Adults, 18–75	Atopic asthma Computer-based instruction	Improved adherence to therapy between computer-assisted instruction and traditional instruction
Peters (1991)	Adults, 22–45	Diabetes Computer-based instruction and decision support	Decreased insulin required
Ogozalek (1993)	Elderly, 65–75	Medication information Leaflets, computer, or interactive videodisk (IVD)	Improved knowledge score with computer and IVD
Turnin (1992)	Adults, 42–47	Diabetes Access to a distributed learning system	Improved knowledge, decreased fat intake, decreased hemoglobin A1
Meyeroff (1994)	Adults, 17–50	Diabetes Glucose meter with data storage	Improved hemoglobin A1c
Osman (1994)	Adults, 48–51	Asthma Computer-generated books	Decreased hospital admission
Liao (1996)	Adult, average, age 61	Coronary artery disease Interactive video	Increased confidence in treatment choices
Madoff (1996)	Adult, average age 35	Psychiatric patients Computer-based instruction	Medication knowledge ($p < .08$)
Petersen (1996)	Children, 9–16	Oncology blood counts	Improved knowledge Computer-based instruction
Brown (1997)	Children, 8–16	Diabetes Educational game	Communication with parents about diabetes, self-care rating scale
Clark (1997)	Adults, "middle age"	Hyperlipidemia Computer-based instruction	Decreased plasma cholesterol level
Evans (1998)	Children, 8–10	Nocturnal enuresis Computer-based instruction	Improved knowledge score

Consumer Health Information Applications

Given the hypothesis that information can support health behavior change and result in positive health outcomes, it follows that consumer health informatics applications hold the greatest promise when they are designed to facilitate the learner's interaction with the content, not just to deliver it. In that context, information technology provides powerful tools for the delivery of consumer health information. We describe a few selected successes in the areas of learning interventions, on-line connections, and nursing information systems.

Learning Interventions

The most common consumer health informatics applications, learning intervention programs are generally disease specific, although some have been developed for health promotion and wellness. Program outcomes include knowledge transfer, skill development, and health behavior change (Lewis, 1999). Using healthcare information technology as a learning tool offers a number of advantages: "just-in-time" availability, a private learning environment, support for the decision-making process, potential for individualization of the information presented, and the ability to simulate life experiences (Lewis, 1999).

Many notable learning intervention programs exist. The applications listed in Table 24.1 have documented significant changes in health outcomes. So too has Diabeto, an application for diet self-monitoring found to have a significant and long-lasting impact on dietetic knowledge and dietary habits for persons with non-insulin dependent diabetes (Turnin et al., 1992). Osman et al. (1994) found that computer-generated booklets distributed to adult patients with asthma resulted in decreased hospital admissions. Sweeney and Guliano (1988) developed a touchscreen multimedia program that was used successfully to provide prenatal education for rural southwest families in a clinic setting.

Information technology has also been used successfully to support skill development and patient decision-making. Shepperd et al. (1995) found that a touchscreen interactive video program was useful in helping patients with hypertension and benign prostatic hypertrophy make healthcare choices. Nishimoto et al. (1994) developed a computer-based patient education program to teach clients skills needed to use the Novo-Pen© insulin delivery device. In this study, computer-based learning intervention supported active participation in the learning process and reduced the time required for learning by as much as 40 percent, thereby allowing the diabetes care provider more time for individualized instruction.

Consumer health information applications are being developed that focus on health promotion and disease prevention. HealthTouch and Health O'Vision are two such programs. Both deliver tailored health information based on an individualized consumer health assessment. Health-Touch delivers wellness information in a family practice clinic setting (Williams et al., 1995), and Health O'Vision (Table 24.2) provides health information and focused disease prevention information in public kiosk settings. These systems have been shown to encourage patients to think about their health and enhance their readiness to interact with care providers (Skinner etal., 1993; Williams et al., 1995).

Virtual reality programs accommodate persons with both physical and cognitive disabilities. These programs provide patients with opportunities for enhanced social interaction, diminished feelings of isolation, and improved self-esteem. Participants use these virtual learning environments to acquire knowledge and skills that can be transferred to the real world (Meredith, 1996; Moline, 1999; Van Biervliet & Gest, 1995; Wilson et al., 1997).

On-line Connections

Consumers often seek healthcare information at a time when they are facing life changes or health challenges that will significantly alter their current lifestyle. Applications have been developed that extend beyond the transfer of information or knowledge to consider the emotional impact of the consumer who is facing a life-altering health condition. The advent of the Internet made it possible to provide information in the context of an on-line social network. ComputerLink was developed to provide caregivers of Alzheimer's disease patients with on-line access to nurses for consultation and support. This system also provided information and decision support tools (Brennan et al., 1992). Initial research results indicated that the on-line approach was successful in promoting collaboration with health team members and in providing access to information. A later study included persons with AIDS, and this group, who used the system even more than the caregivers of patients with Alzheimer's disease, found that access to private support with other AIDS patients as well as nurses for consultation were particularly valuable (Brennan, 1993).

The Computerized Health Enhancement Support System (CHESS) (Gustafson et al., 1992) was developed as an on-line interactive computer-based system to provide information, referral, and support for patients. Target populations for CHESS included adult children of alcoholics, patients with HIV, patients with breast cancer, and victims of sexual assault. Research and usage statistics revealed that the system was found to be most useful for patients with HIV and patients with breast cancer (Gustafson et al., 1992). Tetzlaff (1997) provided a similar system for parents of children with leukemia. This system included clinic-based education, on-line information, and electronic communication with healthcare providers. The parents who participated were most enthusiastic about the use of on-line education in supporting the care that their children were receiving at home (Tetzlaff, 1997).

TABLE **24.2.** Consumer health information resources.

The Comprehensive Health Enhancement Support System (CHESS)
http://chess.chsra.wisc.edu/Chess/
CHESS is a computer-based system of integrated services designed to help individuals cope
with a health crisis or medical concern. The CHESS system provides access to
information, social support, decision-making, and problem-solving tools. Information is
tailored and presented in language that is comprehensible to people at most educational
levels.

Columbia University College of Physicians and Surgeons Complete Home Medical Guide
http://cpmcnet.columbia.edu/texts/guide/
A consumer health medical book offering information on diseases, diagnosis, and treatment
and includes other topics such as diagnostic tests, medications, and first aid and safety.
Topics such as getting a second opinion, talking to your doctor, and checking a doctor's
qualifications are covered in the sections on making certain you get the best medical care
possible.

Healthfinder™
http://www.healthfinder.gov/
A gateway consumer health and human services information website. Provides links to
selected on-line publications, clearinghouses, databases, websites, and support and self-
help groups, as well as government agencies and not-for-profit organizations that produce
reliable information for the public.

Health O'Vision
http://hov.cancer.med.umich.edu/
The goal of the Michigan Interactive Health Kiosk Demonstration Project is to provide
access to customized, accurate and motivating preventive health information presented in
public kiosks using interactive multimedia health software design.

HealthTouch®—Online for better health
http://www.healthtouch.com/
One-stop resource for health information and health services that includes Medi-Span for
drug information, a health resource directory, and up-to-date information on health and
illness.

InteliHealth—John Hopkins University
http://www.intelihealth.com
Information on topics related to the health of children and adults. This includes diseases and
medical conditions, allergies, asthma, and medications. Users can access drug information
provided by the United States Pharmacopoeia Drug Index (USP DI) Advice for the
Patient. The site, which is searchable, includes top medical news of the day, health risk
appraisal quizzes, pollen reports, and "ask a team of experts."

C. Everett Koop Institute
http://koop.dartmouth.edu/
The C. Everett Koop Institute at Dartmouth is dedicated to the improvement of human
health. This website is designed to provide information and access to resources in order to
enhance the health of individuals, families, and communities.

TABLE **24.2.** *Continued.*

Mayo Clinic Health Oasis
http://www.mayohealth.org/
The Mayo Clinic Health Oasis is directed by a team of Mayo physicians, scientists, writers,
and educators. It is updated every weekday to bring the most relevant health information.
Provides "Ask the Mayo Doctor" and "Ask the Mayo Dietitian," which is supported by
staff at the Mayo Clinic. Visitors can e-mail questions or view answers to questions
submitted by other visitors.

NetWellness Home Page
http://www.netwellness.org
Produced by the University of Cincinnati Medical Center Libraries, this resource is a well-
developed site for consumer health. It contains full text information about major health
problems or issues. Consumers can search for topics of interest or ask health-related
questions.

OncoLink
http://oncolink.upenn.edu/
An award winning site for cancer information for health professionals and patients, this site
includes cancer news; a list of cancer-related journals with some abstracts and full-text
articles; clinical trials information; and information about financial issues for cancer
patients. It has textword searching capability. The artwork on the home page changes
weekly and is donated by cancer patients.

Nursing Information Systems

A limited number of research studies document the use of consumer health
applications in clinical nursing practice. Nursing information systems that
incorporate consumer health information have generally been limited to
printable patient information sheets or treatment instructions (Korn &
Wieczorek, 1995).

Consumer telehealth applications are being developed to provide information and nursing interventions in a distributed environment. The Interactive Home Health Care Program in rural Missouri provides audio and
video connectivity that links elderly clients with a telehealth nurse. Evaluation studies of this system are underway (Lindberg, 1997).

In a few cases, theoretical frameworks have been cited in the development of consumer informatics projects. These include behavior change
models, learning theory, and crisis intervention models. Rogers' Diffusion
of Innovation Model (Brennan et al., 1992), Fischbein and Ajzen's Theory
of Reasoned Action (Kinzie, 1993), Becker's Health Belief Model (Skinner
et al., 1993; Wetstone et al., 1985), Prochask's Stages of Change Model
(Skinner et al., 1993), Orem's Self-Care Nursing Theory (Huss et al., 1991),
and Banduras' Self-Efficacy Theory (Boberg et al., 1997; Clark et al., 1997;
Kinzie et al., 1993; Rubin et al., 1986) have been cited as contributing to
the development of consumer informatics interventions. When theoretical

models are provided for consumer informatics, programs are usually described as combining elements of several of the noted theories.

Challenges

The delivery of consumer health information poses a number of issues: security and privacy, quality of available information, access to consumer information resources, cost to the consumer and the healthcare system, and acceptance by healthcare providers. The technology available can provide strategies for meeting these challenges.

Some experts provide evidence that information technology in consumer health care provides easier access to clinical data and improved documentation, whereas others note issues with data compatibility, standardization, and security (Adderly et al., 1997; General Accounting Office, 1996). These incompatibilities are particularly problematic when systems need to exchange information. Different media may not communicate effectively, making it difficult to share health-related data. Security may also be compromised during data transfer. Efforts are underway to establish standards for the safe and efficient transfer of electronic information.

Patient Centered Access to Secure Systems Online (PCASSO) is an example of one such project (Masys & Baker, 1997). It provides Web-based access to sensitive clinical data. The system requires user authentication to ensure access control, privacy and confidentiality, and integrity of information. The PCASSO project provides consumers with access to their own personal health information, and it issues e-mail alerts concerning changes in their health record. Actions allowed by the system are authenticated by roles (i.e., patients have different access control and rights than their healthcare providers). Multiple layers of sensitivity ensure the confidentiality of sensitive information by creating access levels. For example, a psychiatric diagnosis would be at a different level than cholesterol results, and only appropriate users would be permitted access (Masys & Baker, 1997).

A related issue with electronic communication is privacy. Participants in public e-mail lists are at risk of becoming unknowing research subjects. Some individuals may also lurk and misrepresent themselves as members of a consumer group (Gannon-Leary, 1997; Klemm & Nolan, 1998). Projects like ComputerLink and CHESS address these issues by restricting access to identified clients. For public e-mail lists, it is recommended that persons with legitimate research interests contact the list owner for permission to request individual consents from list members to use their e-mail posts. In academic settings, institutional policies for the ethical conduct of research should address research participants who are members of these virtual communities.

The rapid proliferation of information via the Internet raises concerns about the quality and volume of the information being presented. The Internet provides access to a staggering assortment of formal and informal information. This information can be overwhelming and often difficult to interpret. Moreover, its value as a source of high-quality health information is frequently questioned (Anonymous, 1997; Floridi, 1996).

Although it is important to make information available, guiding providers and patients to use it in educationally appropriate ways is equally important. To avoid on-line consumer health misinformation, guidelines have been developed that educate providers and consumers (Lewis, 1998). Healthcare providers should caution consumers to be skeptical until information has been verified. In addition, providers should counsel consumers to

- Read the website's introductory information to determine where it originates. Although it is difficult to always determine the origin of websites, data retrieved from governmental and educational institution websites (.gov or .edu) are likely to be credible and accurate. Websites that provide peer review or an editorial review process are also likely to be reliable.
- Review the information provided and discuss questions with healthcare providers to determine if it is accurate and if it applies to the individual's healthcare situation. Determine if the website provides references to research findings.
- Verify the date of the website and the information provided to ensure that the information is up-to-date.

One way to address concerns about Internet quality is to develop edited websites that provide an interdisciplinary approach to the delivery of high-quality health information (Lewis, 1998). Two examples, OncoLink and NetWellness, are described in this chapter, and additional examples are included in Table 24.2. Because websites change rapidly, the examples cited are illustrative only; they are not meant to be a definitive listing.

OncoLink is a multimedia Internet resource focusing on cancer information for both the healthcare professional and the patient. OncoLink objectives include the rapid collection and dissemination of information relevant to the field of oncology. To ensure the quality of material presented, OncoLink has a rigorous review process. All material is peer reviewed by an editorial board before Internet release (Benjamin et al., 1996; Buhle et al., 1998).

NetWellness, a Web-based consumer health knowledge service, brings together teams of nurses, pharmacists, physicians, and allied health experts to collaborate with information professionals to identify, select, evaluate, and present consumer health content. These teams also answer consumers posting health questions on "Ask an Expert" bulletin boards with a 24 to 48 hour turnaround time. Such teams might consist of a nurse from the University of Cincinnati, a physician from the Ohio State University, a pharmacist from Case Western Reserve University, or any other combination of professions and affiliations. Consumers interact with NetWellness from home or office, via the Web, or through over 6,000 computers in 700 public library locations throughout Ohio (Engstrom, 1997; Morris et al., 1996).

Factors Affecting Success of Interventions

Access to consumer information technologies impacts the consumer, the healthcare organization, and the individual provider. Consumer issues are related to the costs of information technology or to the barriers imposed by the consumer's demography or social living circumstance. Issues related to costs of consumer information applications are usually seen as affecting the consumer's use of informatics in terms of the expenses associated with purchasing software and hardware and fees for using online services (General Accounting Office, 1996).

Demographics of information technology users are distributed unevenly across race and ethnic boundaries. Individuals who are of lower socioeconomic status or who are rural, African-American, or Hispanic are less likely to own computers (Eng et al., 1998; Mandl et al., 1998). In fact, the average computer user is 41 years of age, has a college degree, and has an average annual income of $61,000 (Miller & Reents, 1999). This suggests that a large number of consumers who are at higher risk for heath-related problems may have limited access to these information resources.

However, young children, the elderly, persons from rural and economically disadvantaged economies, those with diverse ethnicity, and clients with disabilities have successfully used information technology to produce positive health outcomes (Eng et al., 1998; Lewis, 1999). Consumer informatics studies that include these populations with high-risk characteristics are limited, but they generally report that when consumer informatics applications are provided for individuals in these groups, positive findings result (Lewis, 1999).

We need to think creatively about reaching consumers where they live and work by adapting electronic access to reach a more diverse community. Some proposed solutions for overcoming the barriers for high-risk consumer groups include access through community organizations (e.g., free health clinics or shelters and public libraries) or through retail stores, malls, and other public access sites. With more than 98 percent of households in the United States owning televisions, television may prove to be a powerful medium for the delivery of consumer health information in the future (CBS MarketWatch, 1999). A recent development, WebTV, provides access to the Internet through the consumer's television set. Although WebTV is limited to browsing the Internet and e-mail, it may be a less costly and useful alternative for those who cannot afford a computer or who are intimidated by them (Eng et al., 1998).

Organizational Challenges

Within healthcare organizations, determinants like administration, finances, facilities, and equipment may be affected by and/or affect the adoption of consumer information technology. Research supports distributed health information as a cost-effective strategy to promote health and prevent the onset of complications of disease, but only a few studies (Adderly et al., 1997; General Accounting Office, 1996; Lewis, 1999) specifically address cost-benefit and cost-effectiveness of consumer information technology. Although some managed care organizations and other payors are reimbursing for health information as a way to meet certain patients' unmet information needs, reimbursement for the delivery of consumer health information is not universally covered (Eng et al., 1998).

In the current healthcare environment, decisions to adopt new resources are driven, at least in part, by the financial impact that those resources will have on the institution. Because consumer informatics is a relatively new field, the research has focused on systems development and user satisfaction, not on cost issues. Additional evidence is needed to document the cost impact of using these resources to provide information for consumers. To influence institutional decision-making, we need to establish the cost implications of using consumer health informatics to deliver health information.

Providers

Understanding the concerns of healthcare providers is important in determining how to integrate consumer information technologies into clinical practice. Adoption of consumer informatics is likely to be linked to attitudes about its use and healthcare providers' levels of personal comfort with the technology. Learning to use information technology in healthcare settings is perceived as being time intensive, and extra time is something that many providers do not have. In addition, the informed consumer challenges the provider to reconsider traditional patient–provider roles (Dudley et al., 1996; Lewis, 1999).

The importance of attitudes and beliefs in learning to use new technologies is widely acknowledged. Research suggests that, despite positive attitudes toward technology, many providers may not consider themselves qualified to use it in clinical settings or believe that it has a use in the healthcare environment (Burkes, 1991; Cork et al., 1998; Scarpa et al., 1992; Stronge & Brodt, 1985). Clearly, such attitudes do not promote the integration of consumer information technology into clinical practice as an adjunct to the care process.

Healthcare providers may be concerned that the use of consumer information technology changes the traditional role of the patient from a passive recipient of healthcare information to one who presents with questions and wants an active role in decisions related to his or her health management plan. The idea of an educated consumer who arrives for the healthcare encounter armed with the latest information may be intimidating to providers who do not have the time or resources to stay as current as they would like. Providers may also be so concerned about the misinformation that is available, especially through Internet resources, that they may discourage clients from using technology to access information (Dudley et al., 1996). Consumers' desire for information and their informed interaction with providers will likely encourage reluctant providers to become familiar with these new information resources.

Information that is easily available and appropriately formatted can assist healthcare providers in understanding the best use of consumer health information technology to support the care they are providing.

Future Implications for Nursing

As consumer health information technologies become more widely available, it is important to understand their implications for nursing practice. The increased availability of consumer health information provides an opportunity for increased collaboration and open communication with patients and their families. Informed consumers will likely come to the health encounter with more questions and with an increased desire to participate in health management decisions. Nurses in primary care provider roles may feel a greater challenge to keep up with the latest information while at the same time welcoming the opportunity to share self-management information and communicate electronically with their patients.

Because information delivery is an integral part of the process guiding healthcare decision-making, consumer health information technologies will likely have the greatest influence on nursing practice roles for those whose practice includes healthcare education. Many current chronic disease management and health promotion programs incorporate an interdisciplinary model with a team approach to decision-making that includes the patient, family, and healthcare providers. In those interdisciplinary models nurses are often coordinators of care and the healthcare provider primarily responsible for healthcare education. The following scenario provides an illustration of how the nursing role may evolve with the incorporation of consumer health information technologies.

The Consumer Health Information Center: A Scenario

The following scenario describes a hypothetical family and their introduction to one future application of consumer-oriented healthcare information resources. Sam is a 52-year-old schoolteacher who lives with his wife Susan. During a routine examination, Sam is diagnosed with diabetes mellitus type 2. Dr. Smith, his primary care physician, prescribes an oral diabetes medication and encourages Sam to monitor his blood glucose level every day. Sam and Susan attend a series of four hospital-based diabetes education classes and receive written educational material to take home.

Adhering to the Treatment Plan

In the ensuing weeks, Sam follows his management regimen faithfully, including the medication and diet instructions he received. He tests his blood glucose level before breakfast and at bedtime and records the values on a spreadsheet he created on his home computer. Both Sam and Susan read all the information they had received. They log on to the Internet, but are quickly overwhelmed by the large number of websites that include diabetes information and advice. They wonder how they can be certain that the information they read on the Internet is accurate.

Seeking Additional Information

Six weeks after diagnosis, Sam notices that his blood sugar level is higher than normal at bedtime. He feels well, but wants to improve his diabetes control. Sam's physician, Dr. Smith, recommends the Consumer Health Information Center. Sam calls the center and makes an appointment for the next day. Upon arrival at the center, he and Susan check with the front desk and are quickly seated in the information resource area. The receptionist invites them to try the interactive learning carrel or to browse through the library. Sam and Susan decide to try the carrel. After answering a few brief on-screen questions, they are presented with a menu of learning choices. Sam chooses a vascular complication, specifically impotence. The carrel provides the privacy Sam needs to feel comfortable exploring this topic. He is relieved to learn that his risks for impotence will be low if he keeps his diabetes in good control. The program helps Sam and Susan focus on the questions they will ask when they have their next appointment with Dr. Smith.

When it is time for Sam and Susan's visit, the information resource nurse, Pat, comes to meet them. Pat prints a summary of the information Sam and Susan received while at the carrel and provides a videotape of the interactive session they can review when they return home. Pat reviews Sam and Susan's interactive learning experience with them and validates that they understand the information the program provides. They also discuss Sam and Susan's concerns to help them decide what information is most important for them to have right now.

Decisions To Be Made

Sam and Susan want to know more about high blood sugar. A decision support program called Second Opinion helps them understand how Sam's diet and medication might affect his blood glucose control. They are given time to explore the impact of different therapeutic choices on the glucose control of a patient with characteristics like Sam's. By simulating a typical day in the life of "Virtual Sam," they weigh the risks of therapy and the likelihood of complications given the different treatment plans. They study the economic impact that frequent monitoring and more expensive medications would have on their household income, what portion of the expense would be covered by their insurance, and what out-of-pocket expenses they would incur. Sam is able to consider the time involved in monitoring and meal planning and how that would impact his work day and leisure time.

Personal Attention

Sam and Susan appreciate the time that Pat spends with them making sure that they receive the information they need to make decisions about their health care. Understanding more about Sam's illness, they are better able to focus on the need to control Sam's blood sugars. The personal attention they receive helps them clarify their information needs. Sam has a list of question to ask Dr. Smith during the next visit and an appointment to consult with a dietitian affiliated with the center.

Staying Connected

Sam and Susan spend the last part of their visit learning about the advantages that the center's Web connection can offer them once they return home. They learn that Sam's glucose meter is equipped with a cable that allows him to download his blood glucose data directly to the Online Decision Support System. The system can also incorporate diet, exercise, and medication information that Sam provides, via the electronic logbook, and generate a comprehensive log he can share with Dr. Smith. Sam and Susan are similarly introduced to other options on the center's site:

- The Virtual Patient Education Library provides access to the resources of the Consumer Health Information Library and regular information updates based on Sam's level of education and areas of interest.
- The Diabetes Challenge, an online knowledge test that includes randomly generated quizzes with customized levels of difficulty, allows Sam and Susan to test their understanding of the information they are reviewing.
- The Virtual Patient area continues to give the couple the opportunity to practice dosage adjustment and other management changes to see what the simulated consequences would be.
- A Hotlink provides the most current clinical guidelines and reviews current research.
- A Patient Support Group, moderated by center personnel, ensures that the discussion is focused and that the information provided is accurate.
- An Expert Forum provides periodic "live chats" with expert clinicians.
- E-mail gives links to clinic personnel for specific management questions.

Hope for a Healthy Future

Sam and Susan leave the center feeling connected to a health information resource that will help them successfully manage Sam's illness. Sam's visit to the center is covered by his HMO, and a summary report is e-mailed to Dr. Smith for inclusion in Sam's electronic health record.

Consumer Health Informatics and Nursing

The scenario illustrates how consumer health informatics technologies may provide new opportunities for the delivery of nursing care. Many other possibilities exist. Nurses need to work collaboratively with other clinical and technical colleagues to ensure that nursing's unique perspective is incorporated in the development and integration of consumer health applications in distributed healthcare environments.

Healthcare providers who use these technologies to support the process of health behavior change are enthusiastic about them, but little research has been done to establish that consumers understand the information they receive and incorporate it into their healthcare decision-making. Researchers have focused on short-term learning and not on the evaluation of consumer health information programs over time. Nurse researchers need to become more involved in studies examining the cost-benefits and long-term outcomes related to health behavior change.

Although technology poses many challenges, it provides powerful tools to support the delivery of consumer health information. Education of nursing students and continuing education offerings at professional meetings are important to guide provider understanding of consumer health informatics applications. It is important that students receive the information they need to support their roles as collaborators in the development and delivery of effective consumer health information technology. For this to be accomplished, nursing curricula will need to integrate consumer informatics and information technology as a component of the didactic and clinical practice experience. Nurses specializing in consumer informatics will require preparation in complementary fields like educational technology, computer science, and cognitive science. Nurses in practice need professional development opportunities to gain understanding about these new approaches to consumer health information delivery. Integration of new technologies and changes in practice roles occur over time and will likely come from research documenting the role of consumer health information tools in the process of delivering cost-effective high-quality health care. Only through future research we will understand the impact of consumer health informatics on consumer health outcomes and nursing practice models.

Acknowledgments. The authors wish to acknowledge Dr. Patricia Flatley Brennan for her thoughtful review and Mary Cleat Szczepaniak and Albert Santucci for their helpful editorial comments. This work was supported in part by the Pittsburgh Medical Informatics Training Program grant NLM/NIDR 5T15LM/DE07059-12 by the National Library of Medicine and by The Jewish Healthcare Foundation, Pittsburgh, PA.

Questions

1. Provide some examples for the appropriate use of consumer health informatics as a component of healthcare information delivery.
2. Describe several issues that nurses should consider when implementing consumer health information techniques in a healthcare organization.
3. Characterize the impact of consumer health informatics on patient and provider roles.
4. What are the most important reasons for evaluating consumer health information systems?

References

Adderly D, Hyde C, Mauseth P. The computer age impacts nurses. *Computers in Nursing* 1997;15(1):43–46.

Anonymous. The web of information inequality. *Lancet* 1997;349:1781.

Benjamin I, Dilling BA, Campbell KC, Maraqa A, Liang B, Medbery R, et al. Technical and editorial administration of a world-wide-web site during a period of rapid growth: the OncoLink experience. In: Cimino JJ, ed. *Proceedings of the American Medical Informatics Association Symposium.* Philadelphia: Hanley & Belfus Inc, 1996;398–402.

Boberg EW, Gustafson DH, Hawkins EB, Pingree S, McTavish F, Wise M, et al. CHESS: the comprehensive health enhancement support system. In: Brennan PF, Schneider SJ, Tornquist E, eds. *Information Networks for Community Health.* New York: Springer-Verlag, 1997;171–188.

Brennan PF. Differential use of computer network services. In: Safran C, ed. Patient-Centered Computing. *Proceedings of the 17th Annual Symposium on Computer Applications in Medical Care.* New York: McGraw-Hill, 1993;27–31.

Brennan PF, Moore SM, Smyth KA. Alzheimer's disease caregivers' uses of a computer network. *Western Journal of Nursing Research* 1992;14(5):662–673.

Brown SJ, Lieberman DA, Germeny BA, Fan YC, Wilson DM, Pasta DJ. Educational video game for juvenile diabetes: results of a controlled trial. *Medical Informatics* 1997;22(1):77–89.

Buhle EL, Goldwein JW, Benjamin I. OncoLink: a multimedia oncology information resource for the internet. www.oncolink.upenn.edu/about_oncolink/manuscripts/amia.html (last access November, 1999).

Burkes M. Identifying and relating nurses' attitudes toward computer use. *Computers in Nursing* 1991;9(5):190–201.

CBS MarketWatch. MarketWatch 'Net poll: demographics. www.nab.org/irch/virtual/faqs.asp, March 14, 1999.

Clark M, Ghandour G, Miller NH, Taylor CB, Bandura A, DeBusk RF. Development and evaluation of a computer-based system for dietary management of hyperlipidemia. *Journal of the American Dietetic Association* 1997;97(2):146–150.

Cork RD, Detmer WM, Friedman C. Validation of an instrument to measure physicians' use of, knowledge about, and attitudes towards computers. *Journal of the American Medical Informatics Association* 1998;5(2):164–176.

Council on Competitiveness. *Highway to Health: Transforming U.S. Health Care into the Information Age*. Washington, DC: Council on Competitiveness Publications Office, 1996.

CyberAtlas. The numbers behind e-mail: 81 million Americans get e-mail via Internet. www.cyberatlas.com/big_picture/traffic_patterns/email.html, March 6, 1999.

CyberAtlas. How ordinary Americans view the web: half say Internet not reaching potential. www.cyberatlas.com/big_picture/demographics/cbs.html, Mach 6, 1999.

Dudley TE, Falvo DR, Podell RN, Renner J. The informed patient poses a different challenge. *Patient Care* 1996;30(16):128–138.

Eng TR, Maxfield A, Patrick K, Deering MJ, Ratzan SC, Gustafson DH. Access to health information and support: a public highway or a private road? *Journal of the American Medical Association* 1998;280(15):1371–1375.

Engstrom P. Wide connections: is online healthcare for the privileged few? *Medicine on the Net* 1997;3(5):9–14.

Evans JH, Collier J, Crook I, Garrud P, Harris P, MacKinlay DR, et al. Using multimedia for patient information—a program about nocturnal enuresis. *British Journal of Urology* 1998;81(Suppl 3):120–122.

Floridi L. Brave.net.world: the Internet as a disinformation highway? *Electronic Library* 1996;14(5):509–514.

Gannon-Leary P. "E" for exposed? e-mail and privacy issues. *Electronic Library* 1997;15(3):221–225.

General Accounting Office. *Consumer Health Informatics: Emerging Issues*. Information Resources Management/Health, Education, and Human Services Accounting and Information Management DivisionGAO/T-AIMD-96–134GAO/AIMD-96–134T(511209). Washington, DC: U.S. General Accounting Office, 1996.

Gustafson DH, Bosworth K, Hawkins RP, Boberg EW, Bricker E. CHESS: a computer-based system for providing information, referrals, decision support and social support to people facing medical and other health-related crises. In: Frisse M, ed. *Proceedings of the 16th Annual Symposium on Computer Applications in Medical Care*. New York: McGraw-Hill, 1992;161–165.

Horan PP, Yarborough MC, Besigel G, Carlson DR. Computer-assisted self-control of diabetes by adolescents. *Diabetes Educator* 1990;16(3):205–211.

Huss K, Salerno M, Huss RW. Computer-assisted reinforcement of instruction: effects on adherence in adult atopic asthmatics. *Research in Nursing & Health* 1991;14(4):259–267.

Kinzie MB, Schorling JB, Siegel M. Prenatal alcohol education for low-income women with interactive multimedia. *Patient Education & Counseling* 1993; 21(1–2):51–60.

Klemm P, Nolan MT. Internet cancer support groups: legal and ethical issues for nurse researchers. *Oncology Nursing Forum* 1998;25(4):673–676.

Korn R, Wieczorek RR. Computerization of standards and patient education material. *Journal of Nursing Staff Development* 1995;11(6):307–312.

Lewis D. Computer based patient education: use by diabetes educators. *Diabetes Educator* 1996;22(2):140–145.

Lewis D. The Internet as a resource for healthcare information. *Diabetes Educator* 1998;24(5):627–632.

Lewis D. Computer-based approaches to patient education: a review of the literature. *Journal of the American Medical Informatics Association*, 1999;6(4):272–282.

Liao L, Jollis JG, DeLong ER, Peterson ED, Morris KG, Mark DB. Impact of an interactive video on decision making of patients with ischemic heart disease. *Journal of General Internal Medicine* 1996;11(6):373–376.

Lindberg CS. Implementation of in-home telemedicine in rural Kansas: answering and elderly patient's needs. *Journal of the American Medical Informatics Association* 1997;4(1):14–17.

Madoff SA, Pristach CA, Smith CM, Pristach EA. Computerized medication instruction for psychiatric inpatients admitted for acute care. *MD Computing* 1996;13(5):427–431.

Mandl KD, Katz SB, Kohane IS. Social equality and access to the World Wide Web and e-mail: implication for design and implementation of medical applications. In: Chute CG, ed. *Proceedings of the American Medical Informatics Association Annual Symposium*. Philadephia: Hanley & Belfus, Inc, 1998:215–219.

Masys DR, Baker DB. Patient-Centered Access to Secure Systems Online (PCASSO): a secure approach to clinical data access via the World Wide Web. In: Masys DR, ed. *Proceedings of the American Medical Informatics Association Annual Fall Symposium*. Philadelphia: Hanley & Belfus, Inc, 1997: 340–343.

Meredith W. Virtual reality for patients with spinal cord injury. *MD Computing* 1996;13(5):400–405.

Meyerhoff C, Bischof F, Pfeiffer EF. Long-term experiences with a computerized diabetes management and glucose monitoring system in insulin-dependent diabetic patients. *Diabetes Research & Clinical Practice* 1994;24(1):1–7.

Miller TE, Reents S. *The Health Care Industry in Transition*. Internet Strategies Group: Cyber Dialogue, Inc. www.cyberdialogue.com/pdfs/articles/intel.pdf, 1999.

Moline J. Virtual reality for health care: a survey. U.S. Department of Commerce. http://nii.nist.gov/pubs/vr-medicine.htm, March 3, 1999.

Morris TA, Guard JR, Marine SA, Schick L, Haag D, Tsipis G, et al. Approaching equity in consumer health information delivery: net wellnesss. *Journal of the American Medical Informatics Association* 1996;4(1):6–13.

Nishimoto M, Kobayashii Y, Kuribayashi S, Takabayashi K, Yoshida S, Satomuro Y. Computer assisted instruction for diabetic patients using multimedia environment on a Macintosh computer. In: *Nursing Informatics: An International Overview in a Technological Era* Grobe SJ, Pluyter-Wenting, SP eds. Amsterdam, the Netherlands: Elsevier, 1994;423.

Ogozalek VZ. The "automated pharmacist": comparing the use of leaflets, text-based computers, and multimedia computers to provide medication information to the elderly. *Journal of Medical Education Technologies* 1993;6–11.

Osman LM, Abdalla MI, Beattie JA, Ross SJ, Russell IT, Friend JA, et al. Reducing hospital admission through computer supported education for asthma patients.

Grampian Asthma Study of Integrated Care (GRASSIC). *BMJ* 1994; 308(6928):568–571.

Peters A, Rubsamen M, Jacob U, Look D, Scriba PC. Clinical evaluation of decision support system for insulin-dose adjustment in IDDM. *Diabetes Care* 1991; 14(10):875–880.

Petersen M. What are blood counts? A computer-assisted program for pediatric patients. *Pediatric Nursing* 1996;22(1):21–25, quiz 26–27.

Rubin DH, Leventhal JM, Sadock RT, Letovsky E, Schottland P, et al. Educational intervention by computer in childhood asthma: a randomized clinical trial testing the use of a new teaching intervention in childhood asthma. *Pediatrics* 1986; 77(1):1–10.

Scarpa R, Smeltzer SC, Jasion B. Attitudes of nurses toward computerization: a replication. *Computers in Nursing* 1992;10(2):72–80.

Shepperd S, Coulter A, Farmer A. Using interactive videos in general practice to inform patients about treatment choices: a pilot study. *Family Practice* 1995; 12(4):443–447.

Skinner CS, Siegfried JC, Kegler MC, Strecher VJ. The potential of computers in patient education. *Patient Education & Counseling* 1993;22(1):27–34.

Stronge JH, Brodt A. Assessment of nurses' attitudes toward computerization. *Computers in Nursing* 1985;3:154–158.

Sweeney MA, Gulino C. From variables to videodiscs: interactive video in the clinical setting. *Computers in Nursing* 1998;6(4):157–163.

Tetzlaff L. Consumer informatics in chronic illness. *Journal of the American Medical Informatics Association* 1997;4(4):285–300.

Turnin MC, Beddok RH, Clottes JP, Martini PF, Abadie RG, Buisson JC, et al. Telematic expert system Diabeto. New tool for diet self-monitoring for diabetic patients. *Diabetes Care* 1992;15(2):204–212.

Van Biervliet A, Gest TR. A multimedia guide to spinal cord injury: empowerment through self instruction. *Medinfo* 1995;8 (Pt 2):1701.

von Bertalanffy L. *General Systems Theory*. New York: George Braziller, 1968.

Wetstone SL, Sheehan TJ, Votaw RG, Peterson MG, Rothfield N. Evaluation of a computer based education lesson for patients with rheumatoid arthritis. *Journal of Rheumatology* 1985;12(5):907–912.

Williams RB, Boles M, Johnson RE. Patient use of a computer for prevention in primary care practice. *Patient Education & Counseling* 1995;25(3):283–292.

Wilson PN, Foreman N, Stanton D. Virtual reality, disability and rehabilitation. *Disability & Rehabilitation* 1997;19(6):213–220.

25
Information Management in Home Care

MARGARET M. HASSETT AND MARJORIE H. FARVER

In today's home setting, nurses are experiencing patient care situations that traditionally would have occurred only in an acute care setting. New medical skills and technologies enable patients to recuperate faster and minimize the trauma of surgery, making home care a viable alternative supported by consumer preference and healthcare reform.

Today, a significant number of informational, regulatory, reimbursement, and practice issues remain in delivering expected care services. Information technology can provide the home healthcare professional with data and information at the point of care in a format that improves home care practice, creates clinical documentation, and captures data for billing and payroll.

History and Trends

Home care, the oldest type of healthcare delivery, constituted a small segment of the healthcare delivery system in the United States throughout the nineteenth and most of the twentieth centuries. Today's home care practice has changed radically since its initial growth spurt in 1966 following the initiation of Medicare and Medicaid reimbursable home care benefits. In 1983, with the advent of prospective payment and diagnosis-related groups (DRGs), the home setting was recognized as a viable alternative setting for care that had previously been provided in acute care facilities. As a result, home care is the fastest growing segment of the U.S. provider industry. Revenue has been growing at 20 percent per year and now exceeds $35 billion (Williams, 1998). The Washington, DC–based National Association of Home Care estimates that 2.5 percent of all adult Americans (nearly 6 million people) have received some form of home health care (Murphy, 1997).

Additional trends that have impacted the development and delivery of home care services are

- Changing population demographics. The number of people living at least 65 years will be nearly 35 million by the year 2000, and by the year 2050 20 percent of the population will be elderly, up 12.6 percent from the year 2000 (Rae-Dupree, 1997).
- Reimbursement pressures. Advances in treatments and medical technology, coupled with reimbursement pressures, will make it possible to treat more conditions in an outpatient setting and to send patients home sooner.
- Consolidation. Integrated delivery networks are including home care agencies in their continuum of services. Twenty-seven percent of Medicare-certified agencies are hospital based, and 60 percent of acute care institutions now own home care services (Meyer, 1998). In addition, there is consolidation of such service offerings as infusion therapy, durable medical equipment (DME), and respiratory care and custodial care to better position home care agencies in a competitive market.

HCFA Home Care Definition

Home health care, as defined by the Health Care Financing Administration (HCFA), encompasses skilled nursing, physical therapy, occupational therapy, speech therapy, medical social work, and home health aide services. Ancillary services are identified as respiratory equipment and DME, infusion and pharmacy, and hospice or "palliative" care. The goals of home care are restorative: to increase self-care knowledge and ability and to improve function. Services provided by home health agencies are highly regulated by the *Federal Medicare and Medicaid Programs: Conditions of Participation for Home Health Agencies*. This document dictates "a patient must be homebound, require skilled professional services (not custodial) under a physician's direction, services must be intermittent, and a caregiver must be available" (http://www.medicare.gov; see also Medicare and Home Health Care, 1998).

Home Care Environment and Workflow

The home care provider and acute care professional require similar information in order to deliver necessary patient care and services. Both types of practitioners require patient demographic data, medical history, diagnoses, laboratory and ancillary test results, and treatment plan. In addition, patient teaching materials, policies and procedures, drug and treatment information, technical data, available community services, current on-call lists, and updated phone lists facilitate the delivery of the patient care, either at home or in the acute care setting.

The point of care in a home care practice is the patient's home. However, without information technology, the patient's medical record, teaching materials, policies and procedure books, and clinical reference books are inaccessible because they are kept at the agency office. The practitioner, who is already carrying assessment equipment, dressing supplies, infection control supplies, and other equipment, must also carry any information required for delivering the appropriate care, such as condensed drug and treatment references, copies of the patient's medical record, new procedure documentation, and patient teaching materials.

Collaboration with peers during the delivery of patient care is traditional in the hospital setting but can be a missing link in home care. Care management conferences are necessary to ensure continuity of care between professional disciplines in home care. Scheduling these conferences is often difficult due to variations in work schedules and dependence on staff who work for more than one agency.

A typical home care provider's caseload involves different physicians and practice locations. Frequent communications provide for

- Verification of treatment plans
- Patient status update notification
- Initiation of verbal orders and obtaining physician signatures
- Validation of HCFA 485 forms (content and signatures)
- Notification of patient discharges or service terminations.

Home care delivery is accomplished in distinct stages that require specific information communication, either in written or verbal form.

- Intake or referrals come from a variety of sources, such as discharge planners, insurance company case managers, families, or physicians. Information is obtained that establishes the medical necessity for identified services, identifies patient demographics, and determines the priority of the admission visit in the home.
- Clinical management is the coordination of a variety of resources to provide the required services, such as infusion therapy, hospice, or home medical equipment, and ensure the appropriate staff is assigned to render prescribed care.
- Admission visit collects and verifies patient demographics, assessment, Outcome and Assessment Information Set (OASIS) data, initial treatment plan, and medical necessity.
- Ongoing case management and visit documentation are crucial in the industry, as Medicare is the main payor that reimburses services. Insufficient or incomplete data can cause denial or delay of payments.
- Discharge of the patient is a process defined by HCFA that requires timely discharge assessment, completion of paperwork, and notification to effect payment for services.

Quality documentation is vital to the efficient and effective operation of a home care agency. However, the majority of service documentation and patient assessments are traditionally accomplished outside the agency's office environment, such as in the patient's home, a staff member's car, or another convenient location. The practitioner's ability to deliver documentation to the agency office in a timely fashion is challenged. Information technology is one way an agency can support a home care practitioner's timely communication.

Documentation supports various facets of the home care business (Table 25.1):

- Business and billing requires solid documentation during audits to protect against allegations of fraud and abuse. Patient documentation is key to validating medical appropriateness of services in particular.
- Submission of OASIS information supports an active program of quality monitoring and improvement in clinical practice and patient manage-

Table 25.1. Description of major standard documentation forms.

Documentation	Purpose	Responsible party
485 Form (HCFA), case initiation	• Initial form to establish case in compliance with HCFA guidelines • Must be completed with patient demographic information, treatment plan, and expected date of discharge • Care provider generated 485 for physician signature • Business office usually receives form back from physician and transmits to Medicare	• Care provider must complete • Physician must sign • Business office tracks and sends in signed form
Signed physician orders	• Utilized to establish initial treatment plan and document future changes to the plan • Required by HCFA to be signed by physician within 30 days of verbal order • Must be collected and filed chronologically	• Care coordinator and physician
485 Form (HCFA) and verbal orders	• Used for recertification (60 days after admission and re-admission after 48 hours in acute care facility) • Updated treatment information goes on this form • Generated by care provider and submitted to physician • Changes to the treatment plan by verbal order of the physician must be documented and signed by the physician, in sequence	• Business office staff, with input and signature by care providers and physician

OASIS requirements for local forms	• Structured data set (79 data elements) mandated by HCFA (beginning in 1998) for inclusion in clinical documentation of all adult nonmaternity patients at
	  • Admission
	  • Recertification
	  • Discharge
		• Clinical care provider, IS, and business office

Copyright 1999 First Consulting Group.

ment, as mandated by the Joint Committee on the Accreditation of Healthcare Organizations (JCAHO) and HCFA.

- Analyzing comprehensive clinical information on patients is a key to developing the best patient management practices within reimbursement limits and costs. This information helps to position an agency better in the competitive environment.
- The need for actuarial data for home care services facilitates the capitation of home care (Perry, 1998).

The financial burden of Medicare's documentation requirements has a significant impact on a home care agency's costs. The HCFA 485 forms, which, without technology, require a large amount of time and resources to complete, are now complemented by the Outcome and Assessment Information Set (OASIS). Proposed in 1997 and finalized in January 1998, the OASIS outcomes assessment initiative is a structured data set comprising 79 patient-specific data elements that are integrated into patient assessment on admission, discharge, and transfer. The data are focused on measures for home healthcare outcomes analysis. These data are intended to be used for clinical assessment, care planning, and other internal agency-level applications, as well as for outcome monitoring (Tidd, 1998).

Implementation of OASIS challenges home health agencies to

- Evaluate their manual data capture forms and procedures
- Determine information systems' capabilities for capturing and reporting the OASIS data
- Quantify impacts on fiscal planning, daily operations, and practice flow
- Absorb the cost of integrating necessary changes in forms and procedures within the agency cost structure.

OASIS and ORYX information allow benchmarking of the number of visits and the cost per visit related to clinical outcomes. Information systems installed by HCFA facilitate OASIS data transmission at a national level. Individual states are responsible for collecting data in accordance with HCFA specifications and preparing data for submission to a central HCFA repository (Shaughnessy et al., 1997). As benchmarking information becomes available, efficient quality care will drive the future business for home health agencies. Agencies can then be positioned as preferred providers for healthcare networks (Chin, 1999).

Data Storage and Structures

Hospital information systems are striving to support the continuum of care information needs. This requires linked information, such as a home health agency patient database, a hospital patient database, and a physician practice network. Interfacing the support systems can achieve a seamless electronic discharge of the patient from the hospital and admission to a home healthcare service. Aside from the technological challenges to accomplishing this, structured languages facilitate the formatting of nursing information for entry into any database, which will support administrative staff and clinicians in their decision-making, problem solving, and planning.

Database structures to consider are:

- Outcome and Assessment Information Set (OASIS) (Shaughnessey et al., 1997)
- Nursing Interventions Classification (NIC) (McCloskey & Bulechek, 1996)
- Nursing Outcomes Classification (NOC) (Johnson & Mass, 1997)
- Home Health Classification Method (HHCM) (Saba et al., 1997)
- The Omaha System (Martin & Scheet, 1992)
- North American Nursing Diagnosis Association (NANDA) (Warren & Hoskins, 1995)
- Nursing Minimum Data Set (NMDS) (Werley et al., 1995)

Technology in Home Care

Clinical Technology

Clinical technology has changed home care practice and available services, just as it has changed hospital practice. Intravenous therapy, chemotherapy, pain management, enteral and parenteral nutrition, and respiratory therapies are now routinely delivered in the home. The equipment and technology is portable, simple to use, and reliable. Teaching and support is provided on an as-needed basis by a visiting professional. Emergency service is always available as a back-up, enabling the patient or a caregiver to participate in therapies formerly delivered in an intensive care unit of the hospital.

Telecommunications

During the early 1990s, home care professionals benefited from improved communication with staff in the main office through the use of display beepers and digital phones. Today, portable computers, notebooks, palmtops, and hand-held devices continue to enhance both collection and communication of data and information gathered in the practice area. Telecommunications has improved the delivery of home care by allowing information to be exchanged regardless of location or time of day.

Telecommunications allows the home health professional's day to begin with a patient information download from the agency's main office into a portable computer via a telephone line or wireless remote connection. The downloaded information informs the practitioner not only of daily assignments, previous assessments, actions, and plans prescribed by other professionals involved in a patient's care but also office communications regarding meetings and inservices. In addition to patient care information, the connection provides access to the agency's policy and procedure manual, database with medication teaching materials, and tools to support decision-making in the home setting.

Telecommunication to the agency and the information database gives the clinicians access to current information about their caseloads, especially about new admissions or emergency visits. This can eliminate the need for visiting the home office or jotting information on a scrap of paper during a telephone call. Complete, accurate demographic and clinical information can be accessed in the office, in transit, and at the point of care.

Internet and E-mail

Through Internet communication, both practitioners and patients can review information on a variety of topics from multiple sources. Reliable Internet resources provide healthcare professionals with up-to-date information that previously would not have been available. Patients also use the Internet as an information source and communication medium. It is a resource that

- Is available for access on a 24 hour basis
- Is accessible by the visually and physically impaired
- Links participants locally and worldwide
- Provides resources and information on various topics
- Is anonymous and private.

Electronic mail (e-mail) further enhances the communication abilities of the home care professional by providing communications regarding

- Notices of schedule changes
- Messages from other team members
- Changes in policies or procedures
- Updated case files.

Specific patient information should only be sent via e-mail when specific and dependable security and confidentiality measures are in place. Appropriate measures and adherence to security policies are difficult for organizations to achieve and enforce. Therefore, using e-mail to communicate this kind of information should be avoided.

Applications to Support Home Care

Several major vendors offer comprehensive information systems packages. These systems provide applications that support the information needs of several of the service lines typically included in home care:

- Medicare
- Private duty
- Home medical equipment
- Hospice
- Intravenous therapy.

These systems are also a part of or designed to interface with major hospital information systems. This integration is important in providing cross-continuum care, and it becomes especially important if a home care agency is part of an integrated delivery network (IDN). Communication of discharge summaries, admission, discharge, transfer (ADT) information, and test results are some examples of the information that can be shared.

Evaluation of a comprehensive vendor must include the identification of specific vendor characteristics and services, such as

- Specific clinical applications of interest
  - Ability to support specific home care business lines
  - Functional specifications
  - Technical specifications
  - Architecture
- General company information
  - Vendor contact
  - Competitive position
  - Other product lines
  - Customization services
  - Research and development activities.

Because of regulatory changes that affect the reporting and reimbursement requirements of home care practice, vendors have been racing to develop enhancements for existing products. As a result, the marketplace is dynamic, and systems and vendors should be evaluated carefully (Williams, 1997).

Specialized or Niche Vendors

Many companies that offer information technology systems and solutions to the home care practice do not sell comprehensive systems. Instead, they focus on some component of information technology support. Specialized or niche vendors can be of interest in vendor selection engagements because they

- Support collection of OASIS data
- Facilitate mandatory reporting of outcomes
- Enable the implementation of clinical documentation
- Promote remote data capture

- Provide scanning capabilities
- Enhance scheduling abilities for staff and services.

Not every organization can afford to replace home care legacy systems or install extensive, comprehensive systems. Instead, one or more specialized applications can provide the support to meet new requirements.

Implementation Planning

Analysis of the present information flow (paper or existing computer system) should focus on identifying priorities and redundancies within the workflow. A suggested result of the analysis may be the reengineering of the organization. If reengineering is required, it should be completed before system implementation in order to reduce the amount of stress within the organization and to achieve stable flow of the paper systems (Hammer & Champy, 1993).

Adequate resources, especially personnel, are required in the system implementation process to achieve success. Attention should be given to existing policies and procedures, productivity expectations, documentation flows, and billing informational needs. Temporary staff may be required to perform ongoing work in the agency while full-time employees learn the new system and become familiar with new technology.

Clinical Field Staff Implementation and Training

The most efficient and effective method for training is a phased-in approach that leverages "super users" from within the organization. Super users can be supervisors, team leaders, and influential staff or clinicians. The program includes training the super users initially, enabling them to train other staff later. By scheduling the training for various times during a week and over a period of several weeks, clinical staff (nurses, therapists, and social workers) can complete a number of hours required for training and achieve necessary computer literacy while continuing with their patient visits.

Administrative Implementation

A clinical system that drives the financial modules is ideal, especially in home health. When data are transferred electronically from the clinician's computer to the home health agency system, timeliness and accuracy are no longer problems. Although automation represents a significant capital expense, the clinical and financial records are inexpensive to maintain compared with the manpower needed to manually create and maintain clinical and financial records. A wide range of Quality Assurance (QA) reports can be generated. Clinical or financial reports can be designed based on QA indicators, and the clinical and financial information can be linked.

Electronic claims are required by most payors, including Medicare and Medicaid, and can be processed for half the cost of paper claims. This is far less expensive for the government, insurer, and home health agency. Another benefit to the electronic claims process is the reduction of outstanding days for accounts receivable due to the speed and efficiency of electronic billing, ease of verifying and communicating billing information, and producing legible billing reports.

Conclusion

The benefits of an integrated home health system include complete, timely clinical documentation and improved patient care. Ease of documentation and communication improve employee satisfaction and retention. Physician satisfaction is enhanced due to improved communication and better patient outcomes. Financial impacts include increased reimbursement because of quality and timeliness of clinical documentation, reduced accounts receivable because of electronic billing and payment, and decreased overhead because of the need for fewer branch offices. Automation can provide the marketing edge that can help home health agencies survive the increased competition in health care.

Published benchmarking information regarding efficient quality care will drive future business for home health agencies as preferred providers for healthcare networks. Management and QA flexible reports are readily available, whereas benchmarking information is supported by the collection of the OASIS and ORYX information.

Acknowledgments. The consultation and information provided by Jane Metzger, Barbara Wyse, and Cheryl Shirk were much appreciated in the composition of this chapter.

Questions

1. Discuss the problems associated with the inability to access information on a home care visit. How can information technology be used to enhance each phase of the home care workflow?
2. Describe and summarize various documentation required in the delivery of home care services. How can information technology help process the documentation?
3. Discuss the various data structures used to collect data in the home care environment. What are the benefits of the various efforts that have been made?

4. How do you envision patients and their families being able to use technology in the home to support their care?
5. What types of software packages and applications support information collection and sharing in the home health environment?
6. Discuss some of the implementation planning suggestions that were presented in this chapter. Would they work in your environment?
7. What are the pros and cons of OASIS documentation in the home health agency? Will the cost of collecting this information be covered eventually by bringing more business to the quality agency?

References

Chin TL. Building a consumer brand. *Health Data Management* 1999;7(4):69–70.

Hammer M, Champy J. *Reengineering the Corporation: A Manifesto for Business Revolution*. New York: Harper Business, 1993.

Johnson M, Mass M. *Nursing Outcomes Classification (NOC): the Iowa Project*. St. Louis, MO: Mosby, 1997.

Martin KS, Scheet NJ. *The Omaha System: Applications for Community Health Nursing*. Philadelphia: WB Saunders, 1992.

McCloskey JC, Bulechek GM. *Nursing Interventions Classification (NIC)*, 2nd ed. St. Louis, MO: Mosby, 1996.

Medicare and Home Health Care. http://www/medicare.gov/publications/home.html/, 1–9, 4-8-1998;1–9, HCFA, 1998.

Meyer H. Home care goes corporate. *Hospitals & Health Networks* 1998;71(5):20–26.

Murphy HL. Home is where the health is. *Crain's Chicago Business* 1997 (February 24);H-12.

Perry A. Capitating home health care. *Healthcare Financial Management* 1998;52(3):39–43.

Rae-Dupree J. Stay home, stay healthy. *Buyside* 1997(October 10);1–4.

Saba VK, Pocklington DB, Miller KP, eds. *Nursing and Computers: an Anthology, 1987–1996*. New York: Springer-Verlag, 1997.

Shaughnessy PW, Crisler KS, Schlenker RE. *Medicare's OASIS: Standardized Outcome and Assessment Information Set for Home Care*. Denver: Center for Health Services and Policy Research, 1997.

Tidd CW. From data to information: management tools for home health care clinical directors. *Home Health Care Management Practice* 1998;10:(2)1–10.

Warren JJ, Hoskins LM. NANDA's nursing diagnosis taxonomy: a nursing database. In: Stenvig T, Hudgings C, eds. *Nursing Data Systems: The Emerging Framework*. Washington, DC: American Nursing Publications, 1995;49–59.

Werley HH, Ryan P, Zorn CR. The nursing minimum data set (NMDS): a framework for the organization of nursing language. In: Stenvig T, Hudgings C, eds. *Nursing Data Systems: the Emerging Framework*. Washington, DC: American Nursing Publications, 1995;19–30.

Williams T. There's no place like home healthcare. *Healthcare Informatics* 1998;14:(10)SS3–SS15.

Williams TD. Market directions. In: *Buyer's Guide to Home Health Automation*, 2nd ed. Rockville, MD: Home Health Line, 1997;1–22.

References for Selected Websites

Department of Health and Human Services home page: http://www.hhs.gov/progorg/.

National Association for Home Care home page: http://www.nahc.org/.

Home Care Magazine, a publication about home care products and services: http://www.homecaremag.com/.

OASIS Help Desk referral (private web page maintained by *Get Name*): http://members.aol.com/oasisdesk.

Joint Commission on Accreditation of Healthcare Organizations: http://www.jcaho.org.

Health Care Financing Administration: http://www.hcfa.gov.

Home Care ORYX Timetable: JCAHO Home page: http://www.jcaho.org/perfmeas/oryx/select.htm. Select "news," "press releases," and go to July 22, 1998 release: Joint Commission Introduces ORYX Requirements for Behavioral Health and Home Care Organizations.

Medicare and Health Care: http://www.medicare.gov.

26
The Nurse's Role in Telehealth

SUSAN K. NEWBOLD

Although nurses perceive telehealth as an emerging reality in today's healthcare environment, they still have questions about their role in telemedicine. Some wonder whether telenursing exists, and what nursing's future roles in telehealth will be. These issues are discussed in this chapter, and suggestions are provided about how nurses might use telehealth technology to benefit their patients.

In the 1995 Healthcare Information and Management Systems Society (HIMSS) Leadership Survey on Trends in Health Care Computing, nearly 75 percent of the respondents indicated that telemedicine projects were a priority or that they were already involved in them (Klein & Manning, 1998). Uses identified in this survey that could and do involve nurses included access to remote physicians for consultation (33 percent), tele-imaging of patient records and films (30 percent), and the connection of remote experts with students in a virtual classroom (10 percent).

In 1999, the HIMSS Leadership Survey (www.himss.org) posed two questions about telehealth (Tables 26.1 and 26.2). Responses indicated that limited numbers of organizations were using telehealth for such processes as medical image transmission and patient education (see Table 26.1). Fifteen percent were not using any telemedicine applications.

When asked about technologies that were likely to be initiated through February 2000 (see Table 26.2), only four percent of respondents thought that a telehealth link to patients' homes would be in use. We note, however, that the preoccupation with Year 2000 problems may have been responsible for organizations ignoring telehealth applications.

In this new century, nursing must be ready to assimilate the technology, but will this be accomplished in the next few years? Will telehealth provide tools that will result in better health outcomes and enable reductions in the cost of health care, or is it a technology in search of an application in nursing?

TABLE 26.1. 1999 HIMSS question on telehealth applications.

Question #16: Please indicate which telehealth applications your organization is currently using	Response (%)
Medical image transmission	25
Management or business-related video-conferences	20
Professional continuing education	17
We are not using any telemedicine applications	15
Patient education	10
Patient interviews and diagnoses	8
Don't know	3
Other	2

Definitions Related to Telehealth

Before telehealth is discussed, several key terms must be defined.

- Telemedicine, according to Pushkin et al. (1997), is the use of telecommunications and information technologies to provide clinical care to individuals at a distance and to transmit the information needed to provide that care.
- Telehealth encompasses telemedicine, but it is a broader term that emphasizes the provision of information to healthcare providers and consumers. Milholland (1997) identifies telehealth as "the removal of time and distance barriers for the deliver of healthcare services or related healthcare activities." The *Telemedicine and Telehealth* journal defines telehealth as the infrastructure and environment in which telemedicine services are delivered.
- Telecommunications (Witherspoon et al., 1994) is the use of wire, radio, optical, or other electromagnetic channels to transmit or receive signals for voice, data, and video communications. The media of telecommuni-

TABLE 26.2. 1999 HIMSS question on emerging information technologies.

Question #18: Which of the following emerging information technologies will your organization most likely begin to use over the next 12 months?	Response (%)
Wireless information appliances	21
Web-enabled business transactions (e-business)	18
Voice recognition	17
Data mining	13
Hand-held personal digital assistants for work groups	12
Other	6
Patient record smart cards	5
Don't know	4
Telehealth links to patients' homes	4

cations include telephone, video, and computers, plus a means of transmission including phone lines, fiberoptics, satellites, and microwave systems.

- Telenursing is the use of telecommunications and computer technology for the delivery of nursing care. It is any nursing at a distance, mediated in whole or in part through electronic means (Yensen, 1996).

Issues in Telehealth

Issues and concerns surrounding telehealth fall into several categories: legal, economic, healthcare related, and technology related. According to Klein and Manning (1998), legal issues fall into three categories: traditional medicolegal issues, conflicts in state law (exacerbated when telemedicine connects geographically separate facilities), and unique telemedicine issues. Although they seemed to direct their discussion to physicians, the issues can be easily interpreted for nurses.

Medicolegal issues, notably privacy and confidentiality of healthcare records, are not unique to telehealth. Nurses have a clear responsibility to their clients in these areas. Interstate telehealth raises licensure questions. Are "telenurses" practicing nursing in the remote state? Do they need a license there? Laws and regulations covering nursing practice vary from state to state, and it is not clear which laws apply to nurses providing telehealth services across geographical boundaries.

This issue may soon be resolved. In the United States, the National Council of State Board of Examiners of Nursing is proposing mutual recognition for nursing regulation. This means that the nurse can be licensed in one state but practice in another. Currently, a nurse needs a license for each state in which she or he practices. The goal is to "simplify governmental processes and remove regulatory barriers to increase access to safe nursing care" (National Council of State Boards of Nursing, 1998). Utah is the only state that has adopted this new model, with the rest to follow by the year 2000. Other issues may arise when nurses practice across international boundaries.

The use of telehealth could require that a computer-based patient record (CPR) be transmitted across state lines. Laws vary in the United States as to how states handle confidentiality, privacy, and data protection, but nurses are committed to promoting and maintaining patient privacy and confidentiality. When using telehealth, nurses must be concerned with

- Maintaining and evaluating current confidentiality and privacy protections to see if they are sufficient for the implementation of telehealth
- Informing the patient of potential risks of using telehealth, such as confidentiality risks

- Dealing with the reimbursement of services across state lines, an issue unique to telehealth in the United States. How would patient-to-facility home monitoring be billed?
- Addressing healthcare issues of cost and quality. Can care provided at a distance be viewed as quality patient care with acceptable outcomes and reasonable cost? Can telehealth technology help keep down costs while maintaining confidentiality and privacy of data?

The Position of the Professional Nursing Organizations

A task force from the American Nurses Association (ANA) developed *Competencies for Telehealth Technologies in Nursing* (1999). The ANA views telehealth technologies as tools to provide nursing services. There are no performance criteria for each of the 11 competency statements. The ANA is not a regulating body. The criteria do seem reasonable, but it is not understood why they are any different for the competencies currently developed for the informatics nurse. Also included is a glossary of telehealth terms and a list of sources for more information on telehealth.

The ANA (1997) promoted telehealth by describing what telecommunications technologies, ranging from a simple telephone to sophisticated networks, can enable nurses to do. These include capabilities to

- Participate in peer conferences
- Obtain consultations from other nurse administrators
- Access expanded populations for recruitment into studies
- Collect data from remote sites
- Consult with remote peers and specific clinical expert nurses on issues of clinical practice
- Consult directly with a client's primary care practitioner, pharmacist, and other disciplines as necessary.

The ANA has been actively involved in developing guidelines for telemedical practices since 1996. Professional nurses play critical roles in home care, where telehealth can help deliver quality care to clients in distant, isolated, and underserved rural areas.

Another major nursing organization, the National League for Nursing (NLN), has a Council on Nursing Informatics (CNI) but does not specifically address telenursing or telehealth in written documents. One objective of the CNI is to promote the use of technology for distance education. Its first distance education conference was broadcast over the Web in September 1998. A second program planned for June 1999 was not offered due to equipment and funding constraints.

Telehealth Projects with Nursing Components

Projects in the United Kingdom

Telehealth projects all over the world have nursing components. One U.K. project with a radio-networked virtual nursing home enables communication with elderly, infirm, and disabled clients (www.dis.port.ac.uk/ndtm/Projects/indiv67.htm).

In a second project, nurse practitioners are investigating the feasibility of real-time nurse practitioner use of videosigmoidoscopy at a community clinic utilizing telemedicine. They are also conducting a randomized trial of using the services of the nurse practitioner versus a medical specialist (www.dis.port.ac.uk/ndtm/Projects/indiv58.htm). This, we note, may be outside the domain of nursing in the United States.

A third project is a study of the use of TV and other hardware to bring information to patients and their caregivers (www.dis.port.ac.uk/ndtm/Projects/indiv42.htm). Findings in Belfast suggested that home telenursing using a videophone could save 15 percent of visits.

Projects in the United States

The Carle Foundation in Illinois has sponsored the Carle Rural Telemedicine Network Project since November 1993 (www.nal.usda.gov/orhp/newtmdcs.htm). Interactive video-conferencing connects seven sites, including a nursing home/senior service center. The network and its units provide consultations, educational services, home health, and clinical telemedicine services in a wide range of specialties.

The University of Kentucky Chandler Medical Center sponsors the Kentucky TeleCare project (www.kytelecare.com), begun in 1995. It now links four sites on campus, eight rural hospitals, and two primary care centers. TeleCare uses interactive video-conferencing as well as FarSite and MedVision systems for still-image and store-and-forward applications. In addition to a range of specialties, clinical applications include preoperative anesthesia screening, tumor boards, nutritional counseling, and nurse case management.

In a collaborative project involving the Eisenhower Army Medical Center, the Georgia Institute of Technology, and the Medical College of Georgia, nurses visit patients at home using telemedicine technology. The system, called The Electronic Housecall, transmits blood pressure cuff, oxygen saturation monitors, temperature probes, three lead electrocardiographic monitors, and a stethoscope (Schlachta, 1997).

The Shepherd Center at the Crawford Research Institute in Atlanta, Georgia, is conducting research on postdischarge follow-up of catastrophic injury survivors in their own homes. Simple telephone-based technology is used for accessibility during tele-rehabilitation with various patient populations.

In Wisconsin, the Marshfield Medical Research and Education Foundation hosts the Marshfield Clinic Telemedicine Network (www.nal.usda.gov/orhp/newtmdcs.htm). DS3 and T1 lines link 38 regional sites; plans call for expanded access to two medically underserved communities. Networked functions include e-mail, shared medical records, video-conferencing for business and patient care, and Internet/intranet access. In addition to clinical specialties, telemedicine services include nurse triage and compliance follow-up. Plans call for increased use of video-conferencing for follow-up, initial patient assessment, physician-to-physician urgent consultations, and emergent stabilization of critical patients. Also part of the project are on-line information for patients and professionals and an evaluation of human factors.

In Connecticut, the AmeriCares Free Clinic (1995) initiated a project to provide free specialty consultation to the uninsured and underinsured residents of South Norwalk and surrounding communities. Technical support is provided by Southern New England Telephone and Norwalk Hospital's Beulah Hinds Research Center. Technology links volunteer physicians and nurses at the clinic with volunteer consulting specialists at Norwalk Hospital.

In one advanced telenursing application, a computerized clinical information system (CCIS) supports nursing care for rural cancer patients in their communities. Run on laptop computers, CCIS provides screens for standard recording of demographics, physical examinations, symptoms, and treatments. Advanced practice nurses track patient symptoms over time, noting which treatments are successful in resolving or reducing the problems. Information from patient visits is selected by help menus for inclusion into referral forms, patient care reports, and discharge summaries. The research team uses the combined data set to examine symptom patterns, nursing diagnoses, and treatments that result in improved physical and psychological functioning and symptom resolution.

Telehealth Applications

According to Yensen (1996), there are few citations in the literature related to telenursing. One telemedicine text (Field, 1996) mentions nursing only a few times in over 250 pages. Although telehealth applications vary greatly, many do involve nurses. For example, nurses are primary players in telephone triage programs like "Ask a Nurse" and Telenurse. In two pilot projects headed by Brennan, persons living with AIDS and caregivers of Alzeheimer's disease patients used e-mail communication to access information and communicate with each other (Skiba, 1995).

Home care depends heavily on nurses. Some nurses use a hand-held device at the point of care, known as the Nightingale Tracker. This links nurse users with a clinical data repository, the Web, and expert advisors;

developed by nurses, it is used in over 40 sites in the United States (V. Elfrink, September 24, 1998, personal communication). Although some home health agencies hope that telehealth will result in cost savings, research is inconclusive. "Telemedicine makes home healthcare more effective and convenient, but it is yet to be determined if it is cost-effective," says Rashid Bashshur, Director of Telemedicine at the University of Michigan, Ann Arbor (Saphir, 1998). Still, in reporting that 50 percent of home health nursing visits require only cognitive access, not instrumental or procedural access, the U.S. Department of Defense (1996) concluded that electronic home health calls would be of benefit.

Other applications include distance education. Duquesne University in Pittsburgh, Pennsylvania, now offers a PhD program in nursing completely via on-line distance education (Milstead & Nelson, 1998).

The National Institutes of Health (NIH) provides healthcare professionals and consumers with medical information. The Agency for Health Care Policy and Research (AHCPR) places clinical practice guidelines on-line.

The Future of Telenursing

Despite growing interest in telemedicine as a healthcare delivery system, "explorations on the contributions of nurses and their potential in tele-health/telemedicine has been markedly absent. In fact, little to no information, with the exception of brief anecdotal comments, has been available on the role of nurses in telemedicine/telehealth" (Hudson, 1998).

In some ways, telenursing is still in its infancy. The International Telenursing Association is currently inactive, as is the electronic mailing list they sponsored. The news group sci.med.telemedicine rarely if ever discusses nursing issues.

Still, there are journals that focus on telehealth. These include the *Journal of Medical Systems, Journal of Telemedicine and Telehealth, Journal of the American Medical Informatics Association*, and the *Telemedicine Journal*. On the web, one of the most informative sites is sponsored by the National Library of Medicine at www.tie.telemed.org.

Action Steps for Nurses

Understand the evolving capabilities of technology. Understanding is the base that will allow nurses to use technology creatively to solve healthcare problems. This might mean taking a basic course in nursing informatics offered at the undergraduate level.

Help disseminate healthcare information on the Web. Many organizations have websites, but currently they may be more focused on providing directions than on healthcare information. The nurse is in a unique position to use the Web as a teaching tool for both patients and colleagues. Whatever the activity, nurses can play a key role in helping to ensure the quality of the information disseminated on the Web. Given the lack of standards on the Web, nurses acting as "quality filters" can fill a critical void.

Support the mutual recognition model for nursing licensure. Such licensure is basic to the development of telenursing in the United States. Nurses can become actively involved by contacting the directors of their state boards of nurse examiners. Knowing their state's position is the first step in knowing how to further the mutual recognition model.

Write grants for telenursing projects that support health care. The TIE web site, www.tie.telemed.org, can be a starting place for identifying funding opportunities.

Act as an advocate for telenursing. In addition to taking on research projects, nurses need to actively disseminate their findings in telehealth by publishing in the nursing journals and presenting papers at conferences.

Become involved in research and policy development. Nurses need to help set the agenda here, looking at issues of importance to the profession and those it serves. Nursing can provide valuable insights into efficacy, effectiveness, and evaluation methodologies in telenursing, and nurses have considerable expertise in the client–practitioner relationship along with client assessment and management, to name just a few.

Maintain a database of telenursing activities. Knowing the breadth and depth of telenursing activities will be critical to initiatives ranging from advocacy to evaluation.

Questions

1. Define telenursing. Discuss the use of telecommunications technology by nurses for healthcare applications.
2. What are sources of further information on telehealth?

References

American Nurses Association. *Nursing Trends & Issues* 1997;2(4).

American Nurses Association. *Competencies for Telehealth Technologies in Nursing.* Washington, DC: American Nurses Association, 1999.

AmeriCares Clinic. National Information Infrastructure Awards, 1995. http://www.gii-awards.com/nicampgn/2cca.htm, May 31, 1999.

Field MJ, ed. *Telemedicine: a Guide to Assessing Telecommunications in Health Care.* Washington, DC: National Academy Press, 1996.

Hudson TL. Telemedicine & telenursing: is there a role for army nurses? *Walter Reed Army Medical Center Nursing Informatics Newsletter* 1998(April).

Klein SR, Manning WL. Telemedicine and the Law. *The Journal of the Healthcare Information and Management Systems Society* 1998(Summer).

Milholland DK. Telehealth: a tool for nursing practice. *Nursing Trends & Issues* 1997;2:4.

Milstead JA, Nelson R. Preparation for an online asynchronous university doctoral course. *Computers in Nursing* 1998;16(5):247–258.

National Council of State Boards of Nursing. *National Council Bulletin* 1998 (October 21). Chicago, IL: Author.

Nightingale Tracker. http://www.fitne.net/tracker/trackermain.html, May 31, 1999.

Pushkin DS, Mintzer CL, Wasem C. Telemedicine: building rural systems for today and tomorrow. In: Brennan PF, Schneider SJ, Tornquist E, eds. *Information Networks for Community Health*. New York: Springer-Verlag, 1997;271–286.

Saphir A. Desperate measures. *Modern Healthcare* 1998;28(43):66.

Schlachta L. Telenursing broadens healthcare scope. *Telemedicine and Telehealth Networks* October 1996, www.telemedmag.com/db-area/archives.

Skiba D. Health-oriented telecommunications. In: Ball MJ, Hannah KJ, Newbold SK, Douglas JV, eds. *Nursing Informatics: Where Caring and Technology Meet*, 2nd ed. New York: Springer-Verlag, 1995;40–53.

National Library of Medicine. www.tie.telemed.org, May 31, 1999.

U.S. Department of Defense.
www.matmo.army.mil/pages/natforum/present/ehtc/ehtc9.html, May 31, 1999.

Witherspoon J, Johnstone S, Wasem C. *Rural TeleHealth: Telemedicine, Distance Education, and Informatics for Rural Health Care*. Boulder, CO: WICHE Publications, 1994.

Yensen J. Telenursing: virtual nursing and beyond. *Computers in Nursing* 1996; 14(4):213–214.

www.dis.port.ac.uk/ndtm/Projects/indiv67.htm (short wave radio), May 31, 1999.

www.dis.port.ac.uk/ndtm/Projects/indiv58.htm, May 31, 1999.

www.dis.port.ac.uk/ndtm/Projects/indiv42.htm, May 31, 1999.

www.dis.port.ac.uk/ndtm/Projects/indiv24.htm, May 31, 1999.

www.nal.usda.gov/orhp/newtmdcs.htm, May 31, 1999.

www.himss.org, May 31, 1999.

27
Health-Oriented Telecommunications

DIANE J. SKIBA AND AMY J. BARTON

Many are predicting that the use of telehealth applications, which emphasize the use of telecommunications in healthcare delivery, will increase as managed care becomes a more predominant force. Lindberg and Humphreys (1995) report that "combining computers, communication networks, online medical information, and electronic patient data can improve healthcare decisions, prevent dangerous oversights, increase access to care, and reduce unnecessary costs." Kassirer (1995) concurred that medical care delivered on-line was a growing trend in health care. The development and expansion of the National Information Infrastructure will undoubtedly change the nature of our communications and our access to information and knowledge resources.

The typical telecommunication providers include telephone, cable television, and broadcast and satellite companies—and, more recently, the computer industry. The media of telecommunications include telephone, video, and computers, and the means of transmission include phone lines, fiberoptics, satellites, and microwave systems (Witherspoon et al., 1994). Thus telecommunications applications can include voice, data, and video communications.

Telecommunications to Telehealth: Definitions

There are numerous terms used to describe health-oriented telecommunications applications. One definition of *telecommunications* is the use of wire, radio, optical, or other electromagnetic channels to transmit or receive signals for voice, data, and video communications (Institute of Medicine, 1996; Witherspoon, et al., 1994). It can also be defined as communications at a distance, using electric or optical transmission of audio, video, and/or data between humans or computers (Strammiello, 1993).

Another term commonly associated with the area of telecommunications is *computer-mediated communication* (CMC). Hiltz and Turnoff (1985) define CMC as the use of computers and telecommunications networks to compose, store, deliver, and process communication. These systems support a person's ability to exchange, edit, store, broadcast, and copy any written documents, to send data and messages instantaneously, and to consult electronically. Applications under this rubric include e-mail, computer conferencing, long-distance blackboards, and bulletin board systems. Computer-mediated communication applications are considered a type of data communications.

Another term now associated with telecommunications in health care is the broad concept called *telehealth*. According to Mosby's Medical and Nursing Dictionary (1998), telehealth is the "use of telecommunication technologies to provide healthcare services and access to medical and surgical information for training and educating healthcare professionals and consumers, to increase awareness and educate the public about health related issues, and to facilitate medical research across distances." Telehealth is considered an umbrella term that encompasses telemedicine, telenursing, teleradiology, and telepsychiatry (American Norses Association [ANA], 1997). The ANA (1997) defines telehealth as "delivery of health care services or activities with time and distance barriers removed and using technologies such as telephones, computers, interactive video transmissions." Accordingly, telenursing is considered a form of telehealth in which nursing practice is delivered via telecommunications. Finally, the Institute of Medicine (1996) broadly defined telemedicine as "the use of electronic information and communication technologies to provide and support health care when distance separates the participants."

For this chapter, the telecommunications classification of voice, data, and video serves as our framework for the discussion of health-oriented applications. Given the rapidly changing technology in this area, applications in health care and education are limited to the past five years and serve as examples rather than as an inclusive list of all available applications.

Voice Communications

Voice communications is based on basic telephone service, referred to by the industry as POTS (Plain Old Telephone Service). This telecommunication medium historically provided adequate service for voice communications. The telephone has several major advantages: ubiquity (universal telephone service was a public policy goal set over 60 years ago), relatively low cost for installation, minimal training for proper use, and relatively low cost per use (Witherspoon et al., 1994). Telephone service can be provided via a voice/low-speed data network or a cellular network. Enhancements to telephone service in the past decade have allowed the following services as part of voice communications: telephone conferencing, voice mail, fax machines, computer communication, and picture phones.

As in the past, telephone applications continue to increase in the delivery of health care. Telephone care is used widely in primary care settings and as a supplement to hospital discharge programs (Garland, 1992). According to Malloy (1998), telephone-based health management is a burgeoning area in managed care. Healthcare benefits plans trying to manage demand are primary users of the telephone-based health management services. "Telephonic nursing has become a pivotal service strategy offered by care delivery networks" (Bleich, 1998).

Telephone care can take many forms. Telephone services can range from simple telephone interventions to "state of the art hardware and software configurations that can manage high volumes of patient specific data, store and retrieve a wide range of complex clinical algorithms, and trend clinical and program evaluation outcomes" (Bleich, 1998). Kinsella (1998) provides a useful schema for categorizing telephone care: "keeping in touch" calls, nurse-initiated calls, patient-initiated calls, computer-generated single-purpose calls, and computer-generated interactive calls. What follows are some examples of the uses of voice communications as a healthcare intervention.

One such program is the Telephone Reassurance Program (TRP) established by graduate students at Yale University School of Nursing with the Regional Visiting Nurse Agency (VNA) of Connecticut, Inc. This innovative program (Shu et al., 1996) provided assistance to chronically ill patients who had been discharged from a VNA. The program was designed as both an outreach support program and an incoming consultation service. One of the evening or on-call staff would contact the client and conduct a comprehensive telephone assessment. Based on this assessment, the staff could make one of three decisions: The client is stable and needs no additional services; the client needs additional support and follow-up calls; or the client is in need of direct care services.

According to Shu et al. (1996), TRP offers a unique extension of the VNA services to the elderly and contributes to the cost-effectiveness delivery of quality care.

A similar program called the ParentLine was developed by nurses to "improve the health and developmental status of children from birth to five years old" (Moore & Krowchuk, 1997). ParentLine was a natural extension of an initial study of telephone intervention to reduce low birth weight, during which mothers requested that the telephone consultation be continued after birth. This program combined the use of three strategies to meet their program goals. These strategies included weekly or bimonthly telephone calls, a telephone hotline, and weekly home visits for those parents who lacked telephones.

There are also numerous programs in the area of interactive telephone services. The first example is a disease management telecommunication system called HomeTalk™. This joint venture between the Visiting Nurses Association of Cleveland and Telepractice, Inc, developed "Brief Prevention Services Screening Tools" that allow any client to call from a touch-tone phone to complete the screening. For example, their Elders Screening Tools included hypertension, mammograms, substance abuse, dental care, eye care, immunizations, fire prevention, bereavement, diet/nutrition, physical activity, family relations, and injury prevention (Niles et al., 1997). Telephone screens for families with children included such items as vision and hearing, lead poisoning, car safety, and fire prevention.

As a result of this program, the level of service that the VNA nurses could provide increased. The technology enabled the nurses to assess an additional 341 clients and to provide service an additional 1,000 times in six centers over four months (Niles et al., 1997). Clients reported limited difficulty using the system, and an overwhelming majority (95 percent) would complete the screening process using the technology.

Another example of an interactive telephone service is the REACH (Resources for Enhancing Alzheimer's Caregiver Health) for TLC (Telephone-Linked Care) system (Mahoney et al., 1998). This telecommunications project designed a voice mail bulletin board system based on the work of Brennan et al. (1991). The TLC system uses a telephone network system and an interactive voice response computer network. The caregiver dials into the system and enters a password to reach one of five modules available. Four of the modules are targeted to reduce the caregiver's stress level, and the fifth module is a technical helpline.

The first module, weekly caregiver's conversation, is considered a monitoring and counseling component that queries the caregiver about disruptive behaviors of the Alzheimer's disease patient. If disruptive behaviors have been noted, there is a series of queries to guide and counsel the caregiver. The second module is a personal mailbox where the caregiver can receive personal and confidential information from experts and nurse specialists. The Bulletin Board, the third module, allows caregivers to join a support group. Similar to an asynchronous electronic bulletin board, caregivers can leave voice mail questions or responses. All messages are retrievable, and anonymity is ensured. The last module is the activity/respite conversation designed to engage the person with Alzheimer's disease in simple, nondemanding conversation to distract the person from disruptive behaviors (Mahoney et al., 1998). This 18-minute conversation walks the care recipient through a relaxation exercise to calm them and to prevent the behaviors. A three-year study has begun to assess the efficacy of this telecommunications system.

A final example of a voice interactive computer system is HumaLink™, designed to improve communication between diabetic patients and their healthcare provider. "Interactive voice-response systems are specialized computers that allow a telephone to function as a computer terminal to connect to another computer for data transmission or retrieval" (Pierce, 1998). Patients access the computer through their phone after each blood glucose measurement. They must enter an identification number and follow computer-generated verbal instructions to enter their measurement and answer other questions about their illness. The system verifies each data entry and provides instructions based on the patient's treatment plan. Clinical algorithms are used as a basis for the automated response mode. According to Harris and Blonde (1998), two studies have demonstrated that HumaLink™ was an effective and safe enhancement to diabetic care management.

According to Kinsella (1998) telephone care will be a mainstay of twenty-first century care. Telephone interventions are used with various patient populations to provide social and emotional support, anticipatory guidance, education, advocacy, and consultation. As managed care and home care increases in the United States, there will be an increasing number of tele-health applications using voice communications.

Data Communications

Data communications is one of the fastest growing types of telecommunications applications. Consumers, businesses, and professionals are all connecting to each other via data communications. Data communications are provided through a variety of methods, such as telephone service for access to dial-up lines and specialized private networks for a selected group of individuals and/or institutions. Most connections use a computer, telecommunications software, and a modem.

Data communications allow computers to "talk" or access other computers at a remote location. The introduction of the World Wide Web (WWW) allowed rapid adoption of data communications as a healthcare delivery system. Numerous examples of data communications applications can be found in the healthcare literature. To begin this section, a brief historical perspective is first provided. This is followed by examples to provide the reader with a sense of how telecommunications can be used to support healthcare professionals and consumers.

Historical Perspective

In health care, the beginning of data communications occurred with the development of electronic bulletin boards systems (BBSs) on the hobbyist network called FidoNet. In nursing, numerous BBSs were developed as a means for healthcare professionals or students to talk with each other and to exchange information (Skiba & Warren, 1991). Most electronic BBSs consisted of e-mail facilities, discussion groups, read-only text file access, and downloadable text and program files.

Another major component of BBSs was the development of electronic support groups (Sparks, 1992). The electronic support groups provided 24 hour service in which consumers could selectively participate in discussions around a variety of health problems. This non-face-to-face communication provided a nonthreatening environment in which to ask questions, share feelings, and communicate with others who have experienced similar consequences of their specific health problems.

As an outgrowth of the electronic BBS movement for healthcare professionals, community computing networks (Grundner, 1991) were spawned. Community computing networks, such as the Cleveland and Denver Free-Nets, were different from professional BBSs in that the network was a reflection of the community and allowed public access to information and communication resources. The Denver Free-Net, operated by the University of Colorado Health Sciences Center School of Nursing, provided health information resources for citizens through its connections with the statewide library access network (Skiba & Mirque, 1994). The Cleveland Free-Net served as the core computer network in the pioneering work conducted by Brennan and colleagues at Case Western Reserve University. Two extensive studies examined the use of an electronic network in the provision of care for both Persons Living with AIDS (PLWAs) (Brennan et al., 1991b) and caretakers of Alzheimer's disease patients (Brennan et al., 1991a). In both studies, Brennan and her colleagues investigated the use of an electronic network, ComputerLink, to bring support services into the homes of patients or caretakers. These BBSs and community networks provided a solid foundation for the next generation of data communications applications.

Internet-Based Applications

The Internet and the introduction of the Web served as catalysts for many data communications over the past decade. Healthcare information resources are widely available on the Internet. According to a 1999 Louis Harris & Associates poll, 74 percent of the estimated 97 million U.S. adults now on-line have used the Internet to search for health and medical information. Lindberg and Humphreys (1998) reported that free access to Medline via the Internet has increased searches tenfold, with 75 million searches conducted annually. Waldo (1998) reported that the Internet "can be an effective tool to assist health care organizations in marketing, educating both staff and patients, and enhancing communication and efficiencies throughout an organization."

The explosion of Internet use is well documented in the literature. An estimated 40 to 45 million Americans use the Internet, with 51 percent of those users earning an income under $50,000 (Barunch College Harris Poll, 1998). According to Anderson (1998), the fastest growing segment of the population to use the Internet is between the ages of 55 and 70 years.

There are thousands of health-oriented websites maintained by academic centers, healthcare institutions, professional organizations, healthcare companies, and even individual consumers. The growth of self-help and support groups has increased at a phenomenal pace (Ferguson, 1997). Consumers can access information about almost any healthcare topic and can even investigate the latest information about specific clinical trials. Osheroff (1997) reported that the federal government's on-line health information site had 4.8 million hits during its first month of operation.

One such example of consumer demand is the dramatic increase in the use of electronic mail (e-mail). "Technically minded, electronically equipped health care consumers have accelerated the demand for e-mail access to their health care providers" (Fridsma et al., 1994; Kane & Sands, 1998; Spielberg, 1998). In an ongoing study of physician use of the Internet, Healtheon (1999) found an increase of 300 percent in regular usage in the last two years. Their findings indicated that physician communication with patients via e-mail is dramatically rising. This increase in patient-provider e-mail communication has given rise to many articles exploring the e-mail phenomenon (Borowitz & Wyatt, 1998; Diepgen & Eysenbach, 1998; Widman & Tong, 1997), legal and ethical issues (Spielberg, 1998), a research agenda for patient–provider communication (Mandl et al., 1998), and even the development of Guidelines for the Clinical Use of Electronic Mail with Patients (Kane & Sands, 1998).

Several nursing examples typify the use of Web-based applications to deliver nursing care. An article by Brennan et al. (1998) builds on Brennan's previous research in the area of computer-mediated health care in her new project called HeartCare. This new initiative will investigate the use of personalized Web pages for cardiac artery bypass graft (CABG) patients. The focus of her grant is the delivery of home healthcare recovery services for CABG patients using WebTV for the first three months after surgery. Nurses will create personalized Web pages for different time periods throughout the recovery process. This experimental group will be compared with patients who receive an audiotape-coaching program. The program also includes e-mail communication between patients and their nurse and physician. Programs like HeartCare will have ramifications for the entire healthcare system.

Another example of data communications is NetWellness, an electronic consumer health information service operated by the University of Cincinnati Medical Center and other 35 other healthcare partners. This project, built on the work of community networks, makes use of a regional community Free-Nets and other public access facilities for community access (Morris et al., 1997). Funded from a national Telecommunications and Information Administration grant, this project delivers consumer health information and resources through the Web. NetWellness offers the following features (Hern et al., 1997): Hot Topics (such as aging, breast cancer), In the News (connections to news providers like CNN and Time

Daily), Hopeline (support for substance abuse), Directories (healthcare providers and community services), and Ask An Expert (consumers can ask a question and receive a personalized response within 24 to 48 hours). The Ask an Expert component involves many healthcare professionals, including nursing faculty from the College of Nursing. Nurses provide consultations in the areas of child development and health, pregnancy, breastfeeding and newborn care, and breast cancer. Nursing faculty involvement in this project has facilitated the curriculum shift to a community-focused nursing health patterns model and has served as a mechanism to increase individual nurses' body of professional knowledge (Hern et al., 1997).

Web-based support groups continue to support patients with a variety of health problems. One targeted area, cancer, has multiple resources developed on the Internet by professional organizations (American Cancer Society, Oncology Nursing Society), National Cancer Institute, and university-based sites (OncoLink, University of Iowa Virtual Hospital). It is not surprising that several Internet cancer support groups have been formed and that the numbers are increasing (Klemm et al., 1998). Many support groups are moderated by cancer survivors and are not affiliated with any research studies.

Several studies have examined the use of Internet support groups for cancer patients. One study (Weinberg et al., 1996) examined the use by six women with breast cancer over a three-month time period. They found that women were very willing to share personal information and feelings with each other over the net. Similar results were found by the research team lead by Gustafson et al. (1993) and Sharf (1997). Other studies, like that of Klemm et al. (1998), investigated the content of messages exchanged in an Internet support group for colorectal cancer patients. The content analysis found that messages could be grouped into the following categories: information giving/seeking, personal opinions, encouragement/support, personal experience, thanks, humor, prayer, and a miscellaneous area. Klemm et al. (1998) highlighted the advantages and disadvantages of Internet cancer support groups. Another cancer support article described the creation of a website for people diagnosed with malignant melanoma (Bliss et al., 1998). This website was created as an undergraduate project and emphasized the efficacy of on-line support for patients.

The numerous other examples of Internet-based applications for patient care delivery indicate that the net is an increasingly powerful channel for interactive healthcare communication (Robinson et al., 1998). Interactive health communication (IHC) is defined as the "interaction of an individual—consumer, patient, caregiver or professional—with or through an electronic device or communication technology to access or transmit health information or to receive guidance and support on a health related issue" (Robinson et al., 1998). This article provides the recommendations of the Science Panel on Interactive Communication and Health. The panel states that IHC applications include six specific functions: relay information, enable informed decision-making, promote healthful behaviors, promote peer information exchange and emotional support, promote self-care, and manage demand for healthcare services. The panel recommends the use of an Evaluation Reporting Template for Interactive Health Communications applications. This template is designed to help consumers judge various IHC applications and designers to evaluate their IHC applications and to promote standard reporting of evaluation results of IHC applications. The basis for an evidence-based approach for IHC development and diffusion is addressed in several articles referenced on the SciPICH website (http://www.scipich.org).

Without a doubt, this area of data communications will continue to increase in the number of applications available to consumers and healthcare professionals. The Council on Competitiveness (1996) believes the National Information Infrastructure can serve as a catalyst for positive change in the healthcare market. Both Ferguson (1997) and Waldo (1998) believe that the Internet has the capacity to empower consumers, providers, and organizations that will eventually revolutionize health care. Pinkowish et al. (1999) concluded that patient education and the self-care trends over the past 20 years are being accelerated by the Internet and that consumers will have access to nearly all the same medical information used by physicians.

Video Communications

Video communications is the third class of telecommunications application. The most common video communication is the full-motion broadcast video that one sees on the television. Full-motion broadcast video is a form of one-way communication. The transmission signal is broadcasted from the station to numerous households, but there are no capabilities for households to broadcast back to the stations. In the United States, it takes 525 lines of video scanned 30 times a second to produce the colors, brightness, and motion of the original broadcast (Witherspoon et al., 1994).

A second type of video communication is compressed video, which uses digital technology to send only those portions of the picture that change from frame to frame (Witherspoon et al., 1994). Compressed video does not require 30 frames per second for quality video. The compression of video is more efficient in terms of speed of transmission and necessary bandwidth.

A third type is slow-scan video that allows for the transmission of still pictures over traditional telephone lines. Slow scan trades capacity or bandwidth for time. Instead of 30 frames per second, it might take over a minute for a single frame of video. Slow scan has been used successfully with the transmission of X-ray images and other diagnostic images using traditional telephone lines (Witherspoon et al., 1994).

The two-way transmission of video images between distance locations is the fourth type of video communications. This type is commonly referred to as *interactive video* or *video-conferencing systems*. The real-time interactive component can be either one-way video/two-way audio or two-way video/two-way audio. Two-way video/audio systems are further divided into group systems (larger groups) and desktop systems (one-on-one systems usually connected to desktop computers). Most video-conferencing systems employ video compression techniques.

For many years, telemedicine and telepsychiatry applications were the most common video communications. Telemedicine applications have been in use for the past 30 years and can be categorized into two application levels: store and forward and two-way transmissions. The first level, store and forward, refers to the transmission of still images from one location to another. Radiological images, pathology slides, and dermatology photos are all examples of level one applications. The second level involves real-time interactions with full motion video. These live transmissions form the basis for teleconsultations between providers and patients.

There are numerous programs using teleconsultations, the largest one being the University of Texas Medical Branch. This program conducts 2,000 to 3,000 patient consults for the prison system in the state of Texas (Crump et al., 1997). Despite the many applications, the Institute of Medicine (1996) stated that there was minimal evidence to support the benefits and costs of telemedicine. The Institute of Medicine (1996) suggested a framework for evaluating not only cost effectiveness and efficacy but also the sustainability of telemedicine applications.

In the last few years, telemedicine has moved from the hospital to the home care environment. Managed care and disease management strategies have prompted the use of telehealth applications in the home. This growing interest in home health care also served as a catalyst for the advent of telehealth applications for nursing. In the home care market, low-end systems that use videophones, personal computers, or television sets are commonplace. These first-generation systems allow for healthcare providers to make "video visits." In some instances, video visits traditionally were augmented with vital sign devices with telecommunications capabilities. For example, blood pressure cuffs, glucometers, and transtelephonic electrocardiograph monitors were available for home use (Kinsella, 1998).

Telehealth workstations were also first-generation high-end systems that combined various tools and capture data at the point of care. These higher end systems provided a more comprehensive snapshot of the patient's status through the use of audio, two-way visual capacity, and vital sign measurements (Kinsella, 1998). What follows are examples of first-generation telehealth applications used by nurses in home care.

The Tele-Home Health Project, conducted by Kaiser Permanente's Sacramento department, compared the use of telehealth applications with traditional home visits for a group of patients with advanced medical problems (Johnston et al., 1997). The results of the study indicated that patient satisfaction was greater in the televisit group, visit time was dramatically reduced, and a significant number of hospital days was saved (Barrell, 1997). The Tele-Home Health Project used a first-generation system, an MCI videophone customized by American TeleCare (Rosen, 1997). An electronic stethoscope could be connected to the videophone system, patient isolation decreased, and the number of visits a nurse could do per shift increased. Normally with drive time and actual visit time, nurses made approximately six visits a shift. With the video visits, the nurse could conduct an average of 15 visits per shift (Rosen, 1997).

Schlachta and Pursley-Crotteau (1997) described a disease management project that used telehealth applications. Electronic Housecall was a collaborative effort between Eisenhower Medical Center, the Center for Total Access, the Medical College of Georgia, the Georgia Institute of Technology, and Jones Intercable (Barrell, 1997). This project combines off the shelf technology to conduct a "proof of concept" trial. The study, which involved 25 chronically ill patients linked to their practitioners through the local cable infrastructure, used a personal telehealth system with two-way video, audio, and diagnostic instrumentation. This proof of concept study demonstrated that three inpatient admissions were prevented (Barrell, 1997), and case studies indicated a savings of over $70,000 for five patients over the 10-month period (Schlachta & Pursley-Crotteau, 1997). Based on these cost savings, a second study of 50 patients with chronic obstructive pulmonary disease and congestive heart failure was to begin in 1998. One drawback of this project was the costly modification of the cable system to allow two-way communication.

Another example of a telehealth application used by nurses is a project conducted by the Hays Medical Center in Kansas (Japsen, 1998). This project uses a 13-inch color television equipped with a phone and camera as well as an automatic blood pressure monitor and a tympanic thermometer (Miller, 1998). The results of this pilot project indicated a substantial cost saving. In this case, a home visit to these patients costs approximately $135 for a visit by a registered nurses and $60 for a visit by a certified nursing assistant. A televisit by a registered nurse cost only $36 per visit (The Economist, 1997).

Another first-generation system for the home is the Home Assisted Nursing Care (HANC) device. This system collects and transmits data on heart rhythm, blood pressure, pulse, temperature, and pulse oximetry over the telephone to a central nursing station (Crump et al., 1997). The device also schedules self-care activities, gives medication reminders, provides healthcare instruction, and has the capability to conduct live video visits. HANC provides in-home interactions between the patient and the device. Interactions include instructions, suggestions, and other care-related questions posed to the patient using a voice recognition system. HANC can be programmed to dispense up to 10 medications—on schedule and in proper dosages—for a two-week period (Managed Home Care, 1995). A recent evaluation of the effectiveness of HANC found that 29 of 43 patients were suitable HANC candidates and that the use of HANC could have saved a total of $5000 per patient per admission (Council on Competitiveness, 1996).

A final example of a telehealth system that combines video and data communications is an interactive network called StarBright World, developed to help sick children find help in a cyberspace world (Stephenson, 1995). The interactive network allows children in different hospitals across the country to communicate with each other and share their experiences. Children can also communicate with their families and friends at school through desktop video-conferencing capabilities. This interactive network includes the use of virtual worlds that children can visit as well as video games that teach children about their diseases. Investigators are studying the use of these interventions on such outcomes as pain management, duration of hospital stays, and feelings of isolation and depression. With the telecommunications and multimedia components, this interactive network is expected to help children accomplish goals in the following areas: feelings of empowerment; socialization with peers, family, and healthcare professionals; improved communication and self esteem; pain management; enhanced understanding of healthcare condition; improved medical compliance; and improved body image, sleeping, and eating habits (StarBright Foundation at http://www.starbright.org/about/goals.html).

Summary

Health-oriented telecommunications serve as a powerful and useful tool that will greatly impact the delivery of health care in the United States. A recent evaluation of distance medicine technologies (Balas et al., 1997) indicated that electronic communication with patients appears to result in significant benefits. These distance medicine technologies (computerized communication, telephone follow-up, interactive telephone systems, and after-hours telephone access) enabled greater continuity of care by improving access and supporting the coordination of activities by a clinician (Balas et al., 1997).

In a recent editorial, Brennan (1999) stated that telehealth augments the capability of healthcare delivery systems and delivers health care to the point of living. Telehealth applications are just reaching their second generation and will continue to grow, especially in the areas of home care and disease management (Kinsella, 1998). This chapter barely scratched the surface of all the telecommunications projects available in the areas of voice, data, and video communications. One thing is certain: More lanes will be needed on the information superhighway to handle future health-oriented telecommunications applications.

Questions

1. How could the capabilities of voice communications be maximized in your organization? Would there be benefits in using telephone conferencing, voice mail, fax machines, computer communications, and/or picture telephones?
2. Do you have or know of someone who uses electronic mail in his or her work or personal life? Is the electronic mail internal to the organization and/or connected to the Internet? For what reasons is e-mail used?
3. Explain the difference between electronic bulletin board systems and e-mail.
4. Can you think of a patient or health professional subgroup that would benefit from the use of an electronic support group? How would you go about finding a support group that meets your personal interests?
5. What would be the benefits and disadvantages of taking distance education classes via computer?
6. Discuss any of the telehealth applications presented in this chapter. Can you think of other applications for video technology in the healthcare arena?

References

American Nurses Association. Telehealth: a tool for nursing practice. *Nursing Trends & Issues* 1997;2(4):1–7.

Anderson R. The Internet comes to home care. *Caring* 1998;17(6):26–28.

Balas EA, Jaffrey F, Kuperman GJ, et al. Electronic communication with patients: evaluation of distance medicine technology. *Journal of the American Medical Association* 1997;278(2):152–159.

Barrell J. Telemedicine: you can't do that at home. *Infusion* 1997;4(2):29–35.

Baruch College-Harris Poll. http://www.midiacentral.com/magazines/md/oldarchives/199704/1997042504.html, 1998(October).

Bleich MR. Growth strategies to optimize the functions of telephonic nursing call centers. *Nursing Economics* 1998;16(4):215–218.

Bliss J, Allibone C, Bontempo B, Flynn T, Valvano N. Creating a Web site for on-line social support. *Computers in Nursing* 1998;16(4):203–207.

Borowitz SM, Wyatt JC. The origin, content, and workload of e-mail Consultations. *Journal of the American Medical Association* 1998;280(15):1321–1324.

Brennan P. Telehealth: bringing health care to the point of living. *Medical Care* 1999;37(2):115–116.

Brennan P, Caldwell B, Moore S, Sreenath N, Jones J. Designing Heart Care: custom computerized home care for patients recovering from CABG surgery. In: Chute CG, ed. *Proceedings of the American Medical Informatics Association Annual Symposium*. Philadelphia: Hanley & Belfus, Inc, 1998;381–385.

Brennan P, Moore S, Smyth K. ComputerLink: electronic support for the home caregiver. *Advances in Nursing Science* 1991a;13(4):14–27.

Brennan P, Ripich S, Moore S. The use of home-based computers to support persons living with AIDS/ARC. *Journal of Community Health Nursing* 1991b;8(1):3–14.

Council on Competitiveness. Highway to Health, Transforming U.S. Health Care in the Information Age. http://nii.nist.gpv/pubs/cos_hghwy_to_hlth/chp2.html, 1996.

Crump WJ, Kotte TE, Perednia DA, Sanders JH. Is telemedicine ready for prime time? *Patient Care* 1997;31(3):64–87.

Diepgen G, Eysenbach T. Responses to unsolicited patient e-mail request for medical advice on the World Wide Web. *Journal of the American Medical Association* 1998;280(15):1333–1335.

The Economist. Big Sister is watching you. 1997(January 11);342(7999):27(1).

Ferguson T. Health care in cyberspace: patients lead a revolution. *The Futurist* 1997(November–December);29–33.

Fridsma D, Ford P, Altman R. A survey of patient access to electronic mail, attitudes, barriers, and opportunities. In: Ozbolt JG, ed. *Proceedings of the Annual Symposium on Computer Applications in Medical Care*. Philadelphia: Hanley & Belfus, Inc, 1994;15–19.

Garland M. Discharge follow-up by telephone. *Rehabilitation Nursing* 1992;17:339–341.

Grundner TM. Community Computing at Case Western Reserve University. Community Telecomputing Lab, unpublished, 1991.

Gustafson D, Wise M, McTavish F, et al. Development and pilot evaluation of a computer based support system for women with breast cancer. *Journal of Psychosocial Oncology* 1993;11:69–93.

Harris RI, Blonde L. Automating diabetes care: the new millennium. *Clinical Diabetes* 1998;16(3):105–106.

Hern M, Weitkamp T, Haag D, Trigg J, Guard J. Nursing the community in cyberspace. *Computers in Nursing* 1997;15(6):316–321.

Hiltz S, Turnoff M. Structuring computer mediated communication systems to avoid information overload. *Communication of the ACM* 1985;28(7):680–689.

Institute of Medicine. *Telemedicine: a Guide to Assessing Telecommunications in Health Care*. Washington, DC: National Academy Press, 1996.

Japsen B. House calls: Kansas hospital's experiment in home health telemedicine cuts costs, visits. *Modern Healthcare* 1998(March 23);47.

Johnston B, Wheeler L, Deuser J. Kaiser Permanente medical center's pilot tele-home health project. *Telemedicine Today* 1997;8:16–19.

Kane B, Sands D. Guidelines for the clinical use of electronic mail with patients. *Journal of American Medical Informatics Association* 1998;5(1):104–111.

Kassirer JP. The next transformation in the delivery of health care. *New England Journal of Medicine* 1995;332(1):52–54.

Kinsella A. *Home Healthcare, Wired & Ready for Telemedicine . . . the Second Generation*. Sunriver, OR: Information for Tomorrow, 1998.

Klemm P, Reppert K, Visich L. A nontraditional cancer support group: the internet. *Computers in Nursing* 1998;16(1):31–36.

Lindberg D, Humphreys B. Computers in medicine. *Journal of the American Medical Association* 1995;273:1667–1668.

Lindberg D, Humphreys B. Medicine and health on the internet: the good, the bad, and the ugly. *Journal of the American Medical Association* 1998;280(15):1303–1304.

Mahoney D, Tarlow B, Sandaire J. A computer-mediated intervention for Alzheimer's caregivers. *Computers in Nursing* 1998;16(4):208–216.

Managed Home Care. Trial of home telemonitoring device gets rave reviews from agencies, MDs, and MCOs. *Managed Home Care* 1995(July);101–104.

Miller N. Leadership roundtable: success to telemedicine program catches eyes. *Nursing Economics* 1998;16(3):137.

Moore M, Krowchuk H. Parent line: nurse telephone intervention for parents and caregivers of children from birth through age 5. *Journal of the Society of Pediatric Nurses* 1997;2(4):179–187.

Morris T, Guard J, Marine S, Schick L, Haag D, Tsipis G, Kaya B, Stoemaker S. Approaching equity in consumer health information delivery, net wellness. *Journal of the American Medical Informatics Association* 1997;4(1):6–13.

Mosby's Medical, Nursing & Allied Health Dictionary, 5th ed. Anderson KN, Anderson LE, Glanze WD, eds. St. Louis, MO: Mosby, 1998;895E.

Niles S, Alemagno S, Stricklin M. Healthy talk: a telecommunication model for health promotion. *Caring* 1997;16(7):46–50.

Osheroff J. Online health-related discussion groups: what we should know and do. *Journal of General Internal Medicine* 1997;12:511–512.

Pierce G. IVR me ASAP. *Healthcare Informatics* 1998;15:147–154.

Pinkowish M, Allen A, Frisse M, Osheroff J. The Internet in medicine: an update. *Patient Care* 1999;33(i1):30–33.

Robinson T, Patrick K, Eng T, Gustafson D. An evidence-based approach to interactive health communication: a challenge to medicine in the information age. *Journal of the American Medical Association* 1998;280(14):1264–1269.

Rosen E. Twenty minutes in the life of a tele-home health nurse. *Telemedicine Today* 1997(December);12–13.

Schlachta LM, Pursley-Crotteau S. Leveraging technology, telemedicine in disease management and implications for infusion services. *Infusion* 1997;4(2):36–40.

Sharf B. Communicating breast cancer on-line: support and empowerment on the Internet. *Women and Health* 1997;26:65–84.

Shu E, Mirmina Z, Nyström K. A telephone reassurance program for elderly home care clients after discharge. *Home Healthcare Nurse* 1996;14(3):154–161.

Skiba D, Mirque D. The electronic community: an alternative health care approach. In: Grobe S, Plutyer-Wenting ESP, eds. *Nursing Informatics, an International Overview for Nursing in a Technological Era.* Amsterdam: Elsevier, 1994.

Skiba D, Warren C. The impact of an electronic bulletin board to disseminate educational and research information to nursing colleagues. In: Hovenga E, Hannah K, McCormick K, Ronald J, eds. *Nursing Informatics '91. Proceedings of the Fourth International Conference on Nursing Use of Computers and Information Science.* Berlin: Springer-Verlag, 1991, vol 42.

Sparks S. Exploring electronic support groups. *American Journal of Nursing* 1992;92(12):62–65.

Spielberg AR. On call and online, sociohistorical, legal, and ethical implications of e-mail for the patient–physician relationship. *Journal of the American Medical Association* 1998;280(15):1353–1359.

Stephenson J. Sick kids find help in a cyberspace world. *Journal of the American Medical Association* 1995;276(24):1899–1901.

Strammiello E, ed. *Colorado Rural Telecommunications Resource Guide.* Denver: Colorado Advanced Technology Institute, 1993.

Waldo B. It's time to adopt Internet technology. *Nursing Economics* 1998;325–329.

Weinberg N, Schmale J, Uken J, Weasel K. Online help: cancer patients participate in computer-mediated support group. *Health & Social Work* 1996;21:24–29.

Widman LE, Tong DA. Requests for medical advice from patients and families to health care providers who publish on the World Wide Web. *Archives of Internal Medicine* 1997;157(2):209–212.

Witherspoon J, Johnston S, Wasem C. *Rural TeleHealth, Telemedicine, Distance Education and Informatics for Rural Health Care*. Boulder, CO: WICHE Publications, 1994.

Appendices

Appendix A
Electronic Resources for Nursing

Susan K. Newbold

Usenet Newsgroups of Potential Interest to Nurses

Nursing Newsgroups

sci.med.nursing	A general forum for nursing
alt.npractitioners	Nurse practitioners
bit.listserv.snurse-l	Student nurses

Medical/Health-Related Usenet Newsgroups

alt.abuse.offender.recovery	Recovery for abuse offenders/ perpetrators
alt.abuse.recovery	Recovery from all types of abuse
alt.abuse.transcendence	Alternate models of dealing with abuse
alt.abuse-recovery	Moderated version of alt.sexual.abuse.recovery
alt.health	General health issues
alt.health.biofeedback	Biofeedback
alt.health.cfs	Chronic fatigue syndrome
alt.health.diabetes	Diabetes
alt.health.hmo	Health maintenance organizations
alt.health.oxygen-therapy	Oxygen therapy
alt.health.policy	Health policy
alt.infertility	Causes and treatments of infertility
alt.med.allergy	Allergy
alt.med.cfs	Chronic fatigue syndrome
alt.med.cure-paralysis	Paralysis
alt.med.ems	Emergency medical services (ambulance, fire)
alt.med.endometriosis	Endometriosis
alt.med.equipment	Durable medical equipment

alt.med.outpat	Outpatient services
alt.med.outpat.clinic	Outpatient clinic
alt.med.software	Medical software
alt.med.urum-outcomes	Utilization review/management outcomes
alt.psychology.help	General help with psychological problems
alt.psychology.personality	Personality taxonomies/assessment/ models
alt.recovery	General topics in recovery
alt.recovery.aa	Alcoholics anonymous
alt.recovery.addiction.alcoholism	Alcohol addiction
alt.recovery.addiction.gambling	Gambling addictions
alt.recovery.addiction.sexual	Recovering from sexual addictions
alt.recovery.codependency	Codependency
alt.recovery.compulsive-eat	Recovery from overeating
alt.recovery.nicotine	Recovery from nicotine addiction
alt.recovery.panic-anxiety.self-help	Self-help for anxiety panic attacks
alt.recovery.religion	Recovery from the effects of religion
alt.sexual.abuse.recovery	Recovery from sexual abuse
alt.support	Other support topics and questions not covered by existing groups
alt.support.addiction	Support for those with addictions
alt.support.abuse-partners	Partners of childhood sexual abuse survivors
alt.support.addisons	Addison's disease
alt.support.adoption.advocacy	Advocates of adoption
alt.support.agoraphobia	Agoraphobia support
alt.support.aids.partners	AIDS partner support
alt.support.alzheimers	Alzheimer's disease caretakers support
alt.support.amputee	Amputee support
alt.support.anxiety-panic	Anxiety and panic disorders
alt.support.arthritis	Arthritis
alt.support.asthma	Asthma
alt.support.ataxia	Ataxia support
alt.support.attn-deficit	Attention-deficit disorders
alt.support.bells-palsy	Bell's palsy
alt.support.big-folks	Fat acceptance with no dieting talk
alt.support.breastfeeding	Breast-feeding support
alt.support.breast-implant	Breast-implant support
alt.support.cancer	Cancer
alt.support.cerebral-palsy	Cerebral palsy
alt.support.chronic-pain	Chronic pain

alt.support.crohns-colitis	Crohn's disease and ulcerative colitis
alt.support.depression	Depression and mood disorders
alt.support.dev-delays	Developmental delay
alt.support.diabetes.kids	Parents and family of children with diabetes
alt.support.diet	Dieting/losing weight/nutrition
alt.support.diseases	Support for subjects not identified individually
alt.support.diseases.autoimmune	Autoimmune diseases (rheumatoid arthritis, lupus, multiple sclerosis)
alt.support.disorders.neurological	Neurological disorders
alt.support.dissociation	Persons with disassociative disorders (e.g., multiple personality disorder)
alt.support.divorce	Divorce/marital breakups
alt.support.domestic-violence	Domestic violence
alt.support.drug-abuse	Drug abuse
alt.support.food-allergies	Food allergies
alt.support.eating-disord	Eating disorders (e.g., anorexia, bulimia)
alt.support.epilepsy	Epilepsy
alt.support.glaucoma	Glaucoma
alt.support.grief	Grief and loss
alt.support.grief.suicide	Grief from suicide
alt.support.headaches.migraine	Migraine and headache ailments
alt.support.hearing-loss	Hearing loss
alt.support.heartburn	Heartburn and reflux
alt.support.heart-defects	Heart defects
alt.support.hemophilia	Hemophilia
alt.support.hepatitis-c	Hepatitis C
alt.support.herpes	Herpes
alt.support.hiatal-hernia	Hiatal hernia
alt.support.impotence	Impotence
alt.support.incest	Incest
alt.support.incontinence	Incontinence
alt.support.inter-cystitis	Intercystitis
alt.support.jaw-disorders	Temporomandibular joint (TMJ) and other jaw disorders
alt.support.kidney-disease	Kidney disease
alt.support.kidney-failure	Kidney failure
alt.support.leprosy	Leprosy
alt.support.loneliness	Loneliness
alt.support.lupus	Lupus
alt.support.marfan	Marfan's syndrome
alt.support.menopause	Menopause

alt.support.menopause.husbands	Support for significant others of menopausal women
alt.support.ms-recovery	Multiple sclerosis
alt.support.mult-sclerosis	Multiple sclerosis
alt.support.musc-dystrophy	Muscular dystrophy
alt.support.myasthe-gravis	Myasthenia gravis
alt.support.narcolepsy	Narcolepsy
alt.support.non-smokers	Effects of second-hand smoke
alt.support.obesity	Obesity
alt.support.ocd	Obsessive-compulsive disorder
alt.support.osteogenesis.imperfecta	Osteogenesis imperfecta
alt.support.ostomy	Ostomy
alt.support.parkinsons	Parkinson's disease
alt.support.post-polio	Post-polio support
alt.support.premature-baby	Premature baby
alt.support.prostate.prostatitis	Prostatitis
alt.support.psoriasis	Psoriasis
alt.support.pulmonary	Pulmonary support (chronic obstructive pulmonary disease, asthma)
alt.support.rape-survivors	Rape survivors
alt.support.schizophrenia	Schizophrenia
alt.support.scleroderma	Scleroderma
alt.support.short	Issues of interest to short people
alt.support.shyness	Shyness
alt.support.single-parents	Single parents
alt.support.sinusitis	Sinusitis
alt.support.skin-diseases	Skin diseases
alt.support.sleep-disorder	Sleep disorders
alt.support.spina-bifida	Spina bifida
alt.support.step-parents	Help being a step-parent
alt.support.stop-smoking	Stopping or quitting smoking
alt.support.stuttering	Stuttering & other speaking difficulties
alt.support.tall	Issues of interest to tall people
alt.support.thyroid	Thyroid disease
alt.support.tinnitus	Tinnitus/ringing ears/other head noises
alt.support.tourette	Tourette's syndrome
alt.support.trauma-ptsd	Post-traumatic stress disorder
alt.support.tuberculosis	Tuberculosis
alt.support.turner-syndrom	Turner syndrome
alt.support-heart	Cardiology
alt.transgendered	Transgendered, transsexual, intersexed persons

alt.sigma2.height	People far from average height
misc.education.medical	Medical education
misc.health.aids	General discussions about AIDS
misc.health.alternative	Alternative health
misc.health.arthritis	Arthritis
misc.health.diabetes	Diabetes, hypoglycemia
misc.health.infertility	Infertility
misc.kids.health	Children's health issues
sci.cognitive	Perception, memory, judgment, and reasoning
sci.med	Medicine and related products and regulations
sci.med.aids	Medical discussion of AIDS/HIV virus
sci.med.cardiology	Cardiology
sci.med.diseases.als	Amyotrophic lateral sclerosis
sci.med.diseases.cancer	Medical discussion of cancer
sci.med.diseases.hepatitis	Hepatitis
sci.med.diseases.lyme	Lyme disease
sci.med.diseases.osteoporosis	Osteoporosis
sci.med.immunology	Immunology
sci.med.informatics	Informatics
sci.med.midwifery	Midwifery
sci.med.nursing	A general forum for nursing
sci.med.nutrition	Nutrition and diet
sci.med.obgyn	Obstetrics and gynecology
sci.med.occupational	Occupational medicine and therapy
sci.med.orthopedics	Orthopedics
sci.med.pathology	Pathology
sci.med.pharmacy	Pharmacy
sci.med.physics	Physics
sci.med.prostate.bph	Benign prostatic hyperplasia
sci.med.prostate.cancer	Prostate cancer
sci.med.prostate.prostatitis	Prostatitis
sci.med.psychobiology	Psychiatry and psychobiology
sci.med.radiology	Radiology and imaging
sci.med.radiology.interventional	Interventional radiology
sci.med.telemedicine	Telemedicine and related applications
sci.med.transcription	Medical transcription issues
sci.med.vision	Vision, ophthalmology, eye care
sci.psychology	General psychology
sci.psychology.digest	Psychology electronic journal
sci.psychology.research	Research issues in psychology, moderated

Nursing-Related World Wide Web Sites

American Nurses Association

Website for and by the American Nurses Association, related entities, organizational affiliates, and Nursing Organization Liaison Forum (NOLF) groups. Includes information on the American Academy of Nursing, American Nurses Credentialing Center, American Nurses Foundation, State Nurses Association, and so forth. Also contains numerous nursing links, including informatics and technology. This includes the www.nursingworld.org.

CINAHL

A guide to nursing literature (subscription required). Includes information on selected Websites of interest to nursing and allied health professionals, researchers, and students. Sponsored by CINAHL Information Systems. www.cinahl.com

Galaxy Nursing Section

Select topics such as medical informatics and health occupations (leads to nursing research, nursing specialties, or nursing theories). www.galaxy.com

Health on the Net

Principles for evaluating healthcare-related information. Also provides a list of health-related conferences. www.hon.ch/HONcode/Conduct.html

HealthWeb—Nursing

Developed by librarians and information systems professionals to assist health professionals and consumers in meeting information needs. Subject areas include nursing, health informatics, telemedicine, and more. www.healthweb.org

InterNurse

Nursing resources, including the voice of Florence Nightingale. www.internurse.com

Lippincott's Nursing Center

This site offers free e-mail, interactive continuing education offerings, a search capability, as well as information on journals, books, and other Lippincott Williams & Wilkins products and services.
www.nursingcenter.com

Mosby's Medical Surfari

A collection of associations, journals, and lists of nursing sites. This is the list of bookmarks from their *Medical Surfari* publication. Sponsored by Mosby-Year Book, Inc.
www.acmec.org/surfari/nur.htm

NIGHTINGALE

Sponsored by the College of Nursing, University of Tennessee, USA.
nightingale.con.utk.edu:70/0/homepage.html

NURSE

Maintained by the School of Nursing, Warwick University, England.
www.csv.warwick.ac.uk:8000

NurseNet

Includes a Nursing Theory page with information on more than 20 theories used in nursing. Compiled by Judy Norris, PhD, RN.
www.ualberta.ca/~jrnorris/nursenet/nn.html

Nursing and Health Care Resources on the Net

A tremendous amount of information on nursing and health care around the globe. Developed and maintained by Rod Ward, RN.
www.shef.ac.uk/~nhcon/

Nursing-Informatics Net

A site that seeks to define and describe nursing, health, and medical informatics. There are links to nursing informatics, health and medical informatics organizations, nursing and health informatics journals, individuals involved in the development and delivery of nursing informatics, nursing, and health informatics courses, and so forth. It is maintained by Peter Murray, BA, RNG, RNT.
www.nursing-informatics.net

NursingNet

A list of nursing schools, journals, publications, and so forth related to nursing and medicine.
www.nursingnet.org

Nursing Network Forum

First full-forum service network for nurses providing a compendium of nursing resources. Includes on-line chat, nursing resources, nursing organizations, and other information. Maintained by Jo Ann Klein, MS, RN, C.
www.nursingnetwork.com

SpringNet

Resources for nurses and other healthcare professionals. Sponsored by Springhouse Corporation.
www.springnet.com

Susan K. Newbold's Home Page

A compilation of nursing informatics information including frequently asked questions, a list of nursing and healthcare informatics conferences, and a list of nursing informatics special interest groups around the world. Compiled and maintained by Susan K Newbold, MS, RN, C.
www.nursing.umaryland.edu/students/~snewbol/

University of Maryland, Baltimore School of Nursing

Website for the University of Maryland, Baltimore School of Nursing.
www.nursing.umaryland.edu

World Wide Nurse

A wealth of information on nursing associations, nursing jobs, nursing organizations, continuing education, and so forth. Includes the Top 10 Nursing Sites list. Maintained by Brian Short, RN.
www.wwnurse.com

Nursing Informatics Special Interest Groups

AUSTRALASIA

Australian Nursing Informatics Council (ANIC)
hisa@hisa.org.au
www.hisavic.aus.net/

NURSINFO (Hong Kong)
Helen Sit Wing-Fun, sithwf@ha.org.hk

Nursing Informatics New Zealand (NINZ)
exec@ninz.gen.nz

CANADA

Canadian Health Informatics Association (COACH) Nursing Informatics
Special Interest Group
www.nursingsig.coachorg.com/

Nova Scotia Nursing Informatics Group
Nancy McCara, itnem@ge2-hsc.ns.ca

Ontario Nursing Informatics Group (ONIG)
www.onig.on.ca/

ONIG, Ottawa Chapter, Nursing Computers Application Network (NCAN)
www.ncan.on.ca/

ONIG, Southern Ontario Chapter
Shirley Scott, sscott@westpark.org

EUROPE

European Federation for Medical Informatics (EMFI) Working Group Five
(WG5), Nursing Informatics in Europe
www.novasys.ch/NIEurope/index.htm

United Kingdom

British Computer Society Nursing Specialist Group
www.man.ac.uk/bcsnsg

Health Informatics in Education at the Open University (HIE-OU)
Laurence Alpay l.l.alpay@open.ac.uk
Peter Murray p.j.murray@open.ac.uk

Germany

Nursing Informatics Special Interest Group of the Deutsche Gesellschaft
fuer Medizinische Informatik, Biometrie und Epidemiologie (GMDS)
http://www.med.uni-muenchen.de/gmds/gmds.html

Spain

Spanish Society of Nursing and Internet
seei@enfe.ua.es
www.seei.es/

Switzerland

Swiss Special Interest Group Nursing Informatics (SIG-NI)
Patrick Van Gele, pvangele@chuv.hospvd.ch

SOUTH AMERICA

Brazilian Nursing Association Nursing Informatics Group at Brazilian
Nursing Association (GEINE), Sao Paulo
Heimar F. Marin, heimar@denf.epm.br
Christine Cunha, icris@denf.epm.br

Nursing Informatics Center, Federal University of Sao Paulo, Brazil
Heimar F. Marin, heimar@denf.epm.br

UNITED STATES OF AMERICA

National

American Academy of Ambulatory Care Nursing (AAACN) Informatics
Special Interest Group
www.aaacn.inurse.com

American Medical Informatics Association (AMIA) Nursing Informatics
Working Group
mail@amia2.amia.org
www.amia-niwg.org/

American Nurses Association (ANA) Council on Nursing Services and
Informatics
www.nursingworld.org/councils.htm

Health Information and Management Systems Society (HIMSS) Clinical
Systems Special Interest Group
www.himss.org

National League for Nursing (NLN) Council on Nursing Informatics (CNI)
nlninform@nln.org
www.nln.org/info-councils-executive.htm#cni

Regional/Local Groups

American Nursing Informatics Association (ANIA), Southern California
www.ania.org

Boston Area Nursing Informatics Consortium (BANIC)
Debra Furlong, Chair, DJFurlong@aol.com

Capital Area Roundtable on Informatics in NursinG (CARING),
Washington, DC Area
www.nursing.umaryland.edu/students~snewbol/caring.htm

Connecticut Healthcare Informatics Network (CHIN)
www.vm.uconn.edu/~spl95001/chin.html

Delaware Valley Nursing Computer Network (DVNCN)
James Cannon, cannon2@aol.com

Florida Nurses Association Computer Applications (CAP) Focus Group
Jackie Skeith, skeithj@allkids.org

Healthcare Informatics of New Jersey (HINJ)
Brenda Gazinski, 908-828-3000, ×2125

Informatics Nurses From Ohio (INFO)
www.junior.apk.net/~lqthede/INFO.htm

Maryland Society for Healthcare Information Systems Management (MSHISM)
www.mshism.org/

Michigan Nursing Informatics Network (MNIN)
www.spyglasshill.com/ni/ni.htm

Midwest Alliance for Nursing Informatics (MANI) (Illinois)
www.maninet.org/

Midwest Nursing Research Society (MNRS) Nursing Informatics Research Section
info@mrns.org
www.mnrs.org/

MInnesota Nursing INformatics Group (MINING)
Martha Bergren, bergren@usinternet.com

New Jersey State Nurses Association (NJSNA) Computer Forum on Nursing Informatics
njsna@nsna.org
www.NJSNA@NJSNA.org/

Nursing Informatics Council (Kansas City Metropolitan Area)
Charlotte Gray, grayck@trumed1.trumanmed.org

Nursing Information Systems Council of New England (NISCNE)
www.niscne.org/

North Carolina State Nurses Association Council on Nursing Informatics (CONI)
Sally Kellum, kellu001@mc.duke.edu

Puget Sound Nursing Informatics Group
Debbie Kelly, debk@olypen.com

South West Michigan Informatics
www.spyglasshill.com/ni/ni.htm

Texas Nursing and Healthcare Informatics Association (Dallas/Fort Worth)
www.inc.com/users/tnhia.html

Tri-State Nursing Computer Network (TNCN) (Pennsylvania, Ohio, West Virginia)
www.homepage.third-wave.com/tncn/

Utah Nursing Informatics Network (UNIN)
Laura Heerman, ldlheerm@ihc.com

Wisconsin Computers in Nursing (WICAN)
Judy Murphy, judy.murphy@aurora.org

INTERNATIONAL

International Medical Informatics Association (IMIA) Special Interest
 Group on Nursing Informatics (SIGNI)
Evelyn Hovenga, Australia, Chair, e.hovenga@cqu.edu.au
Ulla Gerdin Jelger, Sweden, Past Chair, ulla.gerdin@hsn.sll.se
Heather Strachan, UK, Secretary
Virginia Saba, Chair-Elect, USA, sabav@gunet.georgetown.edu
Patricia Abbott, USA, pabbott@umaryland.edu
Robyn Carr, New Zealand, robyn@ahsl.co.nz
Helene Clement, Canada, grasp@ix.netcom.com
Margareta Ehnfors, Sweden, margareta.ehnfors@hoe.se
Anneli Ensio, Finland
Majda Fajdetic, Croatia
William Goossen, the Netherlands, W.T.F.Goossen@al.nhl.nl
Jean-Daniel Henchoz, Switzerland
Hugo Leonzio, Argentina
Tekauc Lucia Dipl Orig, Slovenia
Heimar F Marin, Brazil, heimar.denf@epm.br
Iona Moisil, Romania
Rosaleen Murnane, Ireland
Peter Murray, UK, p.j.murray@open.ac.uk
Hyeoun-Ae Park, Korea, hapark@plaza.snu.ac.kr
Rana Pongruengphant, Thailand
K. Premarini, Singapore
Brigitte Schultz, Germany, 101333.576@compuserve.com
Ammann Sigrid, Austria
Lise Therkelsen, Denmark, dsr_lt@dansk-sygeplejeraad.dk
Ingibjorg Thorhallsdottir, Iceland, runark@mmedia.is
Manuel Perez Vallina, Spain
Guy Vanden Boer, Belgium
Estelle Vivier, Republic of South Africa
Helen Sit Wing-Fun, Hong Kong, sithwf@ha.org.hk

L. Zwanger, Israel
Margarete Lorentsen, Norway, margarete.lorentsen@sykepleievit.uio.no

www.infocom.cqu.edu.au/imia-ni/

Nursing-Related Electronic Mailing Lists

An e-mail discussion group (also known as a listserv group) is a type of electronic mailing list (EML) that is a subscription service. Messages are sent to a common address and then redirected to all subscribers of the list. This service provides special interest groups an area to discuss and support their areas of interest. Once you subscribe, mail will come to you automatically.

E-mail lists are managed by computer host machine programs called mailing list managers. Examples are listserver, mailbase, majordomo, martlist, listprocessor, almanac, and TULP.

There are two addresses for a mailing list: the list manager address for subscribing and unsubscribing (e.g., listserv@internetaddress) and the mail list manager (the name of the list, e.g., NursingNetwork@internetaddress) for posting messages to the list. It is important to use the correct mailing address.

To subscribe to any mailing list, send a message to the administrative address (LISTSERV@place.where.list.lives) with the following line, and nothing else, in the *body* (not in the subject line) of the message:
    SUB LISTNAME   Yourfirstname   Yourlastname
(substituting in the appropriate values, of course). The list name is the part before the @ sign in the list address. To unsubscribe from any LISTSERV list, send a message to the administrative address with the following line, and nothing else, in the body of the message:
    UNSUB LISTNAME

Most e-mail group lists offer archives of messages organized in files by day, month, or subject. This differs from group to group, and directions for accessing these features are available to users at the time they subscribe to the e-mail group.

Make sure to save the e-mail group list instructions in case you want to unsubscribe from the list or stop mail while you are away. Remember that belonging to a list can result in hundreds of e-mail messages a day based on the activity of that particular list.

The material that follows has been excerpted from the promotional materials and welcome messages distributed by the list owners.

CAREPL-L

CAREPL-L is a list dedicated to the storage and retrieval of nursing care plans. Anyone can submit a care plan for review. After the care plan is approved it will be posted to the list and archived on a monthly basis. The archives are open to retrieval and database searches via LISTSERV database commands by the public. Only care plans will be posted to the list. Discussions about care plans that are archived must take place in another forum such as SNURSE-L. The list uses LISTSERV software.

Administrative address: listserv@ubvm.cc.buffalo.edu
List address: carepl-l@ubvm.cc.buffalo.edu
List owner: Tim Brackett, brackett@essex.hsc.colorado.edu

To submit a care plan, send a copy to CAREPL-L@UBVM.CC.BUFFALO. EDU. Your care plan will be forwarded to the editors of the list for review. It will then be posted to the list.

EM-NSG-L

EM-NSG-L is an information list for emergency nurses. At the time of this writing, there were over 500 members of EM-NSG-L from 16 countries.

Administrative address: listserv@itssrvl.ucsf.edu
List address: Em-Nsg-L@ITSSRV1.UCSF.EDU
List owner: Tom Trimble, RN, Em-Nsg-L-request@itssrvl.ucsf.edu or
    Tom@ENW.org

ER-NURSING

ER-NURSING is a list for news, views, and experiences of hospital Emergency Department nurses. To get more information, mail the command "info ER-NURSING" (without the quotes) to ER-NURSING-info@topica.com. It is an unmoderated list created in March 1999. You must subscribe to Topica at http://www.topica.com/ in order to subscribe to this ER-NURSING list.

GLOBALRN

GLOBALRN (formerly CULTURE-AND-NURSING) is a list for nurses and other healthcare professionals interested in or working in the field of cross-cultural and transcultural nursing and health care. The list allows members to discuss issues of cultural competence, theory, practice, research, and experience in an open and unmoderated forum. As of this writing, there are over 875 members on the list. Recent topics have included the use of interpreters in clinical practice, teaching culturally competent care, and education aides and resources. This list uses the LISTSERV mailing list manager.

Administrative address: listserv@itssrvl.ucsf.edu
List address: globalrn@itssrvl.ucsf.edu
List manager: Chuck Pitkofsky, MS, RN, UCSF School of Nursing, chuckp@itsa.ucsf.edu

To subscribe to GLOBALRN, send the following command in the *body* of the mail message (leave the subject header blank) to the administrative address:
    subscribe GLOBALRN
Please take note that the character after "itssrv" is the number one (1), not the letter "L." Although majordomo is similar to the LISTSERV and list-proc programs, there are a few differences. To receive the command list, send a message containing the single word "help" (without the quotes) to the administrative address.

IVTHERAPY-L

The IVTHERAPY-L list is for communication and mutual support of intravenous therapy nurses and other interested professionals. It uses LISTSERV software.

Administrative address: listserv@netcom.com
List address: ivtherapy-l@netcom.com
List owner, Sarah Kuykendall, RN, BS, Oregon Health Sciences University, sarahk@netcom.com

MIDWIFE

MIDWIFE is a list for discussion of midwifery issues. It is a semiautomated list, administered by Denis Anthony (D.M.Anthony@bham.ac.uk).

Administrative address: midwife-request@csv.warwick.ac.uk
List address: midwife@csv.warwick.ac.uk
List owner: Denis Anthony, D.M.Anthony@bham.ac.uk

To subscribe to the list send a message to the administrative address, asking to be added to the list. Please include your e-mail address and your name in the body of the message. The membership list for MIDWIFE is publicly available, and subscriptions from people who wish to remain anonymous are not accepted. Posts to the list are archived on the NURSE WWW/Gopher service under the heading Midwife List Archives.

NRSING-L

NRSING-L is a list primarily for the discussion of nursing informatics topics. Any and all topics relating to nursing are, however, welcomed. It uses the LISTSERV mailing list manager.

Administrative address: listserv@library.ummed.edu
List address: nrsing-l@lists.umass.edu
List owner: Gordon Larrivee, MS, RN, larrivee@umassmed.ummed.edu

To subscribe to NRSING-L, send a message to the administrative address with a blank subject line and the single line:
    sub nrsing-l   Yourfirstname   Yourlastname
in the body of the message.

NRSINGED

NRSINGED provides a forum for the discussion of topics and issues in nursing education. Discussion is meant to be wide-ranging—from teaching methodologies to philosophical issues—in order to meet the diverse needs of nurse educators. It uses the LISTSERV mailing list manager.

Administrative address: listserv@ulkyvm.louisville.edu
List address: nrsinged@ulkyvm.louisville.edu

The list is not "moderated," but you must be subscribed to the list before LISTSERV will let you post to it.

NURCENS

NURCENS is a forum for issues related to nurse management centers. It does not have many subscribers, nor is active as of this writing.

Administrative address: listserv@gibbs.oit.unc.edu
List address: nurcens@gibbs.oit.unc.edu
List owner: Dr. P. Allen Gray, gray@vxc.ocis.uncwil.edu

NURSENET

NURSENET is an international conference for discourse about diverse nursing issues in the areas of nursing administration, nursing education, nursing practice, and nursing research. It is open and unmoderated and uses the LISTSERV mailing list manager.

Administrative address: listserv@vm.utcc.utoronto.ca
List address: nursenet@vm.utcc.utoronto.ca
List owner: Dr. Judy Norris, Judy.Norris@ualberta.ca

As of this writing, NURSENET is the largest and the most prolific of the nursing lists. List volume can top 50 messages a day, so if you are new to e-mail, be sure you know whether you will be incurring per-message charges with your service provider before you subscribe. The NURSENET archives are available from the University of Toronto gopher and can be viewed and retrieved from that site (gopher.vm.utcc.utotonto.ca).

NURSERES

As mentioned in the text, NURSERES focuses on nursing research and nursing practice. The list underwent a merger with the list GRADNRSE, a list devoted to nursing practice issues, and that list no longer exists. NURSERES uses the LISTSERV software.

Administrative address: listserv@kentvm.kent.edu
List address: nurseres@kentvm.kent.edu
List owner: Linda Q. Thede, RN, lthede@kentvm.kent.edu

NURSE-UK

NURSE-UK is a list for discussion of nursing issues in the United Kingdom. It is a semiautomated list administered by Denis Anthony (D.M.Anthony@bham.ac.uk).

Administrative address: nurse-uk-request@csv.warwick.ac.uk
List address: nurse-uk@csv.warwick.ac.uk
List owner: Dr. Denis Anthony, D.M.Anthony@bham.ac.uk

To subscribe to the list send a message to the administrative address, asking to be added to the list. Please include your e-mail address and your name in the body of the message. The membership list for NURSE-UK is publicly available; subscriptions from people who wish to remain anonymous are not accepted. Posts to the list are archived on the NURSE WWW/ Gopher service under the heading NURSE-UK Archives.

NURSINGNETWORK

NURSINGNETWORK is solely for the dissemination of nursing and healthcare resources such as conferences, jobs, educational resources, clinical resources, healthcare policy, and headlines in the news. A key feature of the mailing list is a daily newsletter of healthcare headlines in the news.

Administrative address: majordomo@majordomo.net
List address: nursingnetwork@majordomo.net
List owner: Jo Ann Klein, MS, RN, C (jklein@nursingnetwork.com)

To subscribe to the list send a message to the administrative address. Leave the subject line of the e-mail message blank. The body of the message should be totally empty except for the words: subscribe nursingnetwork. The membership list for NURSINGNETWORK is not publicly available; submissions from nonmembers to the list are not accepted.

ORNURSESDOWNUNDER

ORNURSESDOWNUNDER was created in April 1999 for Australian operating theatre nurses to discuss all aspects of their work in the operating room. See http://www.angelfire.com/nd/ornursesdownunder/. You must first subscribe to Onelist™, a free mailing list service.

PSYCHIATRIC-NURSING

PSYCHIATRIC-NURSING is a list that is part of InterPsych, an international multidisciplinary organization of people interested in mental heath issues. It uses the mailbase mailing list manager.

Administrative address: mailbase@mailbase.ac.uk
List address: psychiatric-nursing@mailbase.ac.uk

To subscribe, send a message to the administrative address with the following in the body:
   join psychiatric-nursing firstname lastname
   stop

RURAL-NURSING

RURAL-NURSING allows for information exchange about nursing in rural areas. To receive more information, mail the word "help" in the subject line to the administrative address.

Administrative address: rural-nursing@texastown.com
List owner: richard@texastown.com

SCHLRN-L

SCHLRN-L, the School Nurse Network, is a forum for school nurses, school nurse practitioners, school nurse teachers, and school nurse managers. The list encourages networking; helps spread information about research and technological advances, educational and funding opportunities, advanced practice, and professional organizations; and supports those nurses working in isolated educational settings. It uses the LISTSERV software.

Administrative address: listserv@ubvm.cc.buffalo.edu
List address: schlrn-l@ubvm.cc.buffalo.edu
List owner: Martha Dewey Bergren, RN, bergren@usinternet.com

SNURSE-L

SNURSE-L is a global electronic forum for nursing students. This list is open to anyone who would like to join. The topics include nursing issues, student issues, electronic databases and libraries useful to nursing students, and National Student Nursing Association issues and events. It uses the LISTSERV software.

Administrative address: listserv@ubvm.cc.buffalo.edu
List address: snurse-l@ubvm.cc.buffalo.edu
List owner: Tim Brackett, brackett@essex.hsc.colorado.edu

WEB-NSG-L

According to the www site (www.enw.org/Web-Nsg-L.htm), WEB-NSG-L is for nurses who are Web and Internet content providers, website writers, managers, administrators, and/or educators who use the Internet and computing technology to communicate, teach, test, or to interact with patients and families. It uses the LISTSERV software. As of this writing, there are nearly 200 subscribers.

Administrative address: listserv@itssrvl.ucsf.edu
List address: web-nsg-l@itssrvl.ucsf.edu
List owner: Tom Trimble, RN, Web-Nsg-L-Request@ITSSRVl.UCSF.EDU
    or Tom@ENW.org

Appendix B
Healthcare Websites

Jo Ann Klein

The value of the Internet, as a network of networks, is its rich resources. Before the development of the World Wide Web (Web), Internet users were required to go through a hierarchy of databases to find a single resource. This methodology, referred to as "gopher," virtually tunneled through layers within multiple networks resulting in timely searches for a minimal amount of information.

When hypertext markup language (HTML) was developed, it enabled users to "jump" from resource to resource in a seamless manner by direct linkages between these resources and a single document. This development was critical in the evolution of the Internet from a purely educational and scientific tool to an instrument for commercial marketing of goods and services. This is particularly true as the Web advanced from an all-text format to a multimedia graphical user interface.

Today, the Web community consists of more than 50,000,000 domain names, domain names being equivalent to home addresses in cyberspace. With so many resources, the concept of portals has emerged. A portal refers to a single domain where multiple resources, goods, and services pertaining to a single theme can be found. Examples are medical portals, book portals, toy portals, auction portals, even search engine portals. Most portals contain search tools that enable users to explore within that particular community for resources. They may also feature bulletin boards and chat rooms for interactive communication between its users. They are generally rich in content revolving around the portal theme.

As more and more portals emerge, single websites will be more difficult to access. This concept can be compared with the super pharmacy stores, baby stores, and hardware stores. In today's busy world, consumers are generally more interested in finding what they want in one place rather than spending time and resources to go from one small store to another, even if the smaller store has a higher quality product.

As previously mentioned, the healthcare arena, in its attempt to keep pace with the general public, has joined the portal frenzy. Mergers with cable and television media organizations have provided the income necessary to fund the procurement of high-level content and services. Although many of these portals may be popular today, it is likely that they will be bought and merged into other large portals if the trend continues.

The challenge for the Internet user is to find websites that project stability within the dynamic environment of the Internet. Among all the healthcare content sites on the Internet, government sites are the most reliable, unless, of course, there is a change in departments with new administrations.

The following websites are provided as recommended supersites for information of interest. It should be noted that the author has no affiliation with the suggested websites except where otherwise noted and recommends these sites based on the quality and quantity of content pertaining to the defined mission and purpose of each site.

General

Allied Health. Pharmacy, Durable Medical Equipment, Physical Therapy, Occupational Therapy, and Speech Therapy Services.
www.alliedhealth.org

DoseCalc OnLine. Fully-referenced database with over 120 standard chemotherapeutic regimens and an online dosage calculator for oncology professionals. Enter a patient's height and weight, and the software calculates the individual drug dosages for the chemotherapeutic protocol you select.
www.meds.com/DChome.html

Hospice Hands. Comprehensive information on palliative care for healthcare professionals and consumers.
http://hospice-cares.com/hands/hands.html

Occupational/Physical Therapy Internet Directory. Rich resource for links related to occupational therapy, physical therapy, and athletic training.
www.slackinc.com/otpt/otptnet.htm

PharmLinks. A division of *Infonet: Pharmacy Information Network* loaded with links to biotechnology resources, drug information resources, drug research, development and regulatory resources, general medical resources, general pharmaceutical resources, government resources, pharmacy and pharmaceutical associations, pharmacy schools and pharmacy education resources, and pharmaceutical companies on the Internet.
http://pharminfo.com/phrmlink.html

RxList: The Internet Drug Index. Comprehensive resource for healthcare professionals with a private area for consumer education regarding pharmaceuticals.
www.rxlist.com/

Clinical Resources

ACP Home Care Guide for Advanced Cancer. A fully downloadable guide to caring for patients in advanced stages of cancer in the home environment. Topics include care giving, pain control, shortness of breath, communication difficulties, clinical expectations, respite care, dealing with the actual death, coping with death and funerals, and grieving.
www.acponline.org/public/h_care/contents.htm

AIDS—The Body: An AIDS and HIV Resource. Comprehensive site for AIDS/HIV information including more than 30,000 documents and clinical trial information.
www.thebody.com/index.shtml

Alternative and Complementary Medicine. A division of the National Institutes of Health, this Center conducts and supports basic and applied research and training and disseminates information on complementary and alternative medicine to practitioners and the public.
http://altmed.od.nih.gov/

American Academy of Family Physicians. Extensive patient information resource for medical conditions and general healthcare information by body systems.
http://familydoctor.org/

Band-Aids and Blackboards. Tips for doctors, nurses, and teachers in helping children with chronic illness in their activities of daily living.
http://funrsc.fairfield.edu/~jfleitas/contents.html

CancerNet. From the National Institutes of Health, this site offers cancer information for the consumer, health professional, and basic researcher with details about ongoing trials, fact sheets, publications, and a searchable database.
www.cic.nci.nih.gov/

Elder Care Online. Comprehensive consumer site for healthcare resource information for seniors and caregivers of seniors.
www.ec-online.net/

Galaxy's Medical Resources. One of the original sites on the Internet for comprehensive healthcare resource information.
http://galaxy.einet.net/galaxy/Medicine.html

Global Reproductive Health Forum. Bilingual Spanish and English, site that provides women around the world with access to critical information about their health and bodies, in addition to serving as an electronic space where women can come together and voice their opinions in the global debate around reproductive health and rights.
www.hsph.harvard.edu/Organizations/healthnet/

Medical Matrix. Guide to Internet clinical medical resources.
www.medmatrix.org/index.asp

Mental Health Net. Guide to mental health, psychology, and psychiatry on-line.
http://mentalhelp.net/

PedInfo: A Pediatrics Webserver. Indexes pediatric clinical information and resources.
www.pedinfo.org/

Reuter's Health Information Services. Medical news and health information for the professional and consumer.
www.reutershealth.com/

Travel Information Page (CDC). A division of the Centers for Disease Control and Prevention, this site is rich in up-to-date information regarding vaccinations, disease outbreaks, health prevention, and recommendations when traveling outside of the United States.
www.cdc.gov/travel/travel.html

Virtual Medical Center. The site contains over 56,000 multimedia teaching files, 1,475 multimedia tutorials, and 3,550 databases.
www-sci.lib.uci.edu/HSG/Medical.html

Visible Human Project. National Library of Medicine project aimed at producing a system of knowledge structures that will transparently link visual knowledge forms to symbolic knowledge formats such as the names of body parts.
www.nlm.nih.gov/research/visible/visible_human.html

WellnessWeb—The Patient's Network. Excellent resource for clinical information pertaining to conventional medicine, alternative and complementary medicine, nutrition and fitness, and late-breaking medical research. A master alphabetized index of hundreds of topics enables users to easily find a topic of interest.
http://wellweb.com/

Databases, Search Engines, and Reference Resources

Achoo Online Health Care Services. One of the original medical Web portals with comprehensive links to journals, publications, employment opportunities, databases, human health and disease information, organizations, education, and news.
www.achoo.com/

All-in-One Search Page. Over 500 of the Internet's best search engines, databases, indexes, and directories in a single site.
www.allonesearch.com/

Ask Jeeves. Provides Internet database searches by inputting a question into a search engine.
www.askjeeves.com/

CINAHL—Cumulative Index of Nursing and Allied Health Database. Premier database for nursing and allied health for journals and book references within previous five year period. Fee for service.
www.cinahl.com/

Dictionaries Online. Linked to more than 800 dictionaries in 150 different languages. This conveniently organized index includes glossaries of specialized terminology, synonyms, homonyms, and abbreviations with links to an index of on-line grammar pages and several pages of linguistic fun.
www.facstaff.bucknell.edu/rbeard/diction.html

Hardin Meta Directory—Telemedicine. List of telemedicine website links.
www.lib.uiowa.edu/hardin/md/telemed.html

Health A to Z. Search engine for health and medicine with over 50,000 professionally reviewed health and medical Internet resources.
www.healthatoz.com/

Healthfinder^{TM}. Federally funded gateway consumer health and human services information website.
www.healthfinder.gov/

Health on the Net Foundation. An international initiative, Health On the Net Foundation (HON) is a nonprofit organization, headquartered in Geneva, Switzerland. The Foundation is dedicated to realizing the benefits of the Internet and related technologies in the fields of medicine and healthcare. The purpose of the Foundation is to advance the development and application of new information technologies, notably in the fields of health and medicine.
www.hon.ch/

The List^{TM}. Guide to Internet Service Providers—those companies that provide access to the Internet. The List^{TM} allows you to find a provider that offers the access speed and computing services that satisfy your needs and budget. Click one of the search options to use the most comprehensive and accurate directory of Internet service providers.
http://thelist.internet.com/

Liszt—Mailing List Search Engine. Premier site for locating more than 90,000 e-mail groups on the Internet.
www.liszt.com/

MedExplorer. Search engine for healthcare and medicine information.
www.medexplorer.com/

MediDex. Indexed directory of more than 22,000 healthcare providers and medical organizations.
www.medimatch.com/web/mdex/index.htm

Medline Plus. A division of the National Library of Medicine, this site exposes health care professionals and consumers to a carefully selected list of healthcare resources, including MEDLINE database, dictionaries, publications, news, organizations, clearinghouses, and other search engines.
http://medlineplus.nlm.nih.gov/medlineplus/

MedWeb. Search engine for comprehensive list of medical resources on the Internet.
www.medweb.emory.edu/MedWeb/

Mind-It. Allows users to track changes to their favorite Web pages. They can highlight sections of a page to track, watch for the appearance of any keywords of interest, and track links to a page *for free* and be notified when there are changes. It is like having a research assistant track any topic and send an alert as soon as it changes.
www.netmind.com/html/individual.html

Publist.com. Comprehensive directory of information about more than 150,000 publications and more than 8,000 newspapers around the world. It is easy to use, and it is free. PubList.comSM information comes from definitive sources such as Ulrich's™ International Periodicals Directory.
www.publist.com/

Surgical, Medical, and New Terms Glossary. Medical transcription and terminology site offers weekly updates of new medical and surgical terms, medical dictionary, A to Z index of new terminology, word lists, sample operative reports, links to the best medical information on the Web by topic, public forums, free classified ads, and live chat.
www.mtdesk.com/swg.shtml

U.S. Postal Service ZIP + 4 Code Lookup. Feature of the U.S. Postal Service to easily search for ZIP codes by address.
www.usps.gov/ncsc/lookups/lookup_zip+4.html

Virtual Medical Center. The site contains over 56,000 multimedia teaching files, 1,475 multimedia tutorials, and 3,550 databases.
www-sci.lib.uci.edu/HSG/Medical.html

WhoWhere. Locates people by e-mail, phone numbers, addresses, personal home pages, organizations, and employers.
www.whowhere.lycos.com/

ZDNet Software Library. Much freeware and shareware located by search engine.
www.zdnet.com/swlib/

Electronic Journals

Medical Journals. Comprehensive list of links to general and specialty medical journals. In addition to journals, this site is rich in reference resources.
http://www.sciencekomm.at/journals/medicine/med-bio.html

Nursing Journals. Comprehensive list of links to general and specialty nursing journals. In addition to journals, this site is rich in reference resources.
www.sciencekomm.at/journals/medicine/nurse.html

Pharmacy and Toxicology Journals. Comprehensive list of links to general and specialty pharmacy and toxicology journals. In addition to journals, this site is rich in reference resources.
www.sciencekomm.at/journals/medicine/toxic.html

PLE. Over 3,500 links to medical, psychiatric, dental, and veterinary journals.
www.priory.com/

Government Services, Regulatory Agencies, and Funding Resources

AHCPR Guidelines. U.S. government agency for healthcare policy and research. This agency has created guidelines for clinical practice by medical condition, which are available through this website.
www.ahcpr.gov/

Centers for Disease Control and Prevention. With its mission to promote health and quality of life by preventing and controlling disease, injury, and disability, this site is a supersite to 11 U.S. government centers, institutes, and offices. The site includes data and statistics, on-line publications, funding opportunities, and a special section devoted to travelers' health.
www.cdc.gov/

Department of Health and Human Services
http://phs.os.dhhs.gov/

FedStats. More than 70 agencies in the U.S. federal government produce statistics of interest to the public. The Federal Interagency Council on Statistical Policy maintains this site to provide easy access to the full range of statistics and information produced by these agencies for public use.
www.fedstats.gov/

Health Care Financing Administration. (U.S. Department of Health and Human Services). Federal agency that administers Medicare, Medicaid, and

Child Health insurance programs. This site serves beneficiaries, plans, providers, states, and researchers. It also contains legislative and regulatory information related to these programs.
www.hcfa.gov/

HCUPnet. Family of administrative, longitudinal databases, Web-based products, and software tools developed and maintained by the Agency for Health Care Policy and Research (AHCPR) as part of a federal–state–industry partnership to build a standardized, multistate health data system. This tool assists in identifying, tracking, analyzing, and comparing statistics on hospitals at the national level.
www.ahcpr.gov/data/hcup/hcupnet.htm

Joint Commission on Accreditation of Healthcare Organizations (JCAHO). Aimed at improving the quality of health care, this private organization is responsible for developing many of the standards and outcomes measures for healthcare institutions and services.
www.jcaho.org/

Medicare/Medicaid Manuals. HIM 11 and other manuals can be downloaded for viewing.
www.hcfa.gov/pubforms/p2192toc.htm

National Association of Insurance Commissioners. Organization of insurance regulators from 50 states and the District of Columbia. Provides a forum for the development of uniform policy where uniformity is appropriate.
www.naic.org/

National Committee for Quality Assurance (NCQA). Private, not-for-profit organization dedicated to assessing and reporting on the quality of managed care plans. Its mission is to provide information that enables purchasers and consumers of managed health care to distinguish among plans based on quality, thereby allowing them to make more informed healthcare purchasing decisions.
www.ncqa.org/Pages/Main/index.htm

National Guideline Clearinghouse^TM. Public resource for evidence-based clinical practice guidelines. It is sponsored by the Agency for Health Care Policy and Research in partnership with the American Medical Association and the American Association of Health Plans.
www.guideline.gov/index.asp

National Health Law Program. Comprehensive site addressing the legal aspects of health care from advocacy to Medicare and Medicaid.
www.healthlaw.org/

National Institute of Nursing Research (NINR). Part of the National Institutes of Health network, the NINR supports clinical and basic research to

establish a scientific basis for the care of individuals across the lifespan—from management of patients during illness and recovery to the reduction of risks for disease and disability and the promotion of healthy lifestyles.
www.nih.gov/ninr/

National Institute of Standards and Technology (NIST). Research center for the U.S. government designed to work with industry to develop and apply technology, measurements, and standards.
www.nist.gov/

National Library of Medicine. Rich federal resource for consumer and professional health information, including grant information, research, and MEDLINE*plus* with its medical dictionaries, search databases for articles and information, clearinghouse of healthcare literature, directories for finding physicians and hospitals, MEDLINE search engine for journal article abstracts, healthcare organization information, publications and news for reading on-line, and libraries for health consumers.
www.nlm.nih.gov/

Occupational Safety and Health Administration. OSHA's mission is to save lives, prevent injuries, and protect the health of America's workers. This site houses the regulations and standards of the organization.
www.osha.gov/about.html

Robert Woods Johnson Foundation. Resource for health care and resources grant information.
www.rwjf.org/grant/jgrant.htm

US Congress on the Internet. Excellent resource for detailed information about U.S. legislation that can be accessed via a site search engine. Also known as Thomas.
http://thomas.loc.gov/

U.S. Surgeon General's Fact Sheets. These fact sheets present report findings in population-specific format with key messages, physical activity facts and benefits, and suggestions for communities.
www.cdc.gov/nccdphp/sgr/fact.htm

Healthcare Conferences

Medical Conferences and Meetings—Doctor's Guide to the Internet.
www.pslgroup.com/MEDCONF.HTM

Nursing Informatics and Health Care Informatics Conferences. Includes dates, sponsor, subject, and contact information.
http://nursing.umaryland.edu/students/~snewbol/sknconf.htm

SearchCME Medical Conferences. Find information on over 5,000 medical conferences throughout the world.
www.searchcme.com/

Yahoo Search Engine Medical Conferences. Alphabetized with links to complete conference information.
http://dir.yahoo.com/Health/Medicine/Conferences/

Yahoo Search Engine Nursing Conferences. Alphabetized with links to complete conference information.
www.yahoo.co.uk/Health/Nursing/Conferences/

Healthcare Education

CE Connection. Continuing education for nurses, nurse practitioners, nursing managers, and other healthcare providers. Results are instantly processed on-line and certificates are e-mailed to the participant.
www.springnet.com/ce.htm

ceWeb. Accredited as a provider of continuing education in nursing by the American Nurses Credentialing Center's Commission on Accreditation. ANCC accreditation is recognized by most states. Nurses can register through a rapid on-line process, take electronic tests over the Internet, and receive feedback and contact hours immediately.
www.ce-web.com/

Professional Education Center. On-line continuing education programs for healthcare professionals.
http://secure.imconline.net/pec/index.htm

Virtual Medical Center. The site contains over 56,000 multimedia teaching files, 1,475, multimedia tutorials, and 3,550 databases.
www-sci.lib.uci.edu/HSG/Medical.html

Healthcare Employment

Career Path. Over 300,000 employment listings from the nation's top newspapers.
http://new.careerpath.com/

Job Search Assistance. Large listing of links to nursing and general job sites.
www.langara.bc.ca/vnc/jobs.htm

MediMatch. The "managing your career" area features resume submission, classified ads, career fairs, and e-mail notification of matching jobs.
www.medimatch.com/pros/

Monster.com Healthcare Zone. One of the largest career centers on the Internet.
www.medsearch.com/

Healthcare Informatics

American Health Information Management Association (AHIMA). Website serves more than 38,000 specially educated health information management professionals who work within the healthcare industry. The site includes consumer advice, career and education opportunities, and continuing education.
www.ahima.org/

American Medical Informatics Association (AMIA). Site provides conference, education, publication, membership, and employment information.
www.amia.org

Center for Healthcare Information Management (CHIM). Trade association for vendors and consultants in the healthcare information technology industry.
www.chim.org/

Center for Healthcare Information Management Executives (CHIME). Provides job postings in healthcare information systems, reference documents, healthcare information systems database, courses in healthcare information technology architectures, strategies, and management, as well as a CIO Forum.
http://chime-net.org/

Healthcare Informatics Standards. Includes links to standards developers, coding systems, informatics organizations, standards organizations, data sets, Internet and middleware standards, government standards, and clinically specific standards information.
www.mcis.duke.edu/standards/guide.htm

Healthcare Information and Management Systems Society (HIMSS). Not-for-profit organization representing information and management systems professionals in health care, serving members, customers, and industry by providing leadership, education, and networking.
www.himss.org/

International Medical Informatics Association (IMIA). Organization to promote informatics in health care and biomedical research, advance international cooperation, stimulate research, development, and routine application, further the dissemination and exchange of information and to encourage education and responsible behavior. Divided into three different sections: IMIA-LAC (Latin and Central America), EFMI (Europe), and APAMI (Asian and Pacific Region). A fourth section, the African region (HELINA), is in the developmental stage.
www.imia.org

Joint Healthcare Information Technology Alliance (JHITA). Collaborative effort of AHIMA, AMIA, CHIM, CHIME, and HIMSS organizations. The

Alliance monitors national legislative and regulatory activities and reports on those activities to the Alliance membership through routine summaries, advocacy papers on topics of particular interest to the membership, and presentations at selected Alliance member organization events.
www.jhita.org/

Nursing Informatics Links. Includes links to organizations, conferences, education, and journals related to nursing informatics.
www.olypen.com/debk/nursinf.htm

Healthcare News

Doctor's Guide to Medical and Other News. Medical news that can be sorted by subject, week, or month.
www.pslgroup.com/MEDNEWS.htm

Intelihealth Professional Network. Daily healthcare headlines in the news with e-mail news delivery option. Aside from healthcare news, this site provides educational, career, and clinical resources.
http://ipn.intelihealth.com/ipn/ihtIPN/

National Health Law Program News. Headlines with links to articles related to national health law and policy.
http://nhelp.org/headlines.shtml

Online Newspaper Collection. Comprehensive list of links to U.S. and worldwide newspapers found on the Internet.
www.ipl.org/reading/news/

Licensing Information

AMA Physician Select. Provides information on virtually every licensed physician in the United States and its possessions, including more than 650,000 doctors of medicine (MD) and doctors of osteopathy or osteopathic medicine (DO). All physician credential data have been verified for accuracy and authenticated by accrediting agencies, medical schools, residency training programs, licensing and certifying boards, and other data sources.
www.ama-assn.org/aps/amahg.htm

National Council: Boards of Nursing. Comprehensive site listing U.S. Boards of Nursing, contact information for Boards of Nursing, links to Boards of Nursing websites, and licensure requirements and maintenance fees.
www.ncsbn.org/

Medical Ethics

Center for Applied Ethics. Biomedical and healthcare resources including ethics institutions and organizations, publications, and courses.
www.ethics.ubc.ca/resources/biomed/

Nursing Ethics Network. Includes research reports.
www.bc.edu/bc_org/avp/son/ethics/nen.html

Veterans Health Affairs Ethics Center. Resources, information, and research on ethics in the Department of Veteran Affairs.
www.visn1.org/wrj/vhaec.html

Index

Contributors

Patricia A. Abbott, PhD, MSIS, RN, C
Assistant Professor, University of Maryland, Baltimore School of Nursing, Baltimore, MD, USA (pabbott@umaryland.edu)

Kathleen C. Allan, MS, RN
Product Manager, Clinical Products, Shared Medical Systems Corp, Malvern, PA, USA

John Anderson
Technical Systems, Shared Medical Systems Corp., Malvern, PA, USA

Kathleen M. Andolina, MS, CS, RN
Consultant, Bournewood Health Systems, Brookline, MA, USA (kandolina@aol.com)

Marion J. Ball, EdD
Professor, The Johns Hopkins University School of Nursing, Baltimore, MD, USA (mball@fcg.com)

Amy J. Barton
Associate Dean for Practice, University of Colorado Health Sciences Center, Denver, CO, USA (amy.barton@uchsc.edu)

Susan Benjamin, BS
Shared Medical Systems Corp, Malvern, PA, USA

Sue Karen Donaldson, PhD, RN, FAAN
Dean and Professor of Nursing, School of Nursing, Professor of Physiology, School of Medicine, The Johns Hopkins University, Baltimore, MD, USA (suek@son.jhmi.edu)

Judith V. Douglas, MA, MHS
Lecturer, The Johns Hopkins University School of Nursing, Baltimore, MD, USA (jdouglas@fcg.com)

Marina Douglas, MSN, RN
Clinical Practice Director, SAIC, Falls Church, VA, USA (douglasma@ cpmx.saic.com)

R. Marjorie Drury, MN, RN
Assistant Professor, Nursing Department, Faculty of Science, Trinity Western University, Langley, British Columbia, Canada (drury@twu.ca)

Margaret J.A. Edwards, PhD, RN
Margaret JA Edwards & Associates, Inc., Calgary, Canada (edwardsc@ cal.cybersurf.net)

Marjorie H. Farver, MSN, RN, C
Vice President, Medlantic Enterprises Inc./Visiting Nurse Association, Hyattsville, MD, USA (margie@crosslink.net)

Linda Fischetti, MS, RN
Nurse Information Systems Specialist, Veterans Administration Medical Center, Washington, DC, USA (Linda.Fischetti@med.va.gov)

Jeannie M. Fitzpatrick, BS, RN
Shared Medical Systems Corp., Malvern, PA, USA

Charles Friedman, PhD
Center for Biomedical Informatics, University of Pittsburgh, Pittsburgh, PA, USA (cpf@cbmi.upmc.edu)

Carole A. Gassert, PhD, RN
Informatics Nurse Consultant, Department of Health and Human Services, Health Resources and Services Administration, Division of Nursing, Rockville, MD, USA (cgassert@hrsa.gov)

Ulla Gerdin, RN
Senior Project Manager, Swedish Institute for Health Services Development, Stockholm, Sweden (ulla.gerdin@spri.se)

Kathryn J. Hannah, RN, PhD
Professor, Department of Community Health Sciences, Faculty of Medicine, The University of Calgary, Calgary, Alberta, Canada (khannah@ ucalgary.edu)

Barbara A. Happ, PhD, RN
Principal, Birch & Davis Associates, Inc., Falls Church, VA, USA (bhapp@ birchdavis.com)

Bennie E. Harsanyi, EdD, RN
Nursing Consultant, Shared Medical Systems Corp., Malvern, PA, USA

Margaret M. Hassett, MS, RN, C
Senior Consultant, First Consulting Group, Lexington, MA, USA
(mhassett@fcg.com)

Betsy Hersher, BS
President, Hersher Associates, Ltd., Northbrook, IL, USA (hersherb@
hersher.com)

Evelyn J.S. Hovenga, PhD, RN
School of Mathematical and Decision Sciences, Faculty of Informatics and
Communication, Central Queensland University, Rockhampton, Australia
(e.hovenga@cqu.edu.au)

Shirley J. Hughes, RN
Vice President, Clinical Services, MC Informatics, Inc., Griswold, IA, USA
(hughes_s_j@email.msn.com)

Suzanne Jenkins, BSN, RN
Vice President, Professional Services, QuadraMed, Reston, VA, USA
(sjenkins@affinity.ccare.com)

Jo Ann Klein, BSN, RN
President, Mid-Atlantic Network Associates, Inc., Reisterstown, MD, USA
(nurse@clark.net)

Deborah Lewis, EdD, RN
Associate Professor of Nursing, West Virginia School of Nursing, Morgan-
town, WV, USA (dlewis@wvu.edu)

Nancy M. Lorenzi, PhD
Associate Senior Vice President, University of Cincinnati Medical Center,
Cincinnati, OH, USA (lorenzi@uc.edu)

Kathleen A. McCormick, PhD, RN, FAAN
Senior Principal, SRA International, Inc., Falls Church, VA, USA
(kathleen_mccormick@sra.com)

Mary Etta Mills, ScD, RN, CNAA
Associate Professor and Chair, University of Maryland, Baltimore School
of Nursing, Baltimore, MD, USA (mmills@umaryland.edu)

Susan K. Newbold, MS, RN, C
Doctoral Candidate, University of Maryland, School of Nursing, Baltimore,
MD, USA (snewbold@umaryland.edu)

Robert T. Riley, PhD
President, Riley Associates, Cincinnati, OH, USA (rileyrt@rileyai.com)

Elizabeth A. Schofield, MBA, RN
Shared Medical Systems Corp., Malvern, PA, USA

Judith Shamian, PhD, RN
Vice President, Nursing, Mount Sinai Hospital, Toronto, Ontario, Canada
(jshamian@mtsinai.on.ca)

Roy L. Simpson, BS, RN, C, FNAP, FAAN
Vice President, Nursing Affairs, McKesson HBOC, Atlanta, GA, USA
(roy.simpson@hboc.com)

Barbara W. Simundza, MBA
Shared Medical Systems Corp., Malvern, PA, USA

Diane J. Skiba, PhD
Associate Dean for Informatics, University of Colorado Health Science
Center, Denver, CO, USA (diane.skiba@uchsc.edu)

Nancy Staggers, PhD, RN
Associate Professor, Nursing and Health Informatics, University of Utah,
College of Nursing, Salt Lake City, UT, USA (Nancy.Staggers@
nurs.utah.edu)

James P. Turley, PhD, RN
Associate Professor and Vice Chair, Department of Health Informatics,
University of Texas–Houston Health Science Center, Houston, TX, USA
(james.p.turley@uth.tmc.edu)

Carolyn R. Valo, MS
Shared Medical Systems Corp., Malvern, PA, USA

Ann Warnock-Matheron, MN, RN
Patient Care IS Specialist, Peter Lougheed Centre of the Calgary General
Hospital, Calgary, Alberta, Canada (warnock@acs.ucalgary.ca)

Emily M. Welebob, MS, RN
Senior Consultant, First Consulting Group, Beltsville, MD, USA
(ewelebob@fcg.com)

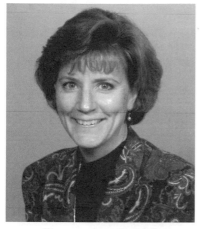

PATRICIA A. ABBOTT

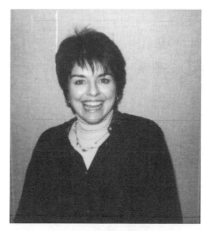

KATHLEEN C. ALLAN

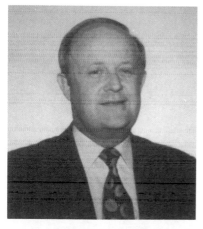

JOHN ANDERSON

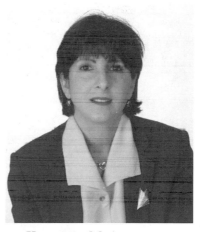

KATHLEEN M. ANDOLINA

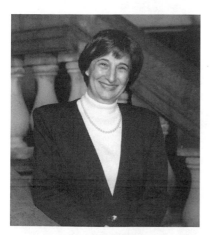

MARION J. BALL

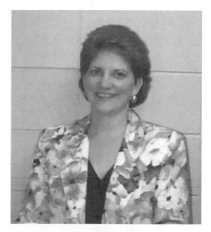

AMY J. BARTON

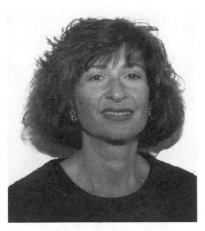

SUSAN BENJAMIN

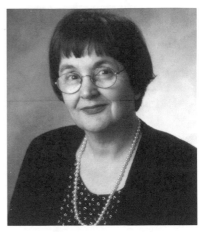

JUDITH V. DOUGLAS

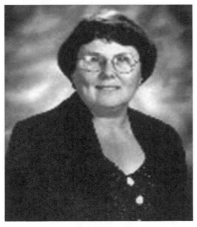

R. MARJORIE DRURY

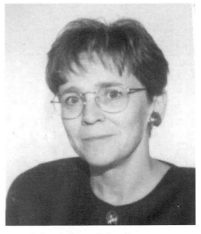

MARGARET J.A. EDWARDS

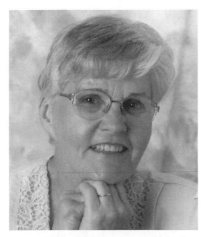

MARJORIE H. FARVER

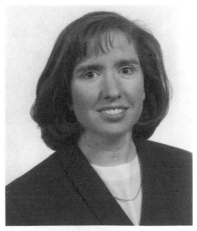

LINDA FISCHETTI

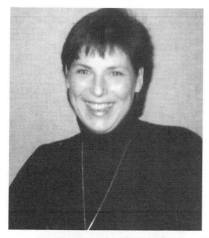

JEANNIE M. FITZPATRICK

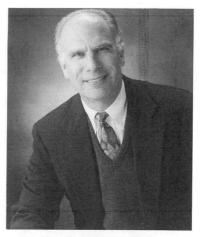

CHARLES FRIEDMAN

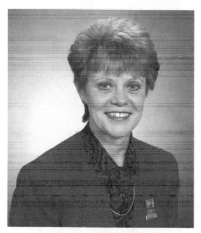

CAROLE A. GASSERT

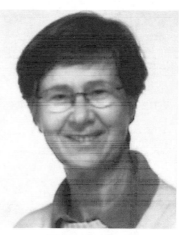

ULLA GERDIN

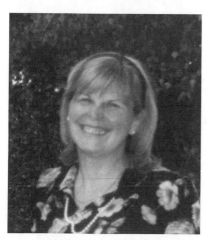

KATHRYN J. HANNAH

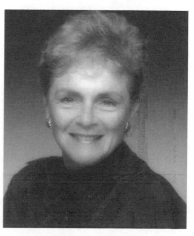

BARBARA A. HAPP

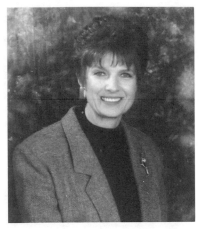

BENNIE E. HARSANYI

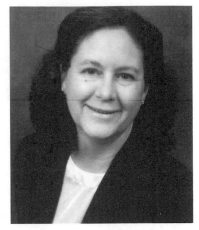

MARGARET M. HASSETT

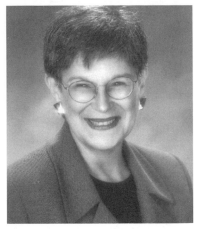

BETSY HERSHER

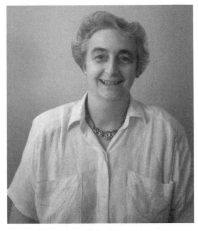

EVELYN J.S. HOVENGA

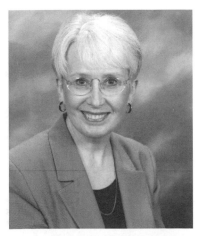

SHIRLEY HUGHES

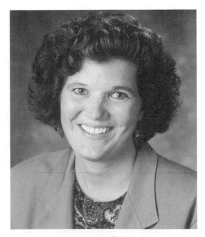

SUZANNE JENKINS

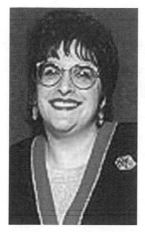

Jo Ann Klein

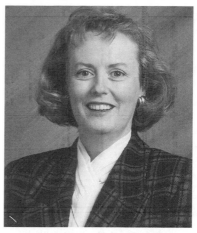

Deborah Lewis

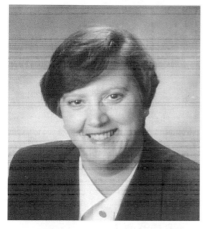

Nancy M. Lorenzi

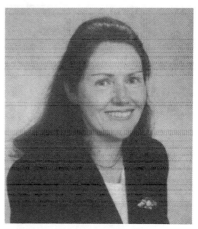

Mary Etta Mills

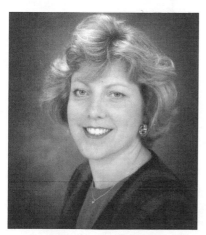

Susan K. Newbold

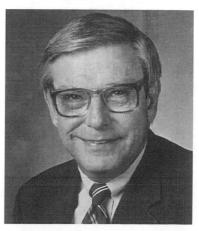

Robert T. Riley

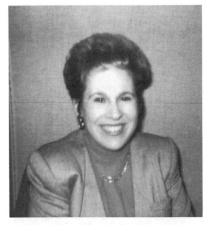

Elizabeth A. Schofield

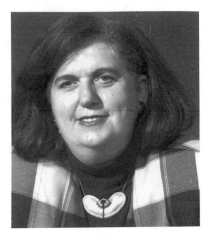

Judith Shamian

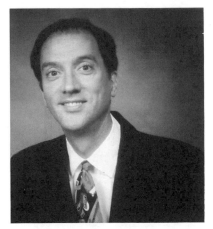

Roy L. Simpson

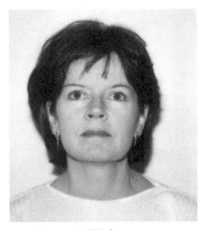

Barbara W. Simundza

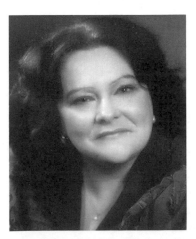

Diane J. Skiba

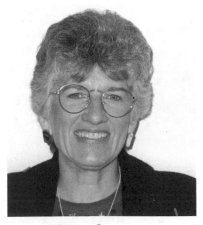

Nancy Staggers

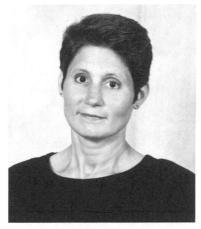

CAROLYN R. VALO

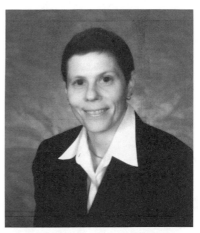

ANN WARNOCK-MATHERON

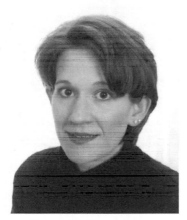

EMILY M. WELEBOB

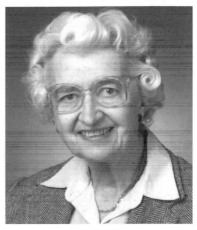

HARRIET H. WERLEY

Health Informatics Series
(formerly Computers in Health Care)

Filmless Radiology
E.L. Siegel and R.M. Kolodner

Clinical Information Systems
A Component-Based Approach
R. Van de Velde and P. Degoulet

Cancer Informatics
Essential Technologies for Clinical Trials
J.S. Silva, M.J. Ball, C.G. Chute, J.V. Douglas, C.P. Langlotz, J.C. Niland, and W.L. Scherlis

Knowledge Coupling
New Premises and New Tools for Medical Care and Education
L.L. Weed